*To the memory of my wife Becky
who encouraged me, sustained me,
helped me, and above all,
believed in me*

Preface

The science of electrocardiology has its greatest application in the diagnosis of coronary artery disease. Not only is the recognition of abnormality essential, but perhaps as important is the distinction of the normal from the abnormal: the recognition of the normal variants which may mimic cardiac disease, and which, in the absence of adequate recognition, can lead to iatrogenic disaster. The literature on the electrocardiographic diagnosis of coronary artery disease is voluminous, and the subject has reached such a complexity, that an organized correlative interpretation for use by all should be available. Such is the aim of this text. It is primarily directed at the clinical electrocardiologist, and consequently deals only with conventional, non-invasive electrocardiography. Although diagrammatic illustrations of the frontal plane vector loop are used, this book is not intended for vectorcardiographic interpretation. Such vector loops are used for the specific purpose of facilitating the electrocardiographic interpretation. Most of the illustrative electrocardiographic studies have application to more than one chapter, and have therefore been grouped together in a single section to facilitate general reference. It is hoped that the form, presentation and character of the book is such that it will have relevance to clinicians at all levels.

Leo Schamroth

The Electrocardiology of

Coronary Artery Disease

The value of experience is not in seeing much, but in seeing wisely.

William Osler

The Electrocardiology of Coronary Artery Disease

Leo Schamroth

M.D., D.Sc., (Witwatersrand), F.R.C.P.(Edin.), F.R.C.P.(Glasg.)., F.A.C.C., F.R.S. (S.Af.)

Professor of Medicine, University of the Witwatersrand,
Chief Physician, Baragwanath Hospital,
Johannesburg, South Africa

BLACKWELL SCIENTIFIC PUBLICATIONS

OXFORD LONDON EDINBURGH MELBOURNE

ISBN 0 632 001275

First Published 1975

Distributed in the United States of America by
J. B. LIPPINCOTT COMPANY, PHILADELPHIA
and in Canada by
J. B. LIPPINCOTT COMPANY OF CANADA LTD. TORONTO

Printed in Great Britain
AT THE ALDEN PRESS, OXFORD
and bound by
WEBB, SON & CO., FERNDALE, GLAMORGAN

Acknowlegements

It is a great pleasure to express my thanks to:

The Editors of the *South African Medical Journal, Circulation*, the *American Journal of Cardiology*, the *Journal of Electrocardiology*, and *Heart and Lung* for permission to reproduce various illustrations from my published papers.

Doctors V.Botoulas, D.Clark, A.Dubb, J.De Kock, H.D.Friedberg, B.Gentin, G.Lapinsky, J.H.Levenstein, Alan Lindsay, H.J.L.Marriott, O.Neurath, M.M.Perlman, D.Pittaway and D.Wilton, for the electrocardiograms they so kindly sent to me (acknowledged specifically in the relevant electrocardiographic studies).

The Photographic Department, Department of Medicine, University of the Witwatersrand for the photographic reproductions.

Leo Schamroth

THE ELECTROCARDIOLOGY OF CORONARY ARTERY DISEASE

Contents

PART ONE

Section I Basic Principles

Section II Myocardial Infarction

Section III Coronary Insufficiency

Section IV Abnormal Rhythms Associated with Acute Myocardial Infarction

PART II

PART ONE

Section 1 Basic Principles

Chapter 1

The Basic Electrocardiographic Manifestations of Impaired Coronary Blood Flow

Coronary artery disease may present electrocardiographically as follows:

A **Myocardial ischaemia**
B **Myocardial injury**
C **Myocardial necrosis**
D **Abnormalities of intraventricular conduction**
E **Abnormal heart rhythms**

The terms *ischaemia*, *injury* and *necrosis* do not have strictly the same connotations as their pathological counterparts. They are rather electropathological expressions which may, to some extent, parallel the histological manifestations. They may be defined in terms of a loss or impairment of the various factors which contribute to, or are responsible for, the maintenance of the cellular electrical potential. These factors are considered further in Chapter 2.

A THE ELECTROCARDIOGRAPHIC EFFECTS OF MYOCARDIAL ISCHAEMIA

The advent of myocardial ischaemia is characterized electrocardiographically by manifestations which affect (1) the **shape**, (2) the **magnitude** and (3) the **direction** of the T wave.

1 CHANGES AFFECTING THE SHAPE OF THE T WAVE

The normal T wave is asymmetrical in shape, the proximal slope being shallower than the distal slope. In other words, the initial angle of the T wave (the angle between the S-T segment and the proximal limb of the T wave) is more obtuse than its terminal angle (the angle between the distal limb of the T wave and the baseline). The apex or nadir is relatively blunt (Diagrams A of Figs. 1 and 2; leads V3 to V6 of Electrocardiographic Study 102A).

The T wave of myocardial ischaemia is characterized by **symmetry** increased **narrowness**, and a **sharper apex**

or **nadir** (Diagrams B and C of Fig. 1; Electrocardiographic Studies 73, 75, 78, 81, 84, 85, 86, 87 and 91).

(a) Symmetry

The T wave tends to become symmetrical, i.e. its initial angle (the angle between the S-T segment and the proximal limb of the T wave) becomes less obtuse and approximates the terminal angle (the angle between the distal limb and the baseline).

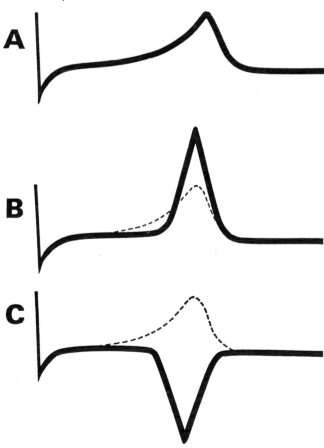

FIG. 1. Diagrams illustrating: A, the normal S-T segment and T wave; and B and C, the T wave of myocardial ischaemia.

5

(b) Increased Narrowness: a More Acute Internal Angle
The angle within the *T* wave, the internal angle, becomes more acute, contributing to the arrow-head appearance of the *T* wave.

(c) A Sharper Apex or Nadir
The apex or nadir of the *T* wave becomes sharply pointed, further contributing to the arrow-head appearance of the *T* wave.

THE CONTRIBUTING EFFECT OF MYOCARDIAL INJURY: THE EFFECT OF THE S-T SEGMENT

The arrow-head and symmetrical appearance of the *T* wave of myocardial ischaemia may be exaggerated by any concomitant effect of coronary insufficiency on the S-T segment (see p. 8). Thus, the normal S-T segment tends to leave the baseline soon after the QRS complex, i.e. it does not hug the baseline for more than 0·12 sec or 3 mm, and merges smoothly, imperceptibly and almost immediately with the proximal limb of the *T* wave (Electrocardiographic Study 93, tracing a). With the progression of coronary insufficiency, the S-T segment tends to become more isoelectric, i.e. it tends to hug the baseline for a longer period (longer than 0·12 sec or 3 mm). There is also the tendency to the development of a sharper, more distinct, initial angle between the S-T segment and the proximal limb of the *T* wave (Diagrams B and C of Fig. 1; see also Diagrams C and D of Fig. 37). All these effects tend to delineate, accentuate or isolate the *T* wave more distinctly, thereby contributing towards the characteristic, symmetrical and arrow-head appearance of the *T* wave, often designated the coronary *T* wave (see, for example, Electrocardiographic Study 87, tracing A and Electrocardiographic Studies 81, 83 and 92).

2 CHANGES AFFECTING THE MAGNITUDE OF THE T WAVE

The *T* wave of myocardial ischaemia is usually increased in magnitude irrespective of whether it is upright or inverted.

3 CHANGES AFFECTING THE DIRECTION OF THE T WAVE

The mean *T*-wave vector of myocardial ischaemia is **directed away from the surface of the ischaemic region** (Diagrams B and C of Fig. 2). It will, for example, be directed posteriorly in anterior wall epicardial ischaemia (Diagram A of Fig. 18), and anteriorly in anterior wall subendocardial ischaemia (Diagram D of Fig. 18).

Leads orientated to the surface of the ischaemia will thus reflect inverted *T* waves, whereas leads orientated to the opposite or healthy surface will reflect upright *T* waves.

Indicative and Reciprocal Changes

Changes recorded by leads which are orientated to the surface of the abnormality are referred to as **indicative changes**. Changes recorded by leads which are orientated to the opposite—normal—surface are known as **reciprocal changes**.

The Mechanism of the T Wave Directional Changes in Myocardial Ischaemia

The *T* wave of myocardial ischaemia is due to an imbalance of repolarization, a disturbance in the orderly sequence of the repolarization of the heart. Repolarization is delayed in the ischaemic area and the *T* wave repolarization forces of the *unaffected* regions of the heart therefore tend to dominate since they are inscribed earlier. Furthermore, the balance of repolarization is thrown out-of-phase since the repolarization forces which normally occur synchronously and thus tend to oppose (nullify) each other, are thrown out of phase. As a result, the repolarization forces of one area, the unaffected area, tend to dominate. The mean vector is thus directed *away* from the ischaemic area—the *T* wave vector is directed away from the region of mischief. The physiological principles governing this change are discussed further in Chapter 2.

The delay in repolarization is due to a delay, a prolongation, in phase 3 repolarization of the transmembrane action potential. It is probably due to a slight diminution in intracellular potassium (Sodi-Pallares, 1970[S114]).

B THE ELECTROCARDIOGRAPHIC EFFECTS OF MYOCARDIAL INJURY

Myocardial injury, in an electropathological sense, reflects a progression or deterioration from the electropathological state of myocardial ischaemia. Pathologically it connotes a greater degree of coronary insufficiency. It is characterized electrocardiographically by (a) **a deviation of the S-T segment** and (b) **a change in the contour of the S-T segment**.

(a) THE DEVIATION OF THE S-T SEGMENT

Myocardial injury results in a **deviation or displacement of the S-T segment towards the surface of injury**. Thus, subepicardial injury is reflected by an elevated S-T segment in leads orientated to the epicardial surface (Diagram E of Fig. 2), and a depressed S-T segment by

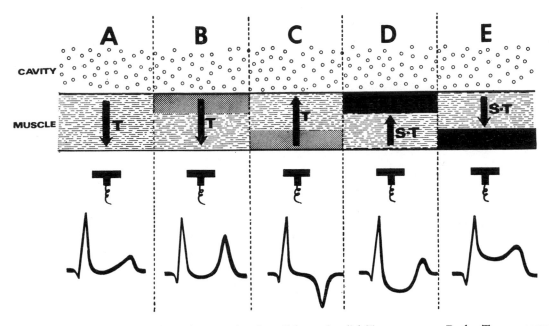

FIG. 2. Diagrammatic illustration of: A, the normal endocardial to epicardial T wave vector; B, the T wave vector of subendocardial ischaemia; C, the T wave vector of subepicardial ischaemia; D, the S-T segment vector of subendocardial injury; and E, the T wave vector of subepicardial injury.

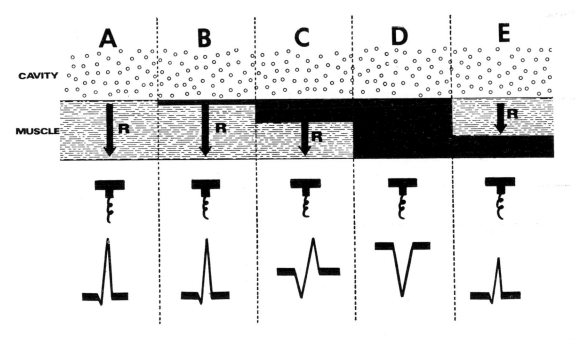

FIG. 3. Diagrammatic illustration of: A, the normal endocardial to epicardial QRS vector; B, the hypothetical unchanged QRS vector associated with minimal subendocardial necrosis; C, the diminished QRS vector (following a pathological Q wave) associated with significant subendocardial necrosis; D, the absent QRS vector associated with transmural necrosis, and E, the diminished QRS vector associated with subepicardial necrosis.

leads orientated to the uninjured endocardial surface. Sub-endocardial injury is reflected by a depressed S-T segment in leads orientated to the epicardial surface, and an elevated S-T segment in leads orientated to the endocardial surface (Diagram D of Fig. 2).

(b)   THE CHANGE IN THE CONTOUR OF THE S-T SEGMENT

The elevated S-T segment may be convex- or concave-upward. The depressed S-T segment is usually concave-upward, but may also have a horizontal configuration, plane depression. The contour of the elevated or depressed S-T segment of myocardial injury is also dependent, in part, upon the shape and direction of the associated *T* wave. If, for example, the elevated S-T segment is associated with an inverted, symmetrical, arrow-head *T* wave of myocardial ischaemia, then the S-T segment will be **coved** or **convex-upward.** The upward convexity tends to be **smooth** and **even,** reflecting a symmetrical parabolic curve. The distal part of the coved S-T segment blends smoothly and imperceptibly with the proximal limb of the inverted *T* wave. This form of S-T segment is characteristic of the fully evolved phase of acute myocardial infarction, and is usually associated with an *R* wave of diminished amplitude or an absent *R* wave (for example, leads V3 to V6 of Electrocardiographic Study 12). If, on the other hand, the elevated S-T segment is associated with an upright *T* wave and a dominantly upright QRS complex, then it is usually concave-upward (Diagram E of Fig. 2). This S-T segment occurs characteristically in acute pericarditis (Electrocardiographic Study 99). The elevated S-T segment may also be asymmetrical with a relatively straight upward slope toward the upright *T* wave. This manifestation is usually seen in the early hyperacute phase of acute myocardial infarction (Diagrams B and C of Fig. 23 and, for example, Standard leads II and III and lead AVF of Electrocardiographic Study 7).

If a depressed segment is associated with an upright *T* wave it usually has a sagging concave-upward appearance, with a symmetrical parabolic curve (Diagram D of Fig. 2, Diagram G of Fig. 60, and, for example, Standard lead II of Electrocardiographic Study 81 and lead V6 in tracing C of Electrocardiographic Study 34).

The S-T segment may also be horizontal, forming a sharp-angled ST-T junction with the upright *T* wave. This is termed **plane depression** (Diagram F of Fig. 60; Electrocardiographic Studies 92, 93 and 94).

If the depressed S-T segment is associated with an inverted *T* wave, it is usually convex-upward (Electrocardiographic Studies 73, 74 and 75).

These manifestations are considered further in Chapters 2 and 3.

The Mechanism of the S-T Segment Abnormalities Associated with Myocardial Injury

The S-T segment abnormalities of myocardial injury are probably due to the development of a *difference in resting potential* between the injured and adjacent healthy cells. This tends to create a continuous current, the current of injury, during the resting, diastolic phase, which is abolished during activation. The phenomenon is considered further in Chapter 2.

C   THE ELECTROCARDIOGRAPHIC EFFECTS OF MYOCARDIAL NECROSIS

Myocardial necrosis, in an electropathological sense, is a state where the myocardial cell can no longer be activated. It is reflected electrocardiographically by a loss of forces, a negative deflection or a loss of normal positive deflection, in a lead orientated to the necrotic region. In other words, the vectorial forces of depolarization are, or tend to be, *directed away* from the area of necrosis. The reasons for this are considered below.

THE BASIC MECHANISM

Depolarization of the ventricles is considered in detail later in this chapter. It is discussed here merely in simplified form for purposes of the ensuing presentation.

Depolarization of the ventricles, the biventricular chamber, begins in the left side of the interventricular septum and spreads through the septum from left to right (arrow 1 in Fig. 4). Depolarization then proceeds outwards *simultaneously* through the free walls of both ventricles from endocardial to epicardial surfaces (arrows labelled 2 in Diagram A of Fig. 4).

The free wall of the left ventricle has a larger muscle mass, and hence a larger potential electrical force, than the free wall of the right ventricle (Fig. 4). Consequently, as depolarization of both free walls occurs simultaneously, the larger left ventricular forces of the left free wall counteract the smaller forces of the right free wall. The result is a single force from right to left (arrow 2 in Diagram B of Fig. 4). Thus, for convenience, depolarization of the ventricles may be represented in a simplified form as a small initial force from left to right through the septum, followed by a larger force from right to left through the free wall of the left ventricle (Diagram B of Fig. 4).

An electrode orientated to the left ventricle will record a small initial downward deflection (a small *q* wave) caused by the spread of the stimulus *away* from the electrode

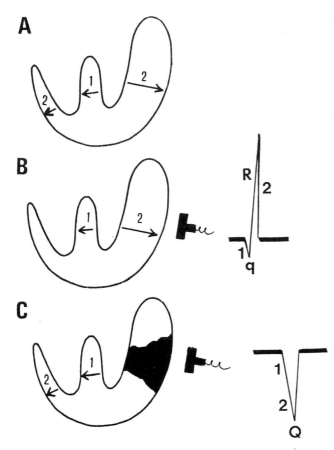

FIG. 4. Diagrammatic representation of normal ventricular activation (Diagrams A and B), as reflected by a qR complex in a lead orientated to the left ventricle, and the ventricular activation associated with transmural necrosis, as reflected by a QS complex in a lead orientated to the left ventricle (C). See text.

through the septum, followed by a larger upward deflection (a tall *R* wave) caused by the spread of the stimulus *towards* the electrode through the left ventricular muscle mass (Diagram B of Fig. 4). The result is a *qR* or a 'left-ventricular' complex (for example, leads V5 and V6 of Electrocardiographic Study 100).

Essentially, myocardial necrosis (infarction) occurs exclusively in the left ventricle (see also p. 13). Consider now the effect of a transmural infarct (one involving the full thickness of the muscle wall) which is situated in the free wall of the left ventricle (Diagram C of Fig. 4). The necrotic material cannot be activated, and the force of the left free wall is consequently abolished within the region of the infarct. In other words, the large right to left force of the left free wall in the region of the infarct is abolished and no longer counteracts the smaller left to right forces of the distant free right wall. An electrode orientated to the necrotic region of the left free wall is, in effect, orientated to and through a window of electrically inert tissue[W51], and will thus reflect firstly, the left to right septal force (Vector 1 in Diagram C of Fig. 4) which is directed *away* from the electrode and hence results in a negative deflection, and secondly, distant left to right forces of the free wall of the right ventricle (Vector 2 in Diagram C of Fig. 4) which are also directed *away* from the electrode and are thus no longer counteracted or cancelled by the lost positive forces in the necrotic area. These distant right ventricular forces also result in a further negative deflection. An electrode orientated to the necrotic area will consequently reflect a deep and wide negative deflection, a pathological Q wave, or a QS deflection.

This pathological Q wave or QS deflection is the expression of a disturbance in the balance of the normal cardiac depolarization forces which have been set out of alignment and reorientated by the effects of necrosis. The electrical centre of gravity has been *shifted away* from the necrotic area.

The characteristics of pathological Q waves are considered further in Chapter 3. It must also be remembered that lesser degrees of infarction may manifest with only a loss of *R* wave amplitude (see Chapter 3).

D ABNORMALITIES OF INTRA-VENTRICULAR CONDUCTION

The abnormalities of intraventricular conduction resulting from impaired coronary blood flow are considered in Chapter 12.

E ABNORMAL HEART RHYTHMS

The abnormal heart rhythms resulting from impaired coronary blood flow are considered in Chapter 17.

Chapter 2
Electrophysiology and Electropathology

THE DIPOLE AND THE DOUBLET

The normal resting, polarized cell has a positive surface charge and a negative intracellular charge (Diagram A of Fig. 5). The charges are of considerable magnitude, being approximately −90 mV within the cell (see below) The charges of equal but opposite polarity on either side of the cell membrane constitute a **dipole**. If a series of such cells, a tissue, are all in the resting state (as illustrated in Diagram A of Figs. 5 and 7), they will all have positive external charges. There is consequently no difference in external potential, and no current flows.

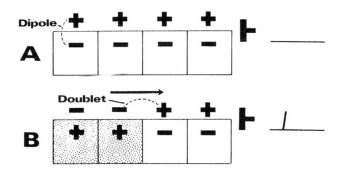

FIG. 5. Diagrammatic representation of: A, a series of 4 cells in the resting, polarized, state; and B, activation—depolarization—of the first 2 cells. A doublet exists between the second and third cells, having a positive head orientated towards the electrode.

Activation, depolarization, of the cell effects a reversal of the resting polarity. The inside of the cell becomes positive and the exterior becomes negative. This is reflected both graphically and qualitatively by the transmembrane action potential (see below), and is illustrated diagrammatically in Diagram B of Fig. 5. The first two cells, the activated or depolarized cells, of the tissue have negative surface charges, whereas the two adjacent polarized or resting cells have positive surface charges. A difference in surface potential thus exists between the second and third cells, and a current flows, having a positive head in the direction of the resting cells and a negative tail in the direction of the activated cells. An electrode orientated to this positive head will consequently reflect a positive, upright, deflection. The presence of *surface* charges of opposite direction on adjacent cells constitutes a **doublet** (Craib, 1927[C51]), and is the basis for current flow. Note that the first doublet in Diagram B of Fig. 5 occurred between the first and second cells of the tissue.

THE TRANSMEMBRANE ACTION POTENTIAL

The electrical events associated with the activation (depolarization) and recovery (repolarization) are due to ionic fluxes, mainly sodium and potassium, across the myocardial cell membrane. These events may be graphically recorded by means of an intracellular microelectrode which constitutes one pole of a bipolar electrocardiographic lead, the other pole of the bipolar lead being a surface electrode.

The recording obtained by such an intracellular electrode is termed the *transmembrance action potential* and has a characteristic form (Fig. 6). At rest, the inside of the cell has a negative potential of approximately −90 mV. This resting phase is termed *Phase 4* of the transmembrane

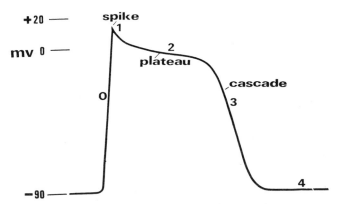

FIG. 6. Diagram illustrating the transmembrane action potential. mv = millivolts. See text.

action potential. Activation, depolarization, of the cell is associated with an abrupt rise (an abrupt reversal of polarity) within the cell which now becomes positive (with reference to the external electrode) to about +10 mV. This phase of activation is termed *Phase 0* of the transmembrane action potential. This abrupt phase of depolarization is followed by a relatively slow period of recovery (repolarization) which may be divided into three phases: *Phase 1*—an early, rapid phase which, because of its appearance, has been termed the *spike*; *Phase 2*—a second, relatively slow phase which, because of its appearance, has been termed the *plateau*; and *Phase 3*—a terminal, relatively fast phase, which will be termed the *cascade*. Although the transmembrane action potential has five phases (0 to 4), they reflect in effect three basic processes or states in the cycle of the excitable cell:

1. The process of activation or depolarization. This is reflected by Phase 0 of the action potential.

2. The process of recovery or repolarization. This is reflected by the Phases 1, 2 and 3 of the action potential.

3. The state of full recovery or polarization. This is reflected by Phase 4 of the action potential.

Electrocardiographic Equivalents of the Transmembrane Action Potential

The transmembrane action potential reflects the electrical events of a single cell, whereas the electrocardiogram reflects the electrical events of cardiac tissue, very many cells. Nevertheless, because of the rapid near-synchronous activation of all the cells, the following approximate correlation exists between the two records:

Phase 0 corresponds to the QRS complex.

Phase 1 corresponds to the J point, the junction of the QRS complex with the S-T segment.

Phase 2 corresponds to the S-T segment.

Phase 3 corresponds to the T wave.

Phase 4 corresponds to the isoelectric baseline of the resting state.

THE PHYSIOLOGY OF NORMAL MYOCARDIAL DEPOLARIZATION AND REPOLARIZATION

Depolarization and repolarization of the ventricles occur transversely, i.e. across the thickness of the ventricular myocardium from endocardial to epicardial surfaces[L49, S41, W48]. This is illustrated in Fig. 7 which, for didactic purposes, depicts a tissue of four cells extending from endocardium to epicardium. Diagram A represents the resting state. All four cells are in the resting state, i.e. they

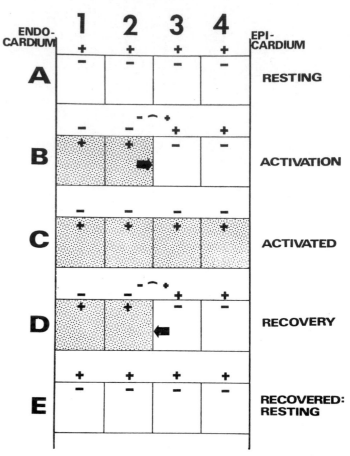

FIG. 7. Diagrams illustrating the process of depolarization and repolarization in a series of four cells hypothetically situated from endocardium to epicardium. Diagram A illustrates all four cells in the resting state. Diagram B illustrates depolarization of the first two cells. Diagram C illustrates depolarization of all four cells. Diagram D illustrates repolarization of the first two cells from the epicardial surface. Diagram E illustrates the fully repolarized, resting, state once again. See text.

are all in Phase 4 of the transmembrane action potential. All the cells of the tissue have positive surface charges and negative internal charges. There is no difference in potential between the cells, and no current flows. Diagram B illustrates the process of normal depolarization from endocardium to epicardium, the cells being activated sequentially from cell 1 to cell 4. Cells 1 and 2 have been activated and are in Phase 0 of the transmembrane action potential; cells 3 and 4 are still at rest and are in Phase 4 of the transmembrane action potential. A doublet exists between cells 2 and 3, the first doublet of the activation process having occurred between cells 1 and 2. The doublet current with a positive head thus flows from endocardium to epicardium, giving rise to a positive QRS deflection in an electrode facing the epicardium. Diagram C reflects the fully depolarized state, all four cells being in the process of recovery. This state corresponds principally to Phase 2 of the transmembrane action potential, the plateau. Since this is a relatively long phase, there is a large measure of overlap between the cells in this state, and sequential differences are usually not evident. Consequently there is no difference in surface potential, and no current flows. The conventional electrocardiogram therefore reflects no deflection, an iso-electric baseline, which corresponds principally to the S-T segment.

Paradoxically, repolarization of the activated cells does not occur in the same sequence as depolarization, but is opposite in direction. In other words, it occurs from epi-cardial to endocardial surfaces instead of from endocardial to epicardial surfaces. The first cell to be depolarized is the last cell to be repolarized, and vice versa. This is probably due to the greater pressure within the endocardial regions compared to the epicardial regions of the myocardium during ventricular systole. This reversed process of re-polarization becomes evident when Phase 3, the cascade of the transmembrane action potential, is reached, for this is a relatively short phase and sequential chronological differences therefore become evident. This is discussed further in the section on 'The Electrophysiology of Myo-cardial Ischaemia' below. The series of cells having been activated or depolarized in the cellular sequence 1, 2, 3, 4 are repolarized in the sequence 4, 3, 2, 1 (as illustrated in Diagram D of Fig. 7). This diagram shows that cells 4 and 3 have already recovered, being fully polarized with positive surface charges. A doublet exists between cells 2 and 3. This is the second doublet in the series. The first doublet occurred between cells 4 and 3. The series of doublets so-to-speak proceeds with a negative head and a positive tail from epicardium to endocardium, giving rise to a positive deflection, an upright T wave in leads orien-tated to the epicardium. If the repolarization or recovery process had occurred in the same sequence as during depolarization, the T wave should have been *opposite* in direction to the QRS complex, i.e. if the normal QRS complex is upright as, for example, the QRS complex normally recorded by lead V5, then the associated T wave should be inverted. Due to the reverse process of repolar-ization, however, the normal T wave is in the *same* direction as the QRS complex, and will be upright in lead V5. Diagram E of Fig. 7 illustrates the resting, fully polarized, state once again. All the cells are in Phase 4 of transmembrane action potential, equivalent to the state illustrated in Diagram A of Fig. 7.

It is important to appreciate that, unlike depolarization, repolarization of a cell is *not* dependent on the state of, or relationship to, the neighbouring cell(s). Furthermore, repolarization requires a much longer time than repolariza-tion for completion.

OBSERVATIONS ON THE ANATOMY AND PHYSIOLOGY OF THE VENTRICLES

The ventricles consist primarily of three muscle masses: (1) *the interventricular septum*, (2) *the free wall of the left ventricle*, and (3) *the free wall of the right ventricle* (Fig. 8). The free wall of the left ventricle and the interventricular septum have thick walls (large muscle masses), and together constitute a uniform ring of muscle or chamber, the anatomical left ventricle (Fig. 8). It is quite evident, from a cross-section of the ventricles, that the interventricular septum and the free wall of the left ventricle constitute an anatomical continuum. The free wall of the right ventricle is, in effect, merely a thin anatomical appendage of the left ventricle (Fig. 8).

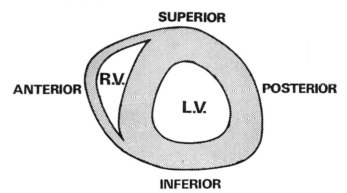

FIG. 8. Diagrammatic representation of a cross-section through the ventricles.

The interventricular septum also contracts functionally with the free wall of the left ventricle, constituting the main haemodynamic pump of the heart. The right ventricle functions principally as a conduit.

From the electrocardiological viewpoint, and particu-larly with reference to the electrocardiology of coronary artery disease, the left ventricle, as constituted by the free wall of the left ventricle and the interventricular septum, is also the dominant chamber. For example, anterior wall myocardial infarction, anterior wall myocardial injury and anterior wall myocardial ischaemia refer principally to infarction, injury or ischaemia of the interventricular septum. The interventricular septum thus, in effect, consti-tutes the electrical anterior wall of the biventricular cham-ber, whereas the thin free wall of the right ventricle constitutes the anatomical anterior wall of the biventricular chamber.

The Electrophysiological Function of the Interventri-cular Septum

The interventricular septum has two endocardial surfaces

and no epicardial surface. The anterior endocardial surface is directed anteriorly and to the right, and forms part of the right ventricular chamber. The posterior endocardial surface is directed posteriorly and to the left, and forms part of the left ventricular chamber. Yet, as indicated above, it is evident from the electrocardiographic manifestations of coronary artery disease that the right, anterior, endocardial surface constitutes, in effect, the *functional* epicardial surface of the interventricular septum; whereas the left, posterior, endocardial surface constitutes, in effect, the *functional* endocardial surface of the interventricular septum This is evident from the following:

1. When an apical or anterolateral infarction extends medially, i.e. to the right, it involves the interventricular septum and not the free wall of the right ventricle (Diagram A of Fig. 9).

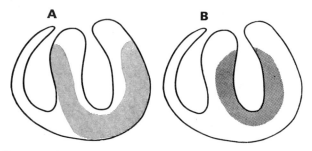

FIG. 9. Diagrammatic representation of: A, an extensive anterior wall myocardial infarction; and B, an extensive anterior wall subendocardial myocardial injury due to coronary insufficiency.

2. When infarction involves the interventricular septum, it is the right side of the interventricular septum which constitutes the principal injured surface. This is evident from the elevated and coved S-T segments which manifest in the precordial leads V1 to V4, an expression of the anterior deviation of the S-T segment vector, i.e. towards the surface of injury, the right endocardial surface.

3. If anterior wall infarction involved solely or principally the right ventricle, the anatomical anterior wall of the heart, then the septal forces (Vectors 1 of Figs. 4 and 11) would not be abolished, and QS complexes or pathological Q waves would *not* be recorded by the precordial leads V1 to V4.

4. In the classic form of angina pectoris, the expression of acute subendocardial injury, the electrocardiogram usually manifests with depressed S-T segments in leads V5 and V6, reflecting acute subendocardial apical coronary insufficiency. When this subendocardial injury extends medially, i.e. to the right, it involves by contiguity the subendocardium of the left or posterior side of the interventricular septum (Diagram B of Fig. 9 and Fig. 61). And

this is evident from the depressed S-T segments in leads V2 and V3, the expression of an S-T segment vector that is directed posteriorly, away from the precordial leads.

The functional electrophysiological division of the interventricular septum into a right, anterior, epicardial side and a left, posterior, endocardial side, is probably related to the higher left intraventricular pressure.

As indicated above, normal ventricular repolarization is the reverse of normal ventricular depolarization, i.e. whereas depolarization occurs from endocardial to epicardial surfaces, repolarization occurs from epicardial to endocardial surfaces. This has been attributed to the higher subendocardial intramural pressure during ventricular systole which delays repolarization. On an analogous basis, the left or posterior side of the interventricular septum has a higher subendocardial surface pressure during ventricular systole than the right or anterior side of the interventricular septum, since systolic pressure within the left ventricular cavity is greater than that in the right ventricular cavity. See also section below on further observations on the polarity of the normal *T* wave.

Further Observations on the Polarity of the Normal T Wave

Although the interventricular septum has approximately the same muscle mass as that of the free left ventricular wall (Figs. 8 and 9), it is the *T* wave of the free left wall which dominates the normal electrocardiographic presentation and, in effect, becomes manifest. Thus, the normal *T*-wave vector is directed posteriorly and to the left, resulting in upright *T* waves in leads orientated to the free left wall. The following postulate is a possible explanation for this phenomenon.

Depolarization of the interventricular septum occurs almost synchronously from either side of the interventricular septum (see p. 17). The resulting vectors thus tend to oppose each other, the vector from the left side being dominant. The resulting *T* wave vectors will consequently also oppose and thereby tend to modify each other's effect. This is an oversimplification, since the genesis of the *T* wave is very complex and dependent upon many factors. Nevertheless, it is probable that repolarization of the interventricular septum has potentially significant neutralizing forces whereas the free left wall has not. This permits the major and largely unopposed *T* wave force of the left free wall to be dominant although, theoretically, it will to some extent be opposed by the very small repolarization forces of the right free wall. In addition, there is a considerable measure of overlap between the initial forces of septal depolarization and the initial forces of free left wall depolarization and repolarization. And since these forces are, or tend to be, opposite in direction, further effective cancellation of the septal forces will tend to occur. The later and unopposed depolarization and repolarization forces of the major part of the left free wall therefore tend to dominate. This further contributes to the reason why the leftward and posteriorly directed T wave force of the left free wall dominates and becomes manifest.

The Question of the 'Silent' Subendocardium

On the basis of depth electrode studies, it has been postulated in the past that a rind of subendocardial muscle is possibly 'silent' electrocardiographically[D47, D48, D49, D50, K18, M28, S108]. These studies were done with stab or plunge electrodes, the experimental animal usually being the dog, although observations in the human have also been made[M28]. It appeared from differential records that part of the subendocardial rind was activated instantaneously or even activated in a reverse, epicardial–endocardial direction. In addition, unipolar records revealed the absence of initial positivity from a variable of the subendocardial rind. Part of the subendocardial rind thus appeared to be electrically 'silent'. The depth of this 'silent' subendocardium was variously estimated as 80 per cent[K18, M28], $66\frac{2}{3}$ per cent[S108] and 40 per cent[D47].

The postulate was interpreted to mean that Purkinje fibres penetrate into the wall of the ventricle. The impulse is initially delivered some distance within the wall of the ventricle, and the resulting excitation fronts then spread transversely to endocardial and epicardial surfaces. It must, however, be emphasized that this intracardiac penetration of Purkinje fibres has not been demonstrated in the human heart.

It has further been demonstrated that a considerable part of the electrical signal related to ventricular depolarization as a whole is not available at the body surface[B38].

It has also been demonstrated experimentally that extensive mechanically induced subendocardial trauma results in only minor changes of the QRS complex[P32].

The postulate of subendocardial 'silence' is controversial and has been challenged. Indeed, improved techniques using high-frequency instrumentation has led to revision of these original estimates. Consequently, Scher and associates (1955)[S44], (1955)[S124], (1957)[S40], Erickson and associates, (1957)[E13] and Durrer and associates, (1954)[D49], (1955)[D50], (1965)[D43] have subsequently estimated that the extent of the 'silent' area was close to o. Furthermore, a positive, almost monophasic, record may be elicited by pressure on the subendocardium by an intracardiac electrode[K40]. This also reflects the absence of 'silence' and a normal or near-normal response of the subendocardial muscle. Moreover, as Durrer [D49, D50] has indicated, the large negative left ventricular cavity potential caused by the early and large magnitude major activation of the left free wall, dominates the cavity potential. Hence, any positivity near the intra-cavity electrode due to subendocardial activation may merely be reflected by a small notch or slur on the down-stroke of the negative cavity potential record. As pointed out by Kossman (1958)[K38], none of these experiments have taken into account the modifications due to boundary effects (see below), the interpretation of results in terms of the conductivity of surrounding media.

The findings have also, to some extent, been extrapolated into the clinical state, for it has been postulated that only the outer part of the myocardial rind contributes towards, or is responsible for, the genesis of the R wave. Hence, the assumption that subendocardial infarction can occur without electrocardiographic manifestations affecting the QRS complex. While this is probably true in some instances, there is nevertheless convincing evidence to prove that this is not always the case[D51, D42, K42, M56]. If such a rind of electrically 'silent' subendocardium does indeed exist, it is not of significant magnitude (Diagram B of Fig. 3).

It would therefore seem that true 'silence' does not occur with respect to a local, small, circumscribed section of tissue. When, however, the subendocardium of the left ventricle as a whole is considered, the formation and merging of multiple wave fronts resulting from instantaneous or near-instantaneous excitation may result in multiple cancellation of forces, both locally and remotely. In addition, the boundary effect of tissues of different resistance and the principles of electrical images (see below) may also have an attenuating effect, particularly during the early stages of depolarization, and thereby contribute to an effective electrical 'silence'.

Boundary Effects: The Significance of the Conducting and Insulating Boundaries

Various factors may attenuate or augment the electromotive forces generated by the heart. These are:

1. Surrounding tissues which constitute conducting media of different resistances.

2. The shape of the boundary dividing the tissues of different resistance and the orientation of the electromotive force to the plane of the boundary dividing the tissues of different resistance.

The Significance of Differential Tissue Resistances

The myocardium is surrounded by tissues of different electrical resistance. Blood has a relatively low specific resistance of about 800 Ω cm, lung a higher resistance of 1000 Ω cm, and fatty tissue a very high resistance of 1500–5000 Ω cm[S59].

A tissue of low resistance (high conductivity) will tend to short-circuit the current from an electromotive force. Consequently blood, which is of low resistance, may reduce the manifest myocardial vector. Experimental observations by Nelson and associates (1956)[N7] indicate that the short-circuiting effect of the contained blood may reduce the manifest heart vector by about 25 per cent. And, as indicated by Kossman (1958)[K39], this correlates well with the fairly common clinical observation that electrocardiographic deflections tend to be diminished in amplitude in a failing heart dilated with blood. The electrocardiographic deflections of the same heart may be increased when it is reduced in size by appropriate therapy.

It has also been shown, for example, that, following experimental induction of a transmural infarction in dogs, there is minimal or no S-T segment deviation from leads situated in the cavity of the heart, but good reciprocal deviation is obtained from leads situated over the epicardial surface[R1]. Similar results were reported by Pruitt and Valencia (1948)[P35].

This would explain the relatively small magnitude of the S-T segment changes reflecting the injury of subendocardial infarction, and the minimal S-T segment deviations recorded by the precordial electrodes in true posterior infarction. In both these instances the short-circuiting effect of the blood plays a major role in diminishing the magnitude of the S-T segment deviations.

The principle would also explain, in part, the reason for the S-T segment elevation in epicardial leads orientated to the transmural myocardial injury of a transmural infarction, and S-T segment depression in endocardial leads orientated to the transmural injury of a transmural infarction, for in a transmural infarction both endocardial and epicardial surfaces are injured. Thus, the relatively high resistance of the tissues overlying the epicardial surface would tend to augment the S-T segment elevation, whereas the relatively low resistance of the blood would tend to diminish the S-T segment elevation. The result would then be an S-T segment deviation towards the epicardial surface.

The Significance of the Boundary Shape and its Relationship to the Orientation of the Electromotive Forces

It has been shown that when a spherical conducting boundary separates tissues of different resistance, for example the boundary between the subendocardium and the blood, the tissue of low resistance will tend to augment the electromotive force which is orientated directly to, perpendicular to, the boundary; but will attenuate those electromotive forces which are tangential to the boundary (Brody, 1956)[B79].

The concept of electrical images is important in this respect. The following description is taken verbatum from Kossman's account (1958)[K39].

The concept of electric images originated with William Thomson (Lord Kelvin)[T10] and was simply compared to virtual optical images by his biographer, S.P.Thompson[T9], quoted by Hecht[H13]. The analogy was given of the well-known example of a candle in front of a mirror and its image, the same distance behind the mirror, giving the equivalent illumination of a candle at each of these sites when the mirror is removed. When the candle is placed in front of a polished silver ball, the image within the ball is smaller and nearer to the surface than the candle itself.

The mathematics of the phenomenon has been reviewed and confirmed by Nelson (1955[N5], 1965[N6]) using the basis of a double-layered electrolytic tank. The method of images was originally applied by Pruitt and Valencia (1948)[P35] to explain the apparent paradoxical behaviour of certain S-T segment deviations associated with myocardial injury.

A generalization of the method of images may be stated as follows (Kossman, 1958)[K39]:

With a source of current, regarded as a charged lamina, at the boundary of any given medium the potential of points between it and its image in a medium of higher resistance will be augmented, and elsewhere in its own medium, attenuated. When the adjacent medium is of lower resistance the reverse effects on the potential of the points under consideration occur. Whether the points will be positive or negative will depend on the orientation of the laminal charges with respect to the media.

As further pointed out by Kossman (1958)[K39], electric images have probably also been inadequately evaluated in the explanation of small R waves in intramural leads near the endocardium. It is true that by the method of images, there should be some augmentation of the R wave if the wave of excitation proceeds outward in normal fashion to the endocardial surface. The ten-times greater rate of conduction in the Purkinje system as compared to the ventricular myocardium makes it certain that some component of mural excitation is tangential to this surface and accordingly will be poorly recorded or not recorded at all. The possible application of the method to this complex problem is cited simply to emphasize that the small or absent R wave in subendocardial leads may have explanations other than that the subendocardial ventricular muscle does not contribute to the electrocardiogram.

ORIENTATION OF THE ELECTRODES

Because the left ventricle constitutes the dominant electrical chamber of the heart, the orientation of the conventional

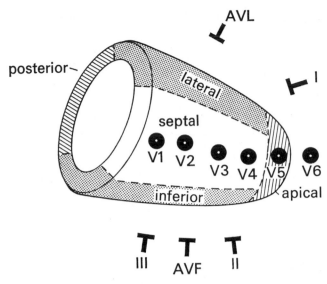

FIG. 10. Diagrammatic representation of the various surfaces of the left ventricular anatomical 'cone', and their relationship to the frontal and horizontal plane leads.

electrodes to this chamber is of particular importance in electrocardiology.

The left ventricle is a cone-shaped structure whose apex is directed downwards and to the left, and whose open base is directed upwards and to the right. It has five principal surfaces (Fig. 10):

1 The anterior or septal surface

This is the interventricular septum, and constitutes the major part of the electrical anterior wall of the heart. It may, from the diagnostic viewpoint, be conveniently divided into upper, middle and lower thirds.

Lead orientation: The principal leads orientated to this surface are leads V1 to V4.

2 The inferior or diaphragmatic surface.

This consists principally of the inferior part of the left free wall.

Lead orientation: The leads orientated to the inferior surface are Standard leads II and III, and lead AVF. Standard lead III is orientated to the right inferior surface and consequently may also be somewhat orientated to the inferior regions of the interventricular septum. Standard lead II is orientated to the left inferior surface and thus also tends to be orientated to the inferior regions of the left lateral or superior wall.

3 The left lateral surface

This is, in effect, the left superior surface and the superior part of the left free wall.

Lead orientation: The principal leads orientated to the left lateral surface are Standard lead I which is orientated to the distal part of the left lateral surface, and lead AVL which is orientated to the proximal part of the left lateral surface.

4 The posterior surface

This is the region of the left free wall between the inferior and lateral (superior) surfaces. It faces the back of the thorax.

Lead orientation: None of the conventional leads are orientated directly to the posterior wall. However, leads V1 to V4 are orientated to the *endo*cardial surface of the posterior wall (Fig. 10; see also Fig. 31), and the electrocardiographic diagnosis of posterior-wall pathology is consequently made from the inverse, or mirror-image, changes in leads V1 to V4.

5 The apical surface

The apex of the left ventricle is, in fact, constituted by an extension of all the aforementioned surfaces. Its proximal boundaries are ill-defined since the base of the apical surface encroaches upon the anterior, inferior, lateral and posterior surfaces.

Lead orientation: The principal leads orientated to the apical surface are leads V5 and V6. However, because of the encroachment of this region upon the other surfaces, it is also orientated to Standard lead I, the lateral (superior) surface, Standard lead II, the inferior surface, and lead V4, the septal surface.

DEPOLARIZATION OF THE VENTRICLES

Depolarization of the ventricles occurs transversely, i.e. across the thickness of the ventricular wall from endocardial to epicardial surfaces[L49, S41, W48]. Depolarization begins in the left side of the midseptal region and spreads transversely from left to right[K22, S41], producing a relatively large left to right force (illustrated as Vector 1a in Diagram A of Fig. 11). Activation of the right side of the interventricular septum begins fractionally, 0·01 sec, later. It begins just below the midseptum at the base of the right papillary muscle close to the trabecular zone. This activation front also spreads transversely, but from right to left, resulting in a relatively small right to left force (illustrated as Vector 1b in Diagram A of Fig. 11). This fractional delay in the activation of the right side of the septum led Wilson (1947)[W54] to conclude that a very minor grade of incomplete right bundle branch block, then, is physiologic.

The two initial septal forces are thus opposite in direction and tend to oppose each other. The larger left to right septal force, however, dominates, and the resultant initial vector is consequently directed from left to right (illustrated as Vector 1 in Diagram A of Fig. 11).

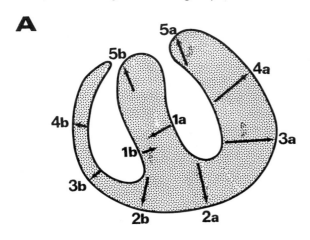

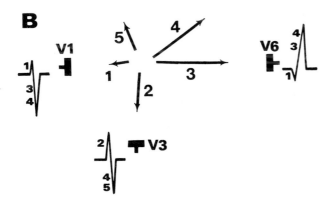

FIG. 11. Diagrammatic illustrations of: A, the sequences of ventricular depolarization; and B, the resultant mean vectors. See text.

Septal activation is followed by activation of both the paraseptal regions (illustrated as Vectors 2a and 2b in Diagram A of Fig. 11). The resultant mean vector is directed anteriorly and inferiorly (illustrated as Vector 2 in Diagram B of Fig. 11).

The initial epicardial breakthrough occurs in the trabecular zone of the right free wall[D43] (Vector 2b in Diagram A

of Fig. 11). This is followed almost simultaneously by epicardial breakthrough in the diaphragmatic surface of the left ventricle (Durrer and associates, 1965[D43], 1966[D44]; Blumenschein and associates, 1969[B59]). This is followed by depolarization of the free right and left ventricular wall spreading transversely from right to left in the left free wall, and from left to right in the right free wall. The forces therefore tend to oppose each other (illustrated by Vectors 3a and b, and Vectors 4a and b in Diagram A of Fig. 11). The larger forces of the left free wall are dominant and the resultant vectors are consequently directed from right to left (Vectors 3 and 4 in Diagram B of Fig. 11). Activation of the relatively thin free right wall of the right ventricle actually begins after, and is completed before, the relatively thick free wall of the left ventricle[S41].

The last regions of the heart to be activated are the base of the left free wall, and then finally the right superior septal surface and adjacent right ventricular outflow tract (illustrated by Vectors 5a and b in Diagram A of Fig. 11) [D43, S39]. This results in a terminal force which is directed to the right, superiorly and inferiorly (illustrated as Vector 5 in Diagram B of Fig. 11).

The Basic QRS Patterns as Reflected by the Precordial Electrodes

The following basic QRS patterns are normally reflected by the precordial electrodes (Diagram B of Fig. 11).

Lead V1: This lead reflects an rS complex. The small initial *r* wave reflects Vector 1 of initial septal depolarization, and the *S* wave reflects Vectors 3 and 4 of ventricular depolarization of the left free wall. Vectors 2 and 5 tend to be directed perpendicularly to the lead axis of lead V1, and hence make little impression on this lead. A small terminal *r'* wave may, at times, appear in lead V1 as a result of Vector 5.

Lead V6: This lead reflects a qR or qRs complex. The small initial *q* wave reflects Vector 1 of initial septal depolarization. The *R* wave reflects the dominant left ventricular depolarization, Vectors 3 and 4. The terminal tiny *s* wave (not always present) reflects Vector 5 of terminal basal activation. Vector 2 tends to be at right angles to the lead axis of lead V6 and thus makes little impression on this lead.

Lead V3 (or leads V2, V3 and V4): This lead reflects an RS complex. The R wave is the expression of Vector 2, reflecting dominant paraseptal depolarization. The S wave reflects Vectors 4 and 5 of dominantly basal depolarization. Vectors 1 and 3 of ventricular depolarization tend to be at right angles to this lead axis, and make very little or no impression on this lead.

THE ELECTROPATHOLOGY OF MYOCARDIAL ISCHAEMIA

The Polarity of the Ischaemic T Wave

Myocardial ischaemia is reflected by a *T wave vector that is directed away from the surface of ischaemia*: a *T* wave vector that is usually opposite in direction to the mean *QRS* vector (see Chapter 1). This manifestation is due to a *delay in repolarization of the ischaemic cells*, the principles of which are considered below.

Myocardial ischaemia results in a *delay in repolarization*, especially Phase 3 of the transmembrane action potential. Consider, for example, the effect of myocardial ischaemia affecting the epicardial region of the heart (Fig. 12 and Diagram B of Fig. 13). Since the epicardial cells are ischaemic, their repolarization is delayed, and the healthy endocardial cells recover first (as illustrated in Diagram D of Fig. 12). The series of doublets now proceeds with negative pole first, from endocardial to epicardial surfaces. An electrode orientated to the epicardial surface will be orientated to the negative pole of the doublet and will consequently reflect a negative deflection, an inverted *T* wave. Furthermore, since the recovery of the epicardial surface occurs late, the neutralizing or balancing, cancellation, effect of earlier opposing *T* wave forces in other remote healthy regions of the heart is lost. The inverted *T* wave of ischaemia is consequently of *greater magnitude*.

These principles of repolarization are illustrated with reference to the transmembrane action potential in Fig. 13. Diagram A illustrates the normal sequence of events. The action potential of the epicardial cell begins later than that of the endocardial cell, since it takes time for the endocardial-epicardial activation process to reach the epicardial surface. Phase 0 of the epicardial cell is consequently inscribed after Phase 0 of the endocardial cell. However, normal repolarization of the epicardial cells begins *before* repolarization of the endocardial cells (as described above).

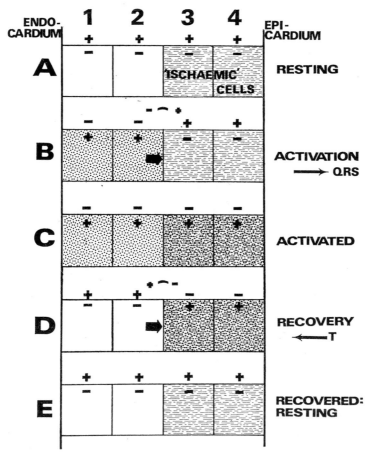

FIG. 12. Diagrams illustrating the process of depolarization and repolarization through a series of transmural cells. The epicardial cells are ischaemic. See text, and compare with Fig. 7.

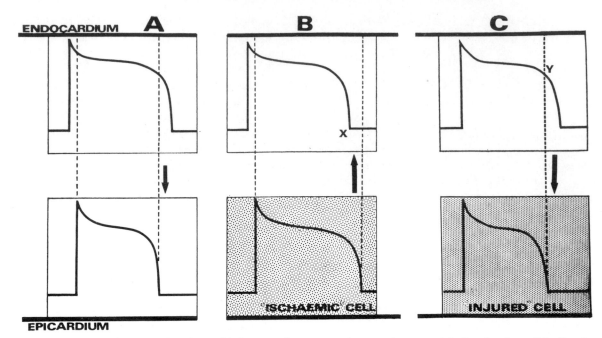

FIG. 13. Diagrams illustrating the relationship between the transmembrane action potential of a subendocardial cell and a subepicardial cell during: A, normal endocardial to epicardial depolarization; B, depolarization in the presence of an ischaemic epicardial cell; and C, depolarization in the presence of an injured epicardial cell.

Therefore, Phase 3 of the epicardial cell is inscribed before Phase 3 of the endocardial cell.

In the event of epicardial ischaemia (Diagram B of Fig. 13), Phase 3 of the epicardial cell is delayed and so occurs later than Phase 3 of the endocardial cell. If the duration of the action potential is delayed in a cell or area, that cell or area will have an *external* charge that is negative or relatively negative to the surrounding tissue with a relatively shorter Phase 3. It is important to note, in the application of this concept, that the action potential reflects the events *within* the cell.

For example, in Fig. 13 at point X the endocardial cell has been completely repolarized and therefore has a negative internal charge and a positive external charge. The ischaemic epicardial cell which has not yet recovered has a positive or relatively positive internal charge and a negative external charge. Since vectors tend to flow from areas that are negative to those which are positive, the repolarization current (arrow) flows from epicardial to endocardila regions. This will result in a negative *T* wave in leads orientated to the epicardial surface. This was also shown to be the case by Mandel and associates (1968)[M11] who used a theoretical electronic repolarization model designed by Harumi and associates (1966)[H10]. It is of interest to note that experimental occlusion of a coronary artery results in a shortening of the transmembrane action potential and then a decrease in the amplitude of the transmembrane action potential in the cells supplied by the coronary artery.

This corresponds to an initial increase in the height of the *T* wave followed by an elevated S-T segment[D7, D41, W39].

THE ELECTROPATHOLOGY OF MYOCARDIAL INJURY

Myocardial injury may present in two phases:

(1) **a hyperacute injury phase,** and
(2) **a subacute injury phase.**

1   The Hyperacute Injury Phase

This occurs in the very early stage of an evolving acute myocardial infarction and in the variant, Prinzmetal's, form of angina pectoris. It is reflected by the following electrocardiographic manifestations:

(a) Acute Injury Block
This is a delay in conduction through the acutely injured tissue resulting in an increase in the ventricular activation time and in an increase in the amplitude of the QRS complex. The principles governing this phenomenon are considered in greater detail in Chapter 12.

(b) Marked Deviation of the S-T Segment, a Slope-elevation Towards the Surface of Injury
The principles governing this phenomenon are considered

in greater detail in the section on subacute injury (see below).

(c) An Increased Amplitude of the T Wave which is also Directed Towards the Surface of Injury

The *T* wave of the early hyperacute phase of myocardial infarction and the variant form of angina pectoris is often taller than normal and directed *towards* the surface of injury. In other words, there is an exaggeration of the *T* wave in leads which normally reflect an upright *T* wave. This would appear to be paradoxical, for the direction is the reverse of that which occurs with myocardial ischaemia where the *T* wave is directed *away* from the surface or area of ischaemia.

A possible mechanism for this phenomenon is a shortening of the refractory period, a shortening of the action potential.

The acute effect of coronary artery occlusion is characterized by a shortening of the Q-T interval. This is followed later by a lengthening of the Q-T interval.

This early shortening of the Q-T interval, an abbreviation of the functional refractory period, is responsible for the deviation of the *T* wave *towards* the surface of injury. This will result in an exaggeration of the normal upright *T* wave in leads orientated to an epicardial injury. The phenomenon is the reverse of that associated with myocardial ischaemia (see above). The underlying mechanism is essentially the same, and is based on the premise that repolarization vectors are directed from areas which are relatively negative to those which are relatively positive. The principle is illustrated in Diagram C of Fig. 13. The epicardial cell is acutely injured. The action potential (refractory period) is shortened. Recovery of the injured epicardial cell occurs before that of the uninjured endocardial cell. For example, at point Y the endocardial cell is still in the process of recovery and has a positive internal charge and a negative external charge, whereas the injured epicardial cell which has fully recovered has a negative internal charge and a positive external charge. The repolarization current will flow from the negative external charge of the uninjured endocardial cell to the positive external charge of the injured epicardial cell (arrow). A lead orientated towards the injured surface will thus reflect an upright *T* wave. And since recovery is earlier than normal, it will no longer be balanced (neutralized or cancelled) by recovery of other cells in remote healthy areas of the heart. Therefore it will be exaggerated in amplitude.

The manifestation of the hyperacute epicardial injury are evident in Electrocardiographic Studies 1, 2, 3, 4, 5, 7, 12, 25, 90 and 91.

This *T* wave change is always associated with the elevated S-T segments of myocardial injury. The manifestation of

depressed S-T segment and inverted increased magnitude *T* waves seen in the precordial leads in cases of subendocardial infarction is essentially the mirror-image of the aforementioned manifestation (Electrocardiographic Studies 73, 74 and 75). The subject is considered further in Chapter 8.

2 The Subacute Injury Phase

The subacute injury phase corresponds to the fully evolved phase of acute myocardial infarction, and is characterized by coved elevation of the S-T segments in leads orientated to the injured surface. In other words, the S-T segment is deviated towards the surface of injury. The deviation is, however, not as marked as that seen in the hyperacute injury phase.

The precise electropathological mechanism of the S-T segment deviation in myocardial injury has not, as yet, been completely elucidated. Several hypotheses have been proposed, and these are considered below.

THE HYPOTHESIS OF DIFFERENTIAL POLARIZATION

Most theories of the S-T segment injury effect are based upon a differential state of polarization between the injured and uninjured surfaces. This is particularly prone to occur during diastole. The basis for this phenomenon is the **inability of the injured cell to maintain the polarized state during diastole.**

The injured myocardial cell is associated with a loss of resting potential. This is due to a loss of intracellular potassium. The resting potential within the cell is reduced, for example, from -90 mV to -70 mV. The balancing positive potential on the surface of the cell is reduced proportionally. The magnitude of the dipole is consequently reduced. A difference in potential will then exist between the normal cell and the injured cell.

There are three hypotheses based on this principle:

HYPOTHESIS 1: DIFFERENTIAL DIASTOLIC POLARIZATION

The injured cell loses its ability to maintain an adequately polarized state. In addition, the cell membrane is injured and is unable to separate the normal internal negativity and external positivity during the resting state[S112]. The cell thus leaks negative ions and the exterior or surface becomes negative or less positive (see below). This is illustrated in Diagram A of Fig. 15. The injured cells develop a negative surface charge, and a doublet consequently develops between the injured and the uninjured cells or zones. This doublet has a negative tail which is directed towards the

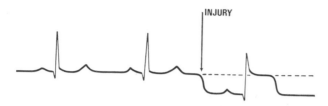

FIG. 14. Diagrammatic representation of the advent of myocardial injury during a continuous electrocardiographic recording.

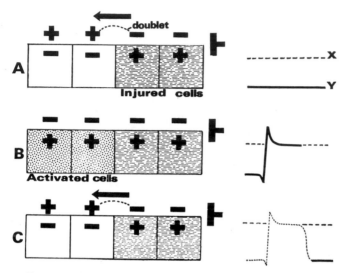

FIG. 15. Diagrams illustrating a possible mechanism of the current of injury. See text.

injured zone and a positive head which is directed towards the uninjured zone. An electrode orientated towards the injured zone (as illustrated in Diagram A of Fig. 15) will be orientated towards a current of negativity, the so-called negative current of injury. This will result in a continuous depression of the baseline (from position X to position Y in Diagram A of Fig. 15). This is, in most cases, inferential and is only evident from the interpretation of subsequent electrocardiographic events (see below). It may, however, be evident experimentally when the precise moment of injury is recorded (arrow in Fig. 14). When this occurs, the injury will manifest by a sudden depression of the baseline recorded by an electrode orientated to the injured surface (Fig. 14). When the healthy cells are activated (as illustrated in Diagram B of Fig. 15), they too will develop a negative surface charge. Thus, during the activated, depolarized state there will be no difference in potential between the injured cells and the uninjured cells. The current of injury is consequently abolished and the depressed baseline returns to normal (as illustrated in Diagram B of Fig. 15, and Fig. 14). This creates the illusion of an elevated S-T segment. Once the healthy, uninjured, cells return to the polarized

or resting state, the current of injury between injured and uninjured tissue is re-established, and the baseline is once again depressed (Diagram C of Fig. 15).

This basic hypothesis assumes that the injured tissue is not depolarized, since cells which have lost their polarity, as evident from a negative surface charge, can no longer be depolarized. It is, however, known that injured tissue can, at times, be depolarized, although such depolarization may be abnormal. For example, the elevated S-T segment reflecting the basic current of injury can be associated with injury block, a *delay* in conduction through the injured tissue. The simplified hypothesis outlined above therefore requires modification to accommodate the associated depolarization of the injured tissue. This is considered in Hypothesis 2.

HYPOTHESIS 2: DIFFERENTIAL DIASTOLIC POLARIZATION

The injured cell is unable to maintain an adequately polarized state, and this is reflected by a *diminution of polarization*; the magnitude of the dipole being diminished. Consequently, although the surface of the injured tissue does not become overtly negative, it becomes *less positive* or *relatively* negative to the adjacent healthy tissue. This is illustrated in Diagram A of Fig. 16. A difference in surface

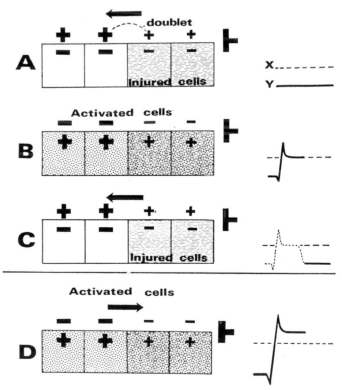

FIG. 16. Diagrams illustrating further possible mechanisms of the current of injury. See text and compare with Figure 15.

potential, a doublet, consequently develops between the injured cell with diminished polarization, and the adjacent healthy cell with full polarization. This too will create a current of injury with a positive head towards the healthy tissue and a relatively negative tail directed towards the injured tissue. This, too, will also result in a depression of the baseline similar to the mechanism described in Hypothesis 1. Depolarization of *both* the injured and uninjured tissues brings about negative surface charges in both the healthy and injured tissues, thereby abolishing the surface potential difference and neutralizing current of injury[N2]. The baseline consequently returns to normal during the activated, depolarized, state, creating the illusion of an elevated S-T segment (Diagram B of Fig. 16). Repolarization results in the re-establishment of the differential surface potential and the current of injury, and this once again results in a depression of the baseline (Diagram C of Fig. 16).

Hypothesis 3: The Systolic Current of Injury

At times it would appear that the elevated S-T segment represents not merely the return of the baseline to its previous isoelectric level, but a true, active, positive displacement. In other words, the S-T segment is actively elevated to a level *higher* than the pre-existing baseline or isoelectric level[E17, S112]. This principle is illustrated in Diagram D of Fig. 16, the equivalent of Diagram B in the same Figure. When depolarization of the injured and healthy tissues occurs, the surface of the healthy cells will, because of their greater initial polarization, become more negative than the adjacent injured surface (Diagrams B and D of Fig. 16).

In other words, the surface of the injured cells are *relatively more positive* than the neighbouring healthy cells. A reverse doublet is thus created between the healthy and injured surfaces (Diagram D of Fig. 16). This doublet has a *relatively* more positive head which is directed towards the injured tissue. This is reflected by an active or true elevation of the S-T segment, i.e. elevation to a level greater than the normal baseline or isoelectric level. Note that the S-T segment in Diagram D of Fig. 16 is elevated to a level higher than the original baseline (dotted line) whereas the S-T segment in Diagram B is not. There is thus a differential potential difference during systole as well as during diastole. The systolic difference in potential actively raises the S-T segment.

It is likely that all the variations of differential polarization and depolarization described above can and do occur. The state reflected by Hypothesis 1 reflects the greatest degree of injury since the injured cells can no longer be depolarized. The state reflected by Hypothesis 2 reflects the least degree of injury since the injured cells can still be depolarized, and the degree of differential depolarization

between injured and healthy tissue is not of sufficient magnitude to create a systolic differential surface potential. The state reflected by Hypothesis 3 reflects a degree of injury intermediate between Hypothesis 1 and Hypothesis 2.

THE HYPOTHESIS OF EARLY REPOLARIZATION

The S-T segment deviations of myocardial injury were investigated by Samson and Scher (1960)[S7] with the aid of stable D-C amplifiers. They observed a lowering of the baseline, the T-Q segment, coincidental with a lowered intracellular resting potential in the injured or anoxic area. The lowered T-Q segment would create the illusion of an elevated S-T segment similar to the mechanism described in Hypothesis 1 above. In addition, and particularly during the later stage of injury, S-T segment elevation was observed which coincided with a shortened repolarization phase in the injured or anoxic area. This S-T segment elevation was thought to be due to differences in repolarization time; earlier repolarization in the injured area would create a difference in potential thereby causing a current flow towards the injured muscle during the S-T interval.

Shortened repolarization of injured tissue is also evident from the conventional electrocardiogram in myocardial infarction. Thus, the mere fact that the R on T phenomenon can occur, i.e. that a ventricular extrasystole can occur with a very short coupling interval (see Chapter 17), indicates that there is a shortening of the refractory period of at least part of the myocardium. This represents a shortening of repolarization. Furthermore, marked fluctuations in the duration of the Q-T interval may be evident during the evolution of myocardial infarction (see p. 140 and Electrocardiographic Study 16). Shortening of the Q-T interval is particularly prone to occur during an exacerbation of pain. Earlier repolarization of injured, anoxic, zones has also been observed by Reynolds and associates (1960)[R7].

THE ELECTROPATHOLOGY OF NECROSIS

With the advent of necrosis, the cell becomes electrically inert. No transmembrane action potential whatsoever can be recorded from the cell. The necrotic tissue represents, in effect, a loss of electrical tissue. This is reflected electrocardiographically by a loss of the forces of depolarization, a loss of QRS deflection, in leads orientated to the necrotic area. This loss of forces also results in a lack of opposition to, or cancellation of, forces in distant viable myocardium, forces which are orientated in the opposite direction. There is consequently a reorientation of electrical forces away from the necrotic tissue. The principle is discussed in Chapter 3.

THE BIOCHEMICAL EXPRESSION

The maintenance of an adequate resting potential, an optimum degree of internal negativity, is dependent upon an adequate level of cellular potassium, a loss of cellular potassium being associated with a loss of resting potential.[S114] The cell becomes inert when the cellular potassium is reduced to 50 per cent of the normal. This has been termed the inertia potential[S28, S31]. Progressive coronary insufficiency is thus associated with a progressive loss of resting potential as reflected by a progressive loss of intracellular potassium[S114] (Fig. 17).

A slight loss of cellular potassium will result in a slight diminution of the resting potential. This results in a delay in repolarization which manifests electrocardiographically by the *T* wave changes of myocardial ischaemia. A further loss of cellular potassium results in a further loss of resting potential which manifests electrocardiographically with the S-T segment changes of myocardial injury. When the cellular potassium is further reduced to 50 per cent of the normal value, the resting potential is reduced to the inertia potential, and the cell becomes electrically dead or necrotic. Depolarization then becomes impossible and the electrocardiogram manifests with a loss of QRS forces resulting in, for example, the pathological *Q* wave of myocardial infarction.

A similar phenomenon has been postulated for the degenerating pacemaking cell[S28], the evolution of ectopic ventricular rhythm being based on a progressive loss of intracellular potassium.

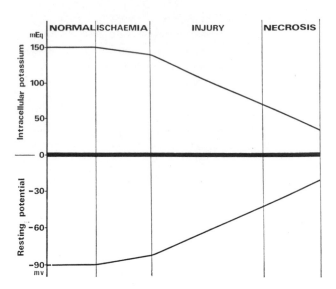

FIG. 17. Diagrammatic representation of the relationship between the intracellular potassium concentration and the resting transmembrane potential. Progressive diminution of the intracellular potassium concentration is associated with a progressive loss of resting potential. The progressive loss passes through the phases of ischaemia, injury and necrosis. See text.

Thus, the evolution of abnormal ventricular rhythms due to degeneration of a pacemaking cell and the abnormalities resulting from the progressive degeneration of non-pacemaking cells, can be based and unified on a similar pathogenesis. **The diseased cell is unable to maintain its resting potential due to a progressive loss of cellular potassium.**

Chapter 3

The Electrocardiographic Syndromes of Myocardial Ischaemia, Injury and Necrosis

THE ELECTROCARDIOGRAPHIC SYNDROMES OF MYOCARDIAL ISCHAEMIA

Myocardial ischaemia is reflected by:

(a) *symmetrical arrow-head* T *waves,*
(b) *an increase in the magnitude of the* T *wave vector, and*
(c) a T wave vector that is *directed away from the surface of the ischaemia.*

There is usually a *prolonged Q-T interval.* These features are described in greater detail in Chapter 1.

The Associations of Myocardial Ischaemia

Myocardial ischaemia may occur as an associated phenomenon or it may be found in association with myocardial injury and myocardial necrosis.

ISOLATED MYOCARDIAL ISCHAEMIA

Isolated myocardial ischaemia manifests with the aforementioned *T*-wave changes only. It may present under the following circumstances:

(a) As an expression of acute coronary insufficiency precipitated by the exercise test (see Chapter 16).
(b) As an expression of angina pectoris.
(c) As an occurrence in an asymptomatic patient with chronic coronary insufficiency.

MYOCARDIAL ISCHAEMIA IN ASSOCIATION WITH MYOCARDIAL INJURY

Myocardial ischaemia may occur in association with myocardial injury. The *T* wave abnormalities of ischaemia will then occur in association with the S-T segment abnormalities of injury. The association usually occurs as a manifestation of acute coronary insufficiency which may be due to angina pectoris or a consequence of the exercise

test. It is also evident at the periphery of an infarction, during the fully evolved phase of acute myocardial infarction. It may, at times, also occur in an asymptomatic patient with chronic coronary insufficiency.

MYOCARDIAL ISCHAEMIA IN ASSOCIATION WITH MYOCARDIAL INJURY AND MYOCARDIAL NECROSIS

Myocardial ischaemia is always present at the periphery of an *acute* myocardial infarction. The *T* wave abnormality of ischaemia then occurs in association with the S-T segment abnormalities of myocardial injury, and the Q waves, QS complexes or diminished *R* wave amplitude of myocardial necrosis (Diagram F of Fig. 23; and Fig. 24).

The Sites of Myocardial Ischaemia

Myocardial ischaemia occurs predominantly in the subepicardial or subendocardial regions of the left ventricle. Ischaemia can also occur in the right ventricle but essentially it may, in effect, be considered to occur exclusively in the left ventricle.

Theoretically the ischaemia can occur at the following sites:

1. The subepicardial region of the anterior wall.
2. The subendocardial region of the posterior wall.
3. The subendocardial region of the anterior wall.
4. The subepicardial region of the posterior wall.
5. The subepicardial region of the inferior wall.
6. The subendocardial region of the inferior wall.

Note: The anterior wall of the left ventricle includes the interventricular septum (see Chapter 2) which constitutes the anterior electrical wall of the heart.

LOCALIZATION OF THE ISCHAEMIC REGIONS

Localization of the ischaemic region is made from the

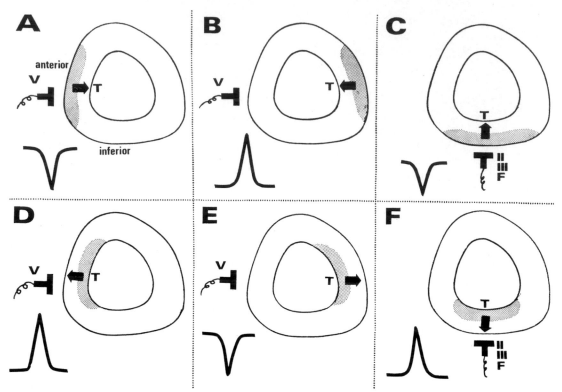

FIG. 18. Diagrams illustrating the theoretical direction of the T wave vectors with epicardial and endocardial ischaemia of the anterior, inferior and posterior wall of the heart. See text.

orientation of the T-wave vector which is *directed away from the surface of ischaemia.*

1   *Anterior-wall Subepicardial Ischaemia*

In anterior wall subepicardial ischaemia the T wave vector is directed posteriorly, resulting in deeply inverted, symmetrical arrow-head T waves in several or all the precordial leads, leads V2 to V6 (Diagram A of Fig. 18).

As with anterior-wall myocardial infarction (Chapter 6), anterior-wall myocardial ischaemia may be subdivided into the following categories which are presented with reference to Fig. 10.

(a)   *Extensive anterior-wall myocardial ischaemia*

The T waves are inverted in all of the precordial leads, especially leads V2 to V6, Standard lead I, lead AVL, and possibly Standard lead II.

(b)   *Anteroseptal myocardial ischaemia*

The T waves are inverted in the right precordial leads, leads V1 to V4. The T-wave vector is directed posteriorly and is perpendicular to the frontal plane. With this localization, similar changes not infrequently appear in the inferiorly orientated leads, Standard leads II and III and lead AVF. The T wave vector is then directed superiorly as

well as posteriorly (see also below, p. 27). *Note*: Low to inverted T waves may also occur in pericarditis. The differential diagnosis is discussed in Chapter 4.

(c)   *Apical myocardial ischaemia*

The T waves are inverted in all three Standard leads and leads V5 and V6. The T wave vector is directed superiorly and to the right.

(d)   *Anterolateral myocardial ischaemia*

The T waves are inverted in Standard lead I and lead AVL, and possibly lead V6. The T wave vector is directed to the right. This manifestation becomes particularly suggestive of myocardial ischaemia when the associated R wave is of low or relatively low voltage; for T wave inversion in the left lateral leads may also be a manifestation of left ventricular hypertrophy and strain when the associated QRS complex is of increased magnitude.

(e)   *High-lateral myocardial ischaemia*

The T wave is inverted in lead AVL but remains upright in the precordial leads. It must, however, be borne in mind that the normal T wave is frequently negative in lead AVL, since a T wave axis between $+60°$ and $+90°$, within the normal range for a T wave axis, will be reflected by a negative *T* wave in lead AVL. Therefore, if the negative *T* wave in AVL is to be significant of high-lateral myocardial ischaemia, it should reflect the following additional characteristics:

(i) The *T* wave should be of the coronary type: symmetrical, sharply pointed, and possibly increased in magnitude.

(ii) There should be a wide QRS-T angle (see Chapter 15, p. 141). The mean manifest frontal plane QRS axis should be deviated somewhat to the left, and the frontal plane QRS-T angle should exceed 60°. The QRS complex will, under this circumstance, be *dominantly upright in lead AVL*.

Note: Low *T* waves may occur as a result of extensive and confluent application of the electrode jelly, which may cause some short-circuiting.

2 Posterior Wall Subendocardial Ischaemia

In posterior wall subendocardial ischaemia the *T* wave vector is theoretically also directed posteriorly, as occurs with anterior wall subepicardial ischaemia. This results in deep, inverted, symmetrical, arrow-head *T* waves in precordial leads V2 to V6, usually leads V2 to V4 (Diagram E of Fig. 18).

It has yet to be established whether this occurs in the clinical setting and, if so, whether it can be recognized electrocardiographically. If indeed it does occur, several factors may lead to the obscurity of the electrocardiographic manifestation. These are: (a) a neutralizing concomitant anterior wall subendocardial ischaemia, (b) the short-circuiting effect of the low-resistant blood which is interspersed between the posterior wall and the electrodes, and (c) the neutralizing boundary effect. These factors are considered in greater detail in Chapter 2.

3 Anterior wall Subendocardial Ischaemia

In anterior wall subendocardial ischaemia the *T* wave vector is directed anteriorly, resulting in tall, symmetrical arrow-head *T* waves in precordial leads V2 to V6 (Diagram D of Fig. 18, and Electrocardiographic Studies 81 to 86). The Q-T interval is usually prolonged.

4 Posterior wall Subepicardial Ischaemia

In posterior wall subepicardial ischaemia the *T* wave vector is directed anteriorly (Diagram B of Fig. 18), resulting in tall, symmetrical, arrow-head *T* waves in the precordial leads. It is doubtful whether this occurs as an isolated phenomenon. The manifestation is usually seen as part of true posterior wall myocardial infarction (Electrocardiographic Studies 31 and 32).

5 Inferior wall Subepicardial Ischaemia

In inferior wall subepicardial ischaemia the *T* wave vector is directed superiorly, resulting in deeply inverted arrow-head *T* waves in leads orientated towards the inferior wall, viz. Standard leads II and III and lead AVF (Diagram C of Fig. 18, and Electrocardiographic Studies 23, 27 and 28). This usually occurs as part of the presentation of the fully evolved phase of inferior wall myocardial infarction.

6 Inferior wall Subendocardial Ischaemia

In inferior-wall subendocardial ischaemia the *T* wave vector is directed inferiorly, i.e. towards Standard leads II and III and lead AVF, resulting in tall, symmetrical *T* waves in these leads (Diagram F of Fig. 18, and Electrocardiographic Study 86).

When myocardial ischaemia occurs in association with myocardial injury and/or necrosis (as in acute myocardial infarction), then precise localization of the ischaemic region presents no difficulty, since the additional parameters of injury and necrosis facilitate the diagnosis. When, however, the ischaemia occurs as the *only* electrocardiographic abnormality, then accurate localization may be difficult. For example, both anterior wall subepicardial ischaemia and posterior wall subendocardial ischaemia are theoretically by a posteriorly directed *T* wave vector, resulting in deep, inverted, arrow-head *T* waves in the precordial leads (Diagram A and E of Fig. 18; see Sections 1 and 2 above). Both anterior-wall subendocardial ischaemia and posterior wall subepicardial ischaemia are theoretically reflected by an anteriorly directed *T*-wave vector, resulting in tall, symmetrical, arrow-head *T* waves in the precordial leads (Diagram B and D of Fig. 18; see Sections 3 and 4 above). Accurate localization under these circumstances may then present some difficulty. The diagnosis, may, however, be facilitated *if there is extension of the myocardial ischaemia to the inferior wall*. This is frequently the case. When this extension occurs, the localization is made on the following theoretical basis. The principle is considered theoretical because posterior wall subendocardial ischaemia has not yet been demonstrated as a definite electrocardiographic entity for the reasons already outlined above. Nevertheless, the theoretical considerations presented below may serve as a useful basis or guide to potential practical localization.

Extension of anterior wall subepicardial ischaemia to the inferior wall must, *ipso facto*, involve the inferior subepicardial wall, and not the inferior subendocardial wall. This results in a *T* wave vector that is directed away from *both* the anterior and inferior subepicardial walls, i.e. a *T* wave directed *posteriorly* and *superiorly*. This will manifest as deeply inverted, symmetrical, arrow-head *T* waves in the precordial leads, as well as in leads orientated to the inferior

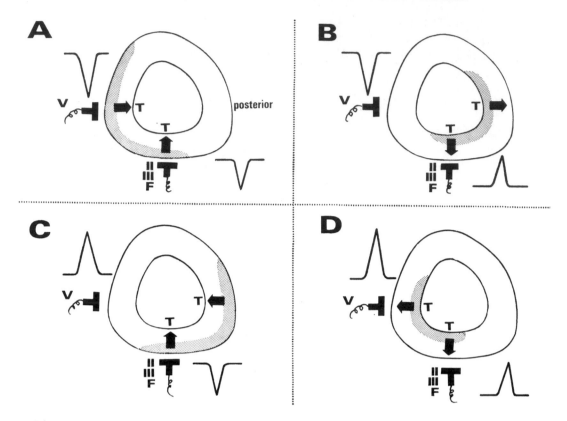

Fig. 19. Diagrams illustrating the combinations of anterior and inferior wall, and posterior and inferior wall, subendo-cardial and subepicardial ischaemia, and their effect on the T wave vectors. See text.

surface of the heart, Standard leads II and III and lead AVF (Diagram A of Fig. 19).

Extension of posterior wall subendocardial ischaemia to the inferior wall must, *ipso facto*, involve the subendo-cardial region of the inferior wall, and not the subepi-cardial region of the inferior wall. This results in a T wave vector that is directed *posteriorly* and *inferiorly*, i.e. a T wave vector directed away from both the posterior and inferior subendocardial walls. (Diagram B of Fig. 19). This will result in deeply *inverted*, arrow-head T waves in the pre-cordial leads, but tall, *upright*, symmetrical, arrow-head T waves in leads orientated to the inferior surface of the heart, viz. Standard leads II and III, and lead AVF. This usually occurs as a concomitant of acute anterior wall myocardial infarction with extension of the ischaemia to the inferior wall (Electrocardiographic Studies 17, 18, 20, 21 and 22).

Thus, the T-wave vector in both anterior walls (sub-epicardial ischaemia and posterior subendocardial ischae-mia) will result in a posteriorly directed T wave vector. However, extension to the inferior wall will facilitate the diagnosis. An upright T wave in Standard leads II and III, and lead AVF indicates subepicardial localization. An inverted T wave in Standard leads II and III and lead AVF indicates subendocardial localization.

Likewise, extension of posterior-wall subepicardial ischaemia to the subepicardial region of the inferior wall will result in a T wave vector which is directed anteriorly and superiorly (Diagram B of Fig. 19). This will result in tall, symmetrical T waves in the precordial leads, but deep, inverted, symmetrical T waves in leads orientated to the inferior wall of the heart, Standard leads II and III and lead AVF. This usually occurs as a concomitant of true posterior wall myocardial infarction with extension of the infarction or the ischaemia to the inferior wall (Electrocardiographic Studies 31 and 32).

Extension of anterior-wall subendocardial ischaemia to a subendocardial region of the inferior wall will result in tall, symmetrical T waves in the precordial leads, and tall, symmetrical T waves in leads orientated towards the in-ferior surface, Standard leads II and III and lead AVF (Diagram D of Fig. 19). It is evident, therefore, that the direction of the T waves in Standard leads II and III and lead AVF help to differentiate between extension from posterior wall subepicardial infarction and posterior wall subendocardial infarction.

The differentiating features are summarized in Table 1.

TABLE 1 Tabular representation reflecting the significance of T wave direction in the theoretical localization of myocardial ischaemia

	T WAVE DIRECTION	
	V leads	*Standard leads II, III and lead AVF*
Anterior wall subepicardial ischaemia:	↓	
Anterior wall subendocardial ischaemia:	↑	
Posterior wall subepicardial ischaemia:	↑	
Posterior wall subendocardial ischaemia:	↓	
Inferior wall subepicardial ischaemia:		↓
Inferior wall subendocardial ischaemia:		↓
Anterior wall subepicardial ischaemia with Inferior wall subepicardial ischaemia:	↓	↓
Posterior wall subendocardial ischaemia with Inferior wall subepicardial ischaemia:	↓	↑
Anterior wall subendocardial ischaemia with Inferior wall subendocardial ischaemia:	↑	↑
Posterior wall subepicardial ischaemia with Inferior wall subepicardial ischaemia:	↑	↓

CORRELATIVE ESSAY

THE DIFFERENTIAL DIAGNOSIS OF TALL T WAVES IN THE PRECORDIAL LEADS

Tall T waves may appear in the precordial leads in the following conditions:

1. Acute anterior wall subendocardial ischaemia.
2. The early hyperacute phase of anterior wall injury or infarction.
3. Acute posterior wall subepicardial ischaemia. This occurs mainly as a concomitant of acute posterior-wall myocardial infarction.
4. Hyperkalaemia.
5. Left ventricular diastolic overload.
6. Acute pericarditis.
7. Recovering inferior wall myocardial infarction.
8. Healthy, vagotonic, individuals.
9. Apical infarction. The tall T waves are then localized to the right precordial leads.
10. The CVA Pattern, for example, acute head injury.

The differentiating characteristics are considered below.

1 Acute Anterior Wall Subendocardial Ischaemia

(a) The T waves are usually tallest in the *mid*-precordial leads, leads V3 to V5 (Electrocardiographic studies 83 to 86).

(b) The T waves may be slightly widened (Electrocardiographic Studies 83 to 86).

(c) The T waves tend to be symmetrical and arrow-head in appearance.

(d) Extension of the ischaemic process to the inferior wall results in the additional manifestations of inferior-wall subendocardial ischaemia, tall T waves in Standard leads II and III and lead AVF (see above; Diagram D of Fig. 19; Electrocardiographic Studies 83 to 86).

(e) There may be associated angina pectoris.

2 The Early Hyperacute Phase of Anterior Wall Injury or Infarction

The tall T waves may manifest as part of the early hyperacute phase of myocardial infarction. The T waves then probably represent the early manifestation of myocardial injury (see Chapter 2). When this occurs, there is associated slope-elevation of the S-T segment (Electrocardiographic Studies 2, 5, 12 and 25), and there are clinical manifestations of acute myocardial infarction.

Similar tall T waves may manifest as part of the presentation of the variant form of angina pectoris: atypical or Prinzmetal's angina (see Chapter 15; Electrocardiographic Studies 90 and 91).

3 Acute Posterior Wall Subepicardial Ischaemia: Acute Posterior Wall Myocardial Infarction

(a) The tall T waves are usually part of the electrocardiographic presentation of true posterior infarction (Electrocardiographic Studies 31, 32 and 33), There are consequently associated tall R waves and possibly depressed S-T segments in leads V1 to V3 (see Chapter 7).

(b) The tall T waves are mainly manifest in the right precordial leads, leads V1 to V3.

(c) Extension of the ischaemic process to the inferior wall is characterized by the additional manifestation of acute inferior wall sub*epi*cardial ischaemia (see above, Diagram C of Fig. 19).

(d) There may be an associated clinical presentation of acute myocardial infarction.

4 Hyperkalaemia

(a) The tall T waves occur mainly in the mid and lateral precordial leads (leads V3 to V6), and in the inferior leads,

Standard leads II and III and lead AVF (Electrocardiographic Study 103).

(b) The *T* waves are usually of considerable amplitude and magnitude, being tall as well as broad. The proximal limb of the *T* wave so-to-speak encroaches upon the S-T segment so that almost the whole of the S-T segment is taken up by the *T* wave. As a result, the QRS complex and *T* wave tend to form a wide, bizarre, multiphasic deflection. In other words, the S-T segment cannot be identified with accuracy.

(c) The QRS complex associated with the tall *T* wave is diminished in amplitude and widened. The widening affects both the initial and terminal deflections of the QRS complex.

(d) The *P* wave may disappear.

5   Left Ventricular Diastolic Overload

In this condition the left ventricle is subjected to excess load or strain during diastole. This is due to increased left ventricular filling during diastole, and results from such conditions as aortic incompetence, mitral incompetence, ventricular septal defect (Electrocardiographic Study 109) and patent ductus arteriosis.

(a) The tall *T* waves manifest in the left precordial leads, leads V5 and V6.

(b) The *T* waves, while relatively tall, do not reach the magnitude nor the width of the *T* waves which occur in hyperkalaemia or acute anterior and posterior-wall infarction.

(c) The associated *R* waves in the left precordial leads are very tall, the expression of left ventricular hypertrophy. There may be an associated delay in the onset of the intrinsicoid deflection.

(d) The associated S-T segments may be slightly elevated.

(e) There is frequently a prominent, though not necessarily pathological, *q* wave in the left precordial leads.

(f) The clinical features of the condition giving rise to the left ventricular diastolic overload may be present.

6   Acute Pericarditis

The *T* waves *may* become slightly taller and pointed in the early phase of acute pericarditis (Electrocardiographic Study 99). This is always associated with elevated concave-upward S-T segments in leads orientated to the external surface of the heart (see section below on 'The Electrocardiographic Syndromes of Myocardial Injury'). It has been suggested that this manifestation is due to myocardial inflammatory hyperaemia secondary to the pericarditis[S114]. The manifestation is usually transient.

TABLE 2   Differential diagnosis between the electrocardiographic manifestations of vagotonia and the epicardial injury of variant angina pectoris, early hyperacute phase of myocardial infarction and acute pericarditis

VAGOTONIA	EPICARDIAL INJURY
Tall, peaked precordial *T* waves.	Tall, peaked precordial *T* waves only in the earliest phase of an acute clinical episode.
Localization mainly in left lateral leads, V2–V4, or inferior limb leads, Standard leads II and III and lead AVF.	Localization may be more general, for example in all the precordial leads, or, for example, in the right precordial leads.
Associated minimal S-T segment elevation rarely exceeds 2 mm in amplitude.	S-T segment elevation usually more marked.
Reciprocal S-T segment depression only in lead AVR.	Reciprocal S-T segment depression common in opposing leads, for example, inferior leads in anterior myocardial infarction. Only present in lead AVR in acute pericarditis.
Associated *R* wave usually very tall.	Associated *R* wave not necessarily tall. May be diminished in amplitude.
Associated *q* waves prominent but narrow.	Associated wide and deep, pathological, Q waves common, except in acute pericarditis.
Associated sinus bradycardia common.	May be associated with sinus bradycardia or sinus tachycardia, more commonly sinus tachycardia. Sinus tachycardia invariable in acute pericarditis.
Presentation stable.	Presentation transient followed by rapid evolution.
Clinical presentation normal.	Clinical presentation markedly abnormal.
Frequent in younger age group: 20–40 years.	More common in older age group: older than 40 years.

7   Recovering Inferior Wall Myocardial Infarction

Tall and symmetrical *T* waves may appear in the precordial leads, particularly the right precordial leads, during the fully evolved phase of inferior wall myocardial infarction and the subsequent regression (Electrocardiographic Study 30). These tall *T* waves may only reach their maximum evolution during the process of regression.

8   Vagotonia

S-T segment elevation is not infrequent in electrocardiograms recorded from normal, usually athletic, individuals who have no evidence of disease[B24, C22, C38, E2, F6, G22, G45, M93, O5, P7, R31, S73, W8]. The condition is not infrequent in the Negro[G22, G45]. The phenomenon is due to increased vagotonia and is associated with a characteristic electrocardiographic presentation. The features are essentially those of left ventricular diastolic overload due to the increased ventricular diastolic filling as a result of the associated sinus bradycardia (see 5 above, and Electrocardiographic Studies 100 and 101).

(a) The *T* wave has the characteristics described under 5 above.

(b) The S-T segment may be minimally elevated, as described under 5 above. This is due to an increased magnitude of the S-T segment vector as a result of early repolarization. The most marked S-T segment deviation is usually evident in those leads with the tallest *T* waves, most commonly leads V4 to V6.

(c) The angle between the mean manifest frontal plane QRS and *T* wave axes is narrow.

(d) The mean manifest frontal plane S-T segment axis is parallel to the mean manifest frontal plane *T* wave axis.

(e) The *T* wave manifestation is usually normalized by mild exercise.

The differential diagnosis between this benign manifestation and the S-T segment and *T* wave abnormalities of such pathological conditions as (a) the variant, Prinzmetal's, atypical form of angina pectoris, (b) the early hyperacute injury phase of myocardial infarction, and (c) acute pericarditis, is presented in Table 2.

9 Apical Infarction

See Chapter 6.

10 The CVA Pattern

See Chapter 15.

THE ELECTROCARDIOGRAPHIC SYNDROMES OF MYOCARDIAL INJURY

Myocardial injury is reflected electrocardiographically by a deviation of the S-T segment towards the surface of injury. The possible electropathological mechanisms governing this phenomenon are discussed in detail in Chapter 2.

The Associations of Myocardial Injury

The myocardial injury may occur as an isolated manifesta-tion, or it may be found in association with myocardial ischaemia and myocardial necrosis.

ISOLATED MYOCARDIAL INJURY

This manifests with S-T segment changes only, and may occur under the following circumstances:

(a) The early stages of myocardial infarction, particularly the early hyperacute phase of myocardial infarction (see page 41, and Electrocardiographic Studies 1, 2, 3, 4, 5, 7, 12 and 25).

(b) Acute subendocardial coronary insufficiency. This is the classic electrocardiographic presentation of angina pectoris and manifests with depression of the S-T segments in the left precordial leads, leads V5 and V6 (see Chapters 15 and 16; Electrocardiographic Studies 92 to 95).

(c) Acute subepicardial coronary insufficiency. This is the electrocardiographic presentation of the variant or atypical form of angina pectoris, Prinzmetal's angina. This is discussed on page 000 (Electrocardiographic Studies 90 and 91).

(d) Acute pericarditis as occurs, for example, in acute rheumatic fever and uraemia, results in an epicardial shell or rind of injured tissue surrounding the heart. This manifests with an S-T segment vector which is directed to the external and dominantly apical surface of the heart. The S-T segment will be elevated in all leads excepting lead AVR (where it is depressed) and lead V1. The dominant elevation occurs in the leads orientated to the apical surface of the heart, leads V4 to V6. The S-T segment vector is directed to +30° on the frontal plane. The associated *T* waves are upright and the S-T segment consequently has a concave-upward configuration in these leads. This occurs particularly in acute rheumatic carditis and uraemia.

(e) Acute subepicardial injury may also occur in acute myocarditis.

MYOCARDIAL INJURY ASSOCIATED WITH MYOCARDIAL ISCHAEMIA

This association manifests with both S-T segment and *T* wave changes, and occurs under the following circumstances:

(a) *In acute myocardial infarction.* The elevated S-T segment is associated with an inverted *T* wave (for example, leads V5 and V6 of Electrocardiographic Study 31).

(b) *In ventricular aneurysm.* The elevated S-T segment is associated with an inverted *T* wave.

(c) *In the hyperacute early phase of acute myocardial infarction* (see p. 42). The elevated S-T segment of acute subepicardial injury is associated with tall symmetrical *T* waves of early injury (Electrocardiographic Studies 1, 2, 3, 4, 5, 7, 12 and 25).

(d) *In the variant form of angina pectoris*, atypical or Prinzmetal's angina (see Chapters 15 and 16). The elevated S-T segment, particularly in the lateral precordial leads, may be associated with the tall *T* waves of early injury or the inverted *T* wave of subepicardial ischaemia.

(e) Acute myocarditis may manifest with the electrocardiographic manifestations of myocardial injury and ischaemia, usually the inverted *T* wave of subepicardial ischaemia.

MYOCARDIAL INJURY ASSOCIATED WITH MYOCARDIAL ISCHAEMIA AND MYOCARDIAL NECROSIS

This combination occurs in the fully evolved phase of myocardial infarction. It may also occur with myocardial aneurysm, although the *Q* waves of necrosis are not necessarily very prominent in this condition and may, indeed, be absent.

The Sites of Myocardial Injury

Myocardial injury occurs predominantly in the subepi-

cardial or subendocardial regions of the left ventricle. Theoretically, the injury can occur in the following sites:

(a) The subepicardial region of the anterior wall.
(b) The subendocardial region of the posterior wall.
(c) The subendocardial region of the anterior wall.
(d) The subepicardial region of the posterior wall.
(e) The subepicardial region of the inferior wall.
(f) The subendocardial region of the inferior wall.

LOCALIZATION OF THE INJURED AREA

Localization of the injury is made from the S-T segment vector which is directed *towards* the injured surface. Thus:

(a)   Anterior Wall Subepicardial Injury
In anterior wall subepicardial injury the S-T segment vector is directed anteriorly, resulting in elevated S-T segments in the precordial leads (Diagram A of Fig. 20).

(b)   Posterior Wall Subendocardial Injury
In posterior wall subendocardial injury the S-T segment vector is also directed anteriorly, resulting in elevated S-T segments in the precordial leads (Diagram E of Fig. 20). This theoretical entity has not yet been definitely recognized, and it is questionable whether this does in fact occur

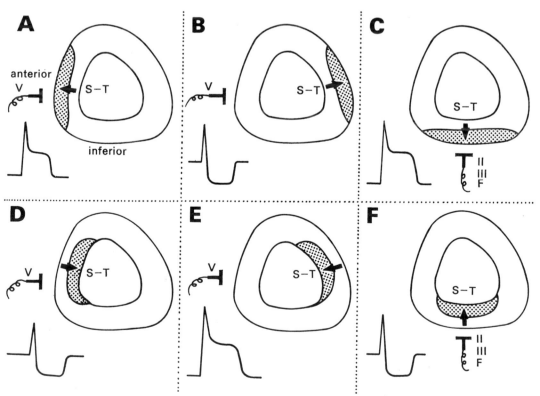

FIG. 20. Diagrams illustrating the theoretical direction of the S-T segment vectors with subepicardial and subendocardial injury of the anterior, inferior and posterior walls of the heart. See text.

electrocardiographically. Several factors may lead to the obscurity of the electrocardiographic manifestation. These are:

   (i) a neutralizing anterior-wall subendocardial injury,
   (ii) the short-circuiting effect of the low-resistance blood which is interspersed between the posterior wall and the precordial electrodes, and
  (iii) the neutralizing boundary effect.

These factors are considered in greater detail in Chapter 2.

(c) Anterior Wall Subendocardial Injury

In anterior-wall subendocardial injury the S-T segment vector is directed posteriorly, resulting in depressed S-T segments in the precordial leads (Diagram D of Fig. 20).

(d) Posterior Wall Subepicardial Injury

In posterior wall subepicardial injury the S-T segment vector is also directed posteriorly, resulting in depressed S-T segments in the precordial leads (Diagram B of Fig. 20). This is the usual manifestation of acute true posterior infarction (see Chapter 7). The deviation is usually minimal as a result of the neutralizing factors described in section (b) above.

(e) Inferior Wall Subepicardial Injury

In inferior wall subepicardial injury the S-T segment vector is directed inferiorly, resulting in elevated S-T segments in the Standard leads II and III and lead AVF (Diagram C of Fig. 20).

(f) Inferior Wall Subendocardial Injury

In inferior wall subendocardial injury the S-T segment vector is directed superiorly, resulting in depressed S-T segments in Standard leads II and III and lead AVF (Diagram F of Fig. 20).

When the myocardial injury is associated with myocardial necrosis and/or ischaemia, then precise localization of the injured region presents no difficulty, since the additional parameters of myocardial ischaemia and myocardial necrosis facilitates the diagnosis. When, however, the S-T segment manifestation of myocardial injury occurs as the only electrocardiographic abnormality, then accurate localization may be difficult. For example, both anterior-wall subendocardial injury and posterior-wall subepicardial injury are reflected by a posteriorly directed S-T segment vector, resulting in depressed S-T segments in the precordial leads (Diagrams D and B of Fig. 20). And both

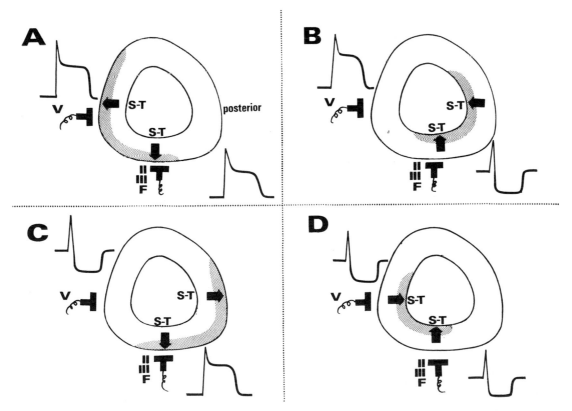

FIG. 21. Diagrams illustrating the combinations of anterior and inferior wall, and posterior and inferior wall, subendocardial and subepicardial injury and their effect on the S-T segment vectors. See text.

anterior-wall subepicardial injury and posterior-wall sub-endocardial injury are reflected by an anteriorly directed S-T segment vector, resulting in elevated S-T segments in the precordial leads (Diagrams A and E of Fig. 20). Accurate localization may, however, be facilitated if there is extension to the inferior wall and this is frequently so. When such extension occurs, the localization may be made on the following theoretical basis.

The principles are considered theoretical because posterior wall subendocardial injury has not yet been recognized as a definite electrocardiographic entity (see above). Nevertheless, the theoretical consideration presented below may serve as a useful basis for potential practical localization.

When there is extension of anterior-wall subepicardial injury to the inferior wall, it must involve the subepicardial region of the inferior wall (Diagram A of Fig. 21) and result in the association of elevated S-T segments in the precordial leads as well as in Standard leads II and III and lead AVF.

When there is extension of the posterior-wall subendocardial injury to the inferior wall, it must involve the subendocardial region of the inferior wall (Diagram B of Fig. 21). This will result in the association of elevated S-T segments in the precordial leads with depressed S-T segment in Standard leads II and III and lead AVF.

When there is extension of the anterior-wall subepicardial injury to the inferior wall, it must involve the subendocardial region of the inferior wall (Diagram D of Fig. 21). This will result in the association of depressed S-T segment in the precordial leads and depressed S-T segments in Standard leads II and III and lead AVF (Electrocardiographic Studies 73, 74, 75 and 76).

When there is extension of posterior-wall subepicardial injury to the inferior wall, it must involve the subepicardial region of the inferior wall (Diagram C of Fig. 21). This will result in the association of depressed S-T segment in the precordial leads and elevated S-T segments in Standard leads II and III and lead AVF (Electrocardiographic Studies 29 and 30).

CORRELATIVE ESSAY

THE CAUSES OF DEPRESSED AND ELEVATED S-T SEGMENTS IN THE PRECORDIAL LEADS

Causes of Depressed S-T Segments in the Precordial Leads

Depressed S-T segments in the precordial leads may occur under the following circumstances:

1 ACUTE SUBENDOCARDIAL ISCHAEMIA

This is discussed in Chapters 15 and 16.

2 ACUTE SUBENDOCARDIAL INFARCTION

This is discussed in Chapter 8.

3 DIGITALIS EFFECT AND DIGITALIS TOXICITY

Digitalis effect and toxicity results in depressed S-T segments which occur predominantly in the left lateral leads, leads V5 and V6, Standard leads I and II. The S-T segment usually has a relatively long downward slope, followed by a sharp terminal rise, the mirror-image of a correction or check mark[S29] (Tracing C of Electrocardiographic Study 87). It may also have a somewhat sagging appearance. The associated Q-T interval is shortened.

If the S-T segment and T wave were normal before the administration of the digitalis, the distal limb of the T wave will rise *above* the baseline following the administration of the digitalis. In other words, there is an important residual of the normally upright T wave. However, in the case of pre-existing abnormal S-T segments or T waves, such as low to inverted T waves associated with depressed S-T segments, the distal limb of the T wave will *not* rise above the baseline following the administration of the digitalis. If the digitalis effect, the depressed S-T segments, occurs in leads with dominantly negative QRS complexes, it is suggestive of digitalis toxicity (Lepeschkin, 1969)[L25].

4 LEFT VENTRICULAR HYPERTROPHY AND STRAIN

This will result in depressed S-T segments with inverted T waves in the left lateral leads. Unlike the manifestation of coronary insufficiency, the S-T segment is minimally convex upward and the T wave is *a*symmetrical with a blunt apex (Tracing B of Electrocardiographic Study 87). The associated R waves are tall. There is an increased ventricular activation time.

5 HYPOKALAEMIA

Advanced hypokalaemia is frequently associated with depressed S-T segments in the left precordial leads and Standard leads I and II. The associated T wave is low or invisible, being absorbed into the S-T segment. The associated U wave is increased in magnitude and may simulate a T wave.

6 QUINIDINE EFFECT

This may also be associated with depressed S-T segments. The Q-T interval is prolonged. The presentation is similar to that of hypokalaemia (see above).

7 ACUTE MYOCARDITIS

Acute myocarditis usually presents with elevated S-T segments in the left lateral leads, a reflection of acute epicardial disease. The brunt of the carditis may, at times, affect the subendocardium, thus presenting with depressed S-T segments in the left lateral leads.

8 ACUTE PULMONARY EMBOLISM

This is discussed in Chapter 5.

9 SHOCK

Acute shock from any cause may result in poor perfusion and subendocardial ischaemia with depressed S-T segments in the precordial leads.

10 RECIPROCAL S-T SEGMENT DEPRESSION IN THE RIGHT PRECORDIAL LEADS IN ACUTE POSTERIOR WALL MYOCARDIAL INFARCTION

Reciprocal depression of the S-T segments may occur with acute inferior wall or true posterior wall infarction (see Chapters 5 and 7).

Causes of Elevated S-T Segments in the Precordial Leads

Elevated S-T segments in the precordial leads may be associated with the following conditions:

1 THE HYPERACUTE PHASE OF ANTERIOR WALL MYOCARDIAL INFARCTION

See Chapter 4.

2 THE FULLY EVOLVED PHASE OF ACUTE ANTERIOR WALL MYOCARDIAL INFARCTION

See Chapter 4.

3 ANTERIOR WALL VENTRICULAR ANEURYSM

See Chapter 4.

4 THE VARIANT FORM OF ANGINA PECTORIS: PRINZMETAL'S ANGINA PECTORIS, ATYPICAL ANGINA PECTORIS

See Chapter 15.

5 VAGOTONIA[C22, C38].

This is discussed in the Correlative Essay on 'The Differential Diagnosis of Tall T Waves in the Precordial Leads' (p. 30 of this chapter).

6 ACUTE PERICARDITIS

See Chapter 4.

7 HYPOTHERMIA

Hypothermia manifests characteristically with a J wave, a hump-like wave which deforms the proximal or junctional part of the S-T segment. The mechanism is speculative, and may be due to early repolarization. The associated manifestations of (a) sinus bradycardia, (b) prolonged Q-T interval, and (c) shivering artifact, facilitate the diagnosis.

THE ELECTROCARDIOGRAPHIC SYNDROMES OF MYOCARDIAL NECROSIS

Myocardial necrosis is reflected electrocardiographically by a loss of positive deflection in leads orientated to the necrotic area. There is, in effect, a reorientation of forces away from the necrotic area. The phenomenon may manifest electrocardiographically as follows:

1 QS deflections

Leads orientated to the necrotic area may reflect deep and wide negative deflections which are not followed by terminal positivities (Diagram D of Fig. 3). This manifestation indicates:

(a) **The presence of a transmural infarction.** This reflects the absence of viable tissue over the surface of the infarcted area (see Chapter 12). The diagnosis of myocardial infarction must not be based on the presence of a single QS complex in the electrocardiographic recording. Such a manifestation may, for example, be the result of incorrect electrode placement. A single QS complex does, however, have significance if it is associated with the S-T segment and T wave parameters of injury and ischaemia.

(b) **The absence of an associated focal or divisional peri-infarction block.** See Chapter 12.

Note: With incomplete or complete left bundle branch block, the right precordial leads (leads V1 to V4) and, at times, the inferiorly orientated leads (Standard leads II and III and lead AVF), may reflect QS complexes. The differential diagnosis of QS complexes in the precordial leads is discussed in Chapter 6, and in the inferiorly orientated leads in Chapter 5, p. 49. The same manifestation may, at times, occur with left anterior hemiblock. This is discussed in Chapter 12.

2   QR or Qr deflections

Leads orientated to the necrotic area reflect deep and wide pathological Q waves which are followed by terminal positivities, r or R waves. The terminal positivity may be due to:

(a) Focal peri-infarction block: delayed, late, activation of remaining viable tissue overlying the surface of the necrotic material (Diagrams C of Figs. 3 and 22). The endo-cardial-epicardial activation process reaches and activates the overlying viable tissue by a circuitous route, thereby resulting in a terminal region. Right bundle branch block and divisional peri-infarction block must be excluded before this conclusion can be reached (see Chapter 12).

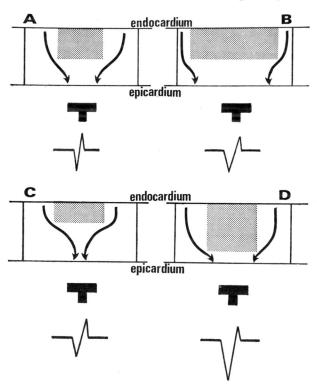

FIG. 22. Diagrams illustrating the effect of variation in length of a subendocardial infarction of constant depth (Diagrams A and B), and the effect of variation in depth of a subendocardial infarction of constant length (Diagrams C and D). See text.

(b) An intraventricular conduction defect such as right bundle branch block or divisional peri-infarction block.

Note: (a) The width-duration of the Q wave is to some extent proportional to the area of necrosis it subtends (compare Diagrams A and B of Fig. 22).

(b) The amplitude of the ensuing R wave (of the QR complex in focal peri-infarction block) is to some extent proportional to the amount of surviving epicardial tissue overlying the region of necrosis[S114] (compare Diagrams C and D of Fig. 22).

(c) The pathological Q wave has the following characteristics:

(i) It appears in leads which do not normally reflect a Qr or QS complex. Thus, a Qr or QS complex in lead AVR is a normal manifestation, and has no special significance.

(ii) The Q wave is larger than 0·03 sec in duration (one millimeter or wider .

(iii) The Q wave usually exceeds 25 per cent of the height of the ensuing R wave. For normal variation and exception to this, see 'Evaluation of a prominent Q wave in Standard lead III' (Chapter 5).

(iv) The presence of a prominent Q wave, exceeding 3 mm in depth, in the left lateral precordial leads is a pointer to the potential presence of infarction. If it is due to infarction, the ensuing R wave will *always* be diminished in amplitude. It may also, for example, be due to left ventricular dominance as in aortic insufficiency or ventricular septal defect (Electrocardiographic Study 109). When this occurs, the ensuing R wave is usually taller than normal.

3   An abnormal sequence in the magnitude of normal Q waves

The q waves of the QRS complexes normally recorded by leads orientated towards the left ventricle (leads V4–V6) usually deepen progressively from leads V4–V6. Failure to show such deepening may indicate the presence of an infarct. For example, a Q wave which is deeper in lead V4 than in lead V6 (Electrocardiographic Studies 13, 23, 38, 40 and 46), or a Q wave in lead V4 which is associated with an absent Q wave in lead V6, indicates a transmural infarction in the lower third of the interventricular septum.

4   Loss of normal q waves

Leads which normally reflect a normal small initial q wave, the left lateral leads V5, V6, AVL and Standard lead I, may show an absence of such q waves (Electrocardiographic Studies 19, 20, 21, 22 and 25). This may constitute corroborative evidence of a septal infarction, provided other causes of absent initial q waves in these leads are excluded. These include left bundle branch block and the Wolff-Parkinson-White syndrome.

5 Loss of Initial Positivity in Leads Normally Reflecting Initial Positivity

The reorientation of forces resulting from myocardial necrosis may manifest with the loss of initial positivity in leads which normally show such initial positivity. For example, myocardial necrosis affecting the middle third of the intraventricular septum is reflected by a loss of the initial small r wave in leads orientated to the right ventricle and right side of the intraventricular septum, leads V1 and V2. The normal rS complex is changed to a QS complex (see p. 76). This does not necessarily connote transmural infarction (see Chapter 8).

6 An Abnormal Sequence or Progression in R Wave Magnitude

There is normally a progressive increase in the magnitude of the r wave from leads V1–V4. Thus leads V1 and V2 reflect a rS complex, whereas leads V3 and V4 usually reflect RS complexes. A lack of such progression, or an irregularity in the progression, may connote the presence of an infarct, provided that the electrode placement has been accurate. For example, if the r waves increase progressively from leads V1–V3 but diminish in lead V4 and increase again in lead V5, it is suggestive of a subepicardial infarction in the lower third of the interventricular septum, the region orientated towards lead V4 (Electrocardiographic Studies 39, 41 and 46).

7 Abnormal Tall R Waves in the Right Precordial Leads

Tall R waves in the right precordial leads may reflect true posterior infarction, the loss of posterior wall forces. This, in fact, represents the mirror-image of the pathological Q wave or QS complex which would be registered by a lead orientated directly to the infarction of the true posterior wall (Fig. 31). When this occurs, the anterior wall forces are no longer balanced by the posterior wall forces, and hence are increased in magnitude. The other causes of a tall R wave in right precordial leads must be excluded,

viz. Type A Wolff-Parkinson-White syndrome, right ventricular hypertrophy, some forms of right bundle branch block, the Duchenne type of muscular dystrophy (Electrocardiographic Study 108).

8 A Loss of Dominant R Wave Amplitude

Leads which normally reflect a dominant R wave, for example, the qR complex of left lateral leads, V5, V6, AVL and Standard lead I, may become diminished in amplitude (Diagram E of Fig. 3) (Electrocardiographic Studies 14, 15, 17, 20–27).

CORRELATIVE ESSAY

CAUSES OF PROMINENT Q WAVES IN THE LEFT PRECORDIAL LEADS

1 Apical Infarction and Antero-lateral Infarction

2 Left Ventricular Diastolic Overload

(Electrocardiographic Study 109). See p. 30.

3 The Duchenne Type of Muscular Dystrophy.

This condition is associated with a relatively characteristic electrocardiographic presentation. The right precordial leads reflect tall R waves, not unlike that of true posterior infarction or right ventricular dominance, and the left lateral precordial leads as well as the Standard leads reflect deep, prominent, although not necessarily pathological, Q waves (Electrocardiographic Study 108). The presentation has been reviewed by Perlof (1967)[P16].

4 Muscular Subaortic Stenosis

This condition may be associated with (a) prominent abnormal Q waves in the left precordial leads, Standard leads I, II and III, leads AVL and AVF, and (b) tall R waves in the right precordial leads [B73].

5 Vagotonia

(Electrocardiographic Studies 100 and 101). See p. 30.

Section 2   Myocardial Infarction

Chapter 4

The Basic Manifestations and Localization of Myocardial Infarction

THE PHASES OF INFARCTION

The evolution of myocardial infarction may, in an electrocardiographic sense, be divided into three principal phases:

1. The early hyperacute injury phase.
2. The fully evolved acute phase.
3. The chronic stabilized phase.

It must, however, be emphasized that, although the classic features of every phase are easily recognized, each blends almost imperceptibly with the other, so that it is difficult to establish clear-cut separation.

1 The Hyperacute Early Injury Phase of Myocardial Infarction

This phase is characterized by:

(a) **Acute injury block.** This is discussed in Chapter 12.
(b) **Slope-elevation of the S-T segment.**
(c) **An increase in the T wave magnitude.**

These features are illustrated in Fig. 23 and Electrocardiographic Studies 1, 2, 3, 4, 5, 6, 12, 25 and 34. They will be described with reference to transmural infarction or infarction that is dominantly subepicardial.

Changes Affecting the S-T Segment: Slope-elevation of the S-T Segment

The first electrocardiographic sign of acute myocardial infarction is frequently a *straightening of the normal upward concavity of the S-T segment*. The normal S-T segment merges smoothly and imperceptibly with the proximal limb of the *T* wave so that the two cannot be separated. It is usually impossible to tell where the S-T segment ends and where the *T* wave begins (Diagram A of Fig. 23). The earliest evidence of acute myocardial infarction may be the *loss of this upward concavity, a straightening or ironing out of the S-T segment* in leads orientated to

the epicardial surface (Diagram B of Fig. 23; Electrocardiographic Study 6). Since the *T* wave remains upright or may even be increased in amplitude (see below), this S-T segment change results in an indirect concomitant *widening of the* T *wave*. The *T* wave is so-to-speak, taken up or absorbed into the straightened S-T segment. This straightening of the S-T segment is the earliest evidence of S-T segment deviation, the S-T segment elevation.

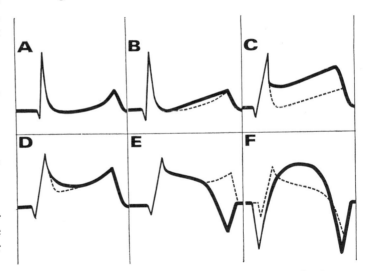

FIG. 23. Diagrams illustrating the evolution of the infarction pattern from normal (Diagram A), through various stages of the hyperacute phase (Diagrams B, C and D), to the fully evolved phase (Diagram F.). See text.

Further evolution of the myocardial infarction results in manifest *elevation of the straightened S-T segment* (Diagram C of Fig. 23; Electrocardiographic Studies 1, 2, 3, 5, 7, 12, 25 and 34). The *T* wave remains upright and thus appears to be even more widened. The *T* wave may also be increased in magnitude (see below). During this stage of evolution the S-T segment usually has an upward slope, since the proximal part is less elevated than the distal part which merges with the *T* wave. This will be termed *slope-elevation of the S-T segment*.

41

At times, the S-T segment may be markedly elevated without the associated straightening, the *S-T segment being elevated with an upward concavity* (Diagram D of Fig. 23; Tracing A of Electrocardiographic Study 4). This concave-upward elevation of the S-T segment in the hyperacute phase of myocardial infarction mimics electrocardiographic manifestations of acute pericarditis. The differential diagnosis is considered on p. 43.

Reciprocal Changes

Leads orientated to the uninjured surface will usually reflect reciprocal S-T segment depression.

Note: Leads which are orientated to the injured surface reflect what is termed the *indicative changes*, whereas leads which are orientated to the uninjured surface reflect *reciprocal changes*.

The magnitude of the S-T segment elevation may, in the early hyperacute injury phase of myocardial infarction, be considerable, reaching amplitudes of 10-15 mm, especially in the mid precordial leads. It may, under this circumstance, dominate the entire electrocardiographic presentation, presenting as a single positive phase deflection, a so-called *monophasic curve* (for example, lead V4 in Electrocardiographic Study 2; lead AVF in Electrocardiographic Study 34).

CHANGES AFFECTING THE *T* WAVE

The early hyperacute injury phase of myocardial infarction is also characterized by an *increase in the magnitude of the* T *wave.* (Electrocardiographic Studies 1, 2, 3, 4, 5, 7 and 12)[D30]. This may, in fact, be the earliest manifestation, and may even appear before the S-T segment changes described above. This is particularly so in the case of anterior-wall myocardial infarction, when prominent precordial *T* waves may herald the impending myocardial infarction (Wasserburger and Corliss, 1965)[W10]. This increase in the *T*-wave magnitude is a true and active process and not merely secondary to the elevation of the S-T segment. There would thus appear to be a *primary* orientation of the *T* wave force towards the surface of infarction. This is also evident from the electrocardiographic manifestations of the hyperacute phase in subendocardial infarction, which may present with depression of the S-T segment in the leads orientated to the epicardial surface, i.e. the S-T segment vector is deviated to the subendocardial surface 'Electrocardiographic Studies 73, 74, and 75). The *T* wave is increased in magnitude, but is frequently inverted 'Electrocardiographic Studies 73, 74 and 75), i.e. it is directed *towards* the injured subendocardial surface. This contrasts with the classic behaviour of the *T* wave vector in subacute myocardial ischaemia, which is deviated *away* from

the surface of the ischaemia 'see Chapters 1 and 2). The phenomenon is analysed in Chapter 2.

Experimentally, too, the early *T*-wave changes of the hyperacute phase of myocardial infarction appear to be paradoxical. For example, the earliest change following the induction of experimental infarction in open-chest anaesthetized animals is *inversion of the* T *wave* [B20]. When, however, experimental infarction is induced in a non-anaesthetized closed-chest animal, the earliest change is an increase in the amplitude of the positive *T* wave[L20], a change which approximates that seen in human infarction.

The classical pathological Q waves of myocardial necrosis do not appear until these large amplitude *T* waves have regressed[D30].

Note: The fully evolved phase of anterior-wall myocardial infarction may, at times be preceeded by the hyperacute phase of *subendocardial* injury (see Chapter 8).

THE SIGNIFICANCE OF THE EARLY, HYPERACUTE, INJURY PHASE OF ACUTE MYOCARDIAL INFARCTION

The early hyperacute injury phase reflects a *critical electropathological and clinical state*, since it is during this phase that the potentially lethal complication of ventricular fibrillation can arise. The reasons are as follows:

(a) Increased ventricular automaticity, ventricular extrasystoles and ventricular tachycardia are generated at the periphery of the injured area. Ectopic ventricular rhythms are favoured by critical diastolic depolarization[S28], and this is particularly prone to occur at the periphery of the infarcted area.

(b) There is marked differential diastolic depolarization of the ventricles. The marked injury represents appreciable diastolic depolarization (see Chapter 2), and a marked differential electropathological, out-of-phase, state exists between the injured and surrounding healthy tissues. Moreover, conduction within the injured area is delayed, resulting in injury block and manifesting with a delay in ventricular activation time or even complete intraventricular block (see Chapter 12). This further contributes to an out-of-phase state.

The association of this differential electropathological state with the increased automaticity which occurs at the periphery of the injury, is conducive to the precipitation of complete electropathological ventricular fragmentation, the state of ventricular fibrillation.

There are indications that the greater the degree of the S-T segment elevation, the worse the prognosis[N11]. This requires further study.

THE DURATION OF THE HYPERACUTE INJURY PHASE

The classic presentation of the hyperacute phase usually lasts but a few hours and commonly reaches its peak on the first or the second day. The manifestation may rarely persist for longer (days or weeks)[G31]. Due to the relative short duration of the hyperacute phase, it is frequently missed, and the electrocardiographic presentation is usually that of the fully evolved phase.

DIFFERENTIAL DIAGNOSIS OF THE HYPERACUTE EARLY MYOCARDIAL INJURY PHASE FROM ACUTE PERICARDITIS

(a) The elevated concave-upward S-T segment of acute pericarditis is usually evident in all leads orientated to the external surface of the heart; the anterior leads (leads V1 to V6), the inferior leads (Standard leads II and III and lead AVF), and the lateral or superior leads (lead AVL and Standard lead I), i.e. all leads except lead AVR and possibly lead V1 (Electrocardiographic Study 99). In acute myocardial infarction, however, the concave-upward and elevated S-T segment is usually seen in one group or set of surface leads only, namely either the inferior leads, the lateral leads, or the anterior leads. At times, with extensive infarction, the elevated S-T segment may present in more than one set of leads (Electrocardiographic Study 2), but even then the change is not as widely distributed as is usually the case in acute pericarditis, and other electrocardiographic features of the hyperacute phase of infarction such as injury block and very tall and widened T waves are usually present.

(b) Acute pericarditis is always associated with sinus tachycardia, whereas acute myocardial infarction may be associated with either sinus tachycardia or sinus bradycardia (see Chapter 17).

(c) Acute myocardial infarction may be associated with first, second and third degree A-V block, whereas these do not occur with acute pericarditis.

(d) Acute pericarditis is usually associated with normal or low-amplitude QRS complexes. The early changes of acute myocardial infarction, however, are usually associated with a possible increase in R wave amplitude or some intraventricular conduction defect.

(e) With the evolution of acute pericarditis the T waves become inverted, and this may mimic the myocardial ischaemia of coronary insufficiency. In pericarditis, however, the QRS complexes are, at this stage, always diminished in amplitude, and the mean manifest frontal plane QRS axis is normally directed to the region of $+40°$ to $+60°$. The frontal plane T wave vector is directed superiorly and to the right.

NORMALIZATION OF THE ELECTROCARDIOGRAPHIC PRESENTATION DURING EVOLUTION FROM THE HYPERACUTE EARLY INJURY PHASE TO THE FULLY EVOLVED PHASE

The evolution from the early hyperacute injury phase to the fully evolved phase of myocardial infarction may sometimes be marked by apparent normalization of the abnormal pattern. For example, the change from the tall T wave of the hyperacute to the inverted T wave of the fully evolved phase may be marked by an apparent normalization of the T wave, since at an intermediate stage the tall T wave will have regressed to one of normal amplitude (Tracing B of Electrocardiographic Study 4).

2 The Fully Evolved Acute Phase of Myocardial Infarction

The fully evolved phase of myocardial infarction is the classic common presentation, and is characterized by the presence of **pathological Q waves or QS complexes, coved and elevated S-T segments and inverted symmetrical arrow-head T waves** (Electrocardiographic Studies 4, 5, 10, 11, 12, 14, 15, 17–23, 25, 27–34). Reciprocal changes S-T segment depression and tall T waves, will occur in leads orientated to the uninjured surface.

The fully evolved phase reflects some regression from the state of dominant injury in the hyperacute phase to one of dominant ischaemia and necrosis. Thus, the T waves in leads orientated to the infarcted epicardial surface become progressively more inverted, eventually becoming deeply inverted, symmetrical and arrow-head in appearance (Diagrams E and F of Fig. 23 and Fig. 24). This contributes

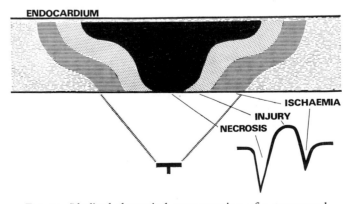

FIG. 24. Idealized theoretical representation of a transmural infarction with lateral subendocardial extension. The infarct is illustrated with the hypothetical sparing of a thin subendocardial rind. See text.

to the coving effect on the S-T segment. The S-T segment, while still elevated, is nevertheless diminished in amplitude from the maximal deviation seen in the hyperacute phase. It is coved, convex-upward and, in the classic presentation, blends smoothly with the preceding pathological Q wave and the ensuing inverted T wave.

The monophasic QRS-T deflection of the hyperacute phase is therefore changed to a deflection that is clearly triphasic in form, the Q wave, the elevated S-T segment, and the inverted T wave, of the fully evolved phase (Diagram F of Fig. 23 and Fig. 24).

Clinically, this change is the desired progression, and reflects a less dangerous phase during the evolution of myocardial infarction.

RESOLUTION OF THE FULLY EVOLVED PHASE

The fully evolved phase gradually resolves during the 3—6 months following its maximal evolution. The S-T segment gradually returns to the baseline, eventually becoming isoelectric. The T wave inversion becomes progressively less marked and, in the event of complete resolution, eventually returns to a normal upright configuration.

Ventricular Aneurysm

If the features of the fully evolved phase, pathological Q wave, elevated and coved S-T segment, and inverted T wave, persists for 6 months or longer, the presence of an acquired ventricular aneurysm should be suspected[E1]. The mechanism of the persistent S-T segment elevation in ventricular aneurysm has not been fully established. The most likely explanation would appear to be earlier repolarization of a ring of viable but injured tissue surrounding the aneurysm[C6, S7]. An acquired ventricular aneurysm is more commonly associated with anterior wall myocardial infarction, and particularly anteroseptal myocardial infarction[C23, D34, L64].

Note: A congenital subvalvular ventricular aneurysm may, by compression of a coronary artery, result in the typical electrocardiographic presentation of myocardial infarction[C24]. The presentation is more commonly one of inferior wall myocardial infarction (Electrocardiographic Study 107).

3 The Chronic Stabilized Phase of Myocardial Infarction: Old Myocardial Infarction

This is the residual phase, and reflects the maximal regression from the fully evolved phase. Complete resolution to normal is uncommon. The QRS complex may reflect a pathological Q wave as part of a QR complex (Electro-

cardiographic Studies 35, 36, 38, 39 and 40). This may be the only evidence of a previous infarction. The R waves may be rather low and not as tall as in the pre-infarction tracing. At times, the end result of multiple infarctions is a generalized diminution in QRS amplitude, a loss of positive QRS deflection (Electrocardiographic Study 39). The S-T segment of the acute transmural or epicardial infarction becomes isoelectric, and the T wave may become upright. Note that although the coved and elevated S-T segment has regressed and become isoelectric, it frequently reflects the manifestations of chronic coronary insufficiency, for example horizontality, sharp angled ST-T junction, or even S-T segment depression (Electrocardiographic Studies 35, 36 and 38; see Chapter 15). Similarly, although the T wave abnormality of the acute phase regresses, it frequently reflects the stigmata of chronic coronary insufficiency (Electrocardiographic Study 38).

Note: It is the presence of the S-T segment and T wave changes which connotes the *acute phases* of myocardial infarction. The only exception to this statement is the presence of a ventricular aneurysm.

SUMMARY

Hyperacute phase	Slope-elevation of the S-T segment. Tall and widened T wave.
Fully evolved acute phase	Pathological Q wave. Elevated and coved S-T segment. Inverted arrow-head T wave.
Chronic phase	Pathological Q wave. S-T segment and T wave are normal or, more likely, reflect the manifestation of chronic coronary insufficiency.

THE LOCALIZATION OF MYOCARDIAL INFARCTION

The localization of myocardial infarction is based on the recognition of the infarction patterns in the specific leads or groups of leads which are orientated to the infarcted area.

The following classification is based on the localization of transmural infarction or infarction that is dominantly subepicardial. The diagnosis and localization of subendocardial infarction is considered in Chapter 8.

The localization of myocardial infarction may be classified on the basis of the three major surfaces of the cone-shaped left ventricle (Fig. 10); the *anterior*, the *inferior* and the *posterior* walls.

1. **Anterior wall myocardial infarction** is recognized from the infarction pattern in several or all of leads V1–V6, Standard lead I and lead AVL (Figs. 10 and 30). The various and arbitrary subdivisions of the anterior infarctions are considered in Chapter 6.

2. **Inferior wall myocardial infarction** is recognized by the appearance of the infarction pattern in the leads orientated to the inferior surface, Standard leads II and III and lead AVF (Fig. 10). (See Chapter 5.)

3. **Posterior wall myocardial infarction** is recognized by the appearance of inverse or mirror-image changes in the right precordial leads, leads V1–V3. See Chapter 7.

The effects of myocardial necrosis, the pathological Q waves or QS complexes—and the other abnormalities of the QRS complex—are usually more circumscribed, localized or restricted than those of injury and ischaemia, and may be localized to but a few specific leads. The effects of myocardial injury and myocardial ischaemia tend to be more extensive. For example, the QS complexes of anteroseptal myocardial infarction may be confined to leads V1, V2, V3 and V4, whereas the associated elevated and coved S-T segment of myocardial injury may be present in leads V1–V6. At the same time, the associated symmetrical T-wave inversion of myocardial ischaemia may extend even further, i.e. it may be present in leads V1–V6 as well as in Standard lead I and lead AVL (Electrocardiographic Studies 15, 17, 18 and 19).

Chapter 5

Inferior Wall Myocardial Infarction

The inferior wall of the heart is constituted by the inferior wall of the left ventricle and is orientated to the *positive electrodes of Standard leads II and III and lead AVF* (Fig. 10). Inferior wall myocardial infarction is thus reflected in these leads.

THE BASIC MANIFESTATIONS

There are three principal phases:

1. An early hyperacute injury phase.
2. The fully evolved phase.
3. The chronic stabilized phase.

THE EARLY HYPERACUTE INJURY PHASE

This is reflected by the following *indicative* changes:

(a) marked elevation of the S-T segments.

(b) upright *T* waves which may be increased in magnitude.

(c) injury block—a delay in intraventricular conduction as reflected by a delay in the inscription of the intrinsicoid deflection and an increase in the amplitude of the *R* wave (see Chapter 12).

Reciprocal Changes
Leads orientated to the anterior wall may reflect reciprocal S-T segment depression, which may be marked.

These features are evident in Electrocardiographic Studies 1, 2, 3, 4, 7 and 34 (Tracing A). This phase is usually present for only a few hours during the early stages of the infarction and is, as a result, frequently missed.

THE FULLY EVOLVED PHASE

The fully evolved phase of inferior-wall myocardial infarction is characterized by the presence of pathological *Q* waves or QS complexes, coved and elevated S-T segments,

and inverted sharply pointed and symmetrical *T* waves in Standard leads II and III and lead AVF. These indicative changes are evident in Electrocardiographic Studies 4, 27–34).

Reciprocal Changes
Leads orientated to the anterior wall may reflect slight reciprocal S-T segment depression and relatively tall symmetrical *T* waves.

THE CHRONIC STABILIZED PHASE

This phase is characterized by residual *Q* wave abnormalities in Standard leads II and III and lead AVF, particularly in Standard lead III and lead AVF (Electrocardiographic Studies 35, 36 and 38). The parameters of injury and ischaemia, the elevated and coved S-T segments and the inverted *T* waves which connote the acute phases, have regressed and disappeared. The S-T segments may, however, still reflect the signs of chronic coronary insufficiency, for example, horizontality or plane depression of the S-T segment. The features of the chronic phase are reflected in Electrocardiographic Studies 26, 35, 36 and 38).

FURTHER OBSERVATIONS ON THE QRS PATTERN

A. The magnitude of the pathological *Q* waves.

B. Variations of the QRS deflections in Standard leads II and III and lead AVF.

C. Evaluation of a prominent *Q* wave in Standard lead III.

A The Magnitude of the Pathological Q Waves

The pathological *Q* waves of inferior-wall myocardial infarction are not usually as deep, nor as wide, as the pathological *Q* waves which occur with anterior wall myocardial infarction (compare Electrocardiographic

Studies 27 and 28 with Electrocardiographic Studies 17, 18, 19 and 20). This is because (a) anterior wall myocardial infarction is reflected by the precordial leads which are proximity leads, and hence reflect complexes of greater magnitude, whereas inferior wall infarction is reflected by extremity leads, and (b) the right precordial leads are dominantly negative, reflecting rS complexes, and the mere disappearance of the initial r wave will result in a deep, wide QS complex (see p. 76).

The pathological Q wave of inferior-wall myocardial infarction is larger in Standard lead III than in lead AVF, and is larger in lead AVF than in Standard lead II (Diagram A of Fig. 25).

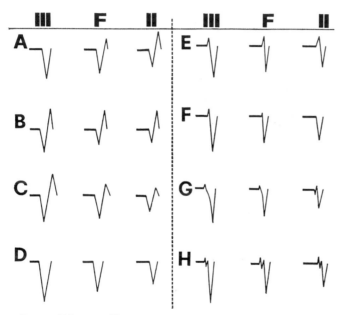

FIG. 25. Diagrams illustrating various presentations of inferior wall myocardial infarction and its complications. See text.

B Variations of the QRS Deflections in Standard Leads II and III and lead AVF

Inferior wall myocardial infarction may manifest with the following variations of abnormal QRS deflections in Standard leads II and III and lead AVF:

1. A dominant QR complex in Standard lead II.
2. QS complexes in all three leads.
3. QR complexes of equal magnitude in all three leads.
4. A dominant QR complex in Standard lead III.

A Dominant QR Complex in Standard lead II
It is uncommon for QS complexes to be recorded by all of the three inferior orientated leads, Standard leads II and III and lead AVF, in cases of uncomplicated inferior wall myo-

cardial infarction. A QS complex is usually present in Standard lead III and less commonly in lead AVF. Standard lead II, however, usually reflects a Qr or QR complex. Lead AVF also frequently reflects a Qr complex (Electrocardiographic Studies 27, 28, 30 and 31; Diagram A of Fig. 25). Even if all these inferior leads reflect a terminal R wave, this terminal R wave, in uncomplicated inferior wall myocardial infarction, is usually tallest in Standard lead II (Electrocardiographic Study 34, Tracing B; Diagram A of Fig. 25).

The possible reasons for this distributional pattern are considered below.

(a) The brunt of the infarction affects the right lateral region of the inferior wall with some sparing of the left lateral region of the inferior wall (Diagram A II of Fig. 26). In other words, extension to the lateral regions of the inferior wall is mainly subendocardial. Consequently, Standard lead III, which is orientated to the right side of the inferior wall, reflects the brunt of the infarction, and hence the largest and widest QS complex (Diagram A I of Fig. 26; Electrocardiographic Studies 27, 28, 29, 30 and 31). Standard lead II, however, is orientated principally to the left lateral region of the inferior wall, and consequently reflects the potentials of some healthy overlying muscle as a terminal R wave. The terminal R wave is, therefore, in all probability an expression of focal peri-infarction block. The infarction extends subendocardially to the left lateral inferior wall, and the overlying healthy tissue is activated by a circuitous activation process from the neighbouring healthy tissue (see Fig. 22 and Chapter 12).

(b) Another possible explanation for the terminal R wave in Standard lead II is the specific orientation of the inferior leads. The right side of the inferior wall is continuous with the anterior or septal wall. The left side of the inferior wall is continuous with the left lateral wall. Hence, a lead orientated to the left lateral wall, Standard lead II, may reflect the late positive potentials of the left lateral wall as a terminal positivity or R wave (Diagram A II of Fig. 26).

These principles are reflected in the vector loop of uncomplicated inferior-wall myocardial infarction[B31, C9, H31, H40, P36, Y4]. The afferent limb of the loop is directed superiorly and is inscribed in a *clockwise* direction (Diagram A of Fig. 26). The returning limb of the vector loop will enter the zone of positivity for Standard lead II first, resulting in a terminal R wave. It may enter the zone of positivity of lead AVF, and it remains in the zone of negativity for Standard lead III. This is illustrated in Fig. 26 and Diagram A of Fig. 47. The zone of positivity for Standard lead II extends from −30° counter-clockwise to +120°. Note that the zone of positivity for lead AVF begins at 0° and extends counter-clockwise to +180°. The

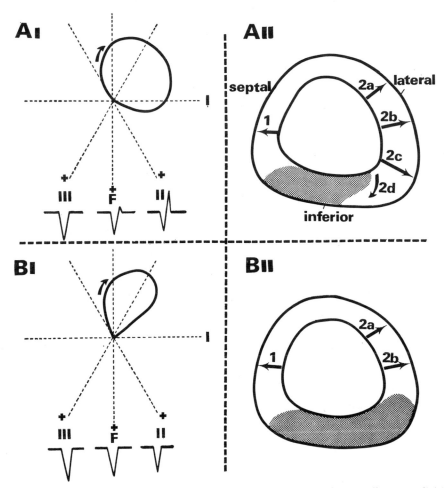

FIG. 26. A is a diagrammatic representation of the frontal plane vector loop in inferior wall myocardial infarction with sparing of the inferolateral wall. B, is a diagrammatic representation of the frontal plane vector loop in extensive inferior wall myocardial infarction.

zone of positivity for Standard lead III begins at $+30°$ and extends clockwise to $-150°$.

QS Complexes in all the Inferior Leads: Standard Leads II and III and Lead AVF.

If QS complexes are present in all three of the leads orientated to the inferior wall, Standard leads II and III and lead AVF, (Diagram D of Fig. 25), the following diagnosis must be considered:

(a) Extensive inferior wall myocardial infarction.

(b) Inferior wall myocardial infarction associated with left anterior hemiblock.

(c) Left bundle branch block associated with left anterior hemiblock, with or without inferior-wall infarction.

Note that all these conditions will result in a left axis deviation. Their differential diagnosis is considered below and further in Chapter 12.

Extensive inferior wall myocardial infarction. There is an extension of the inferior infarction to include the entire inferior wall, and possibly regions of the lateral wall. Under these circumstances, signs of infarction will usually also be present in the laterally orientated leads, particularly leads V5 and V6, since the lateral extension tends to be apical (Electrocardiographic Study 33).

Inferior wall myocardial infarction associated with left anterior hemiblock. The inferior infarction may be superimposed upon, or associated with, a left anterior hemiblock. This will cause the terminal vector to be directed superiorly and to the left, and Standard lead II will, as a result, reflect a terminal negativity instead of the usual terminal positivity. The differential diagnosis from the extensive inferior wall myocardial infarction (as described under (a) above) is made from:

(i) The absence of the S-T segment and *T* wave signs of

acute infarction in the lateral orientated leads, leads V5 and V6.

(ii) The presence of left axis deviation in pre-infarction tracings.

(iii) The persistence of left axis deviation in post-infarction tracings. Standard lead I and lead AVL will usually show rather tall *R* waves (Electrocardiographic Study 29). (See Chapter 12.)

Left bundle branch block with left anterior hemiblock. This will result in QS complexes in Standard leads II and III and lead AVF because:

(i) the left axis deviation results in deep negative deflections in Standard leads II and III and lead AVF.

(ii) the left bundle branch block results in the disappearance of the initial tiny *r* wave (Fig. 53).

The differential diagnosis from inferior wall myocardial infarction is based on the absence of the classical S-T segment and *T*-wave changes of myocardial infarction. The S-T segments are elevated but have a straight or slightly concave-upward slope to an upright *T* wave, in contrast to the coved S-T segment and inverted *T* wave of myocardial infarction. Furthermore, there will be evidence of left bundle branch block in the other leads, for example, in leads V4–V6.

QR Complexes of Equal Magnitude in the Inferior Leads: Standard Leads II and III and AVF
If there are QR complexes in all three of the inferior leads and the terminal *R* waves are of approximately of equal magnitude, the diagnosis of a complicating diaphragmatic peri-infarction block should be entertained (Diagram B of Fig. 25; Electrocardiographic Studies 34, Tracing B, 49 and 50). The terminal *R* wave vector will, under these circumstances, be directed to the region of +90° to +100° on the frontal plane hexaxial reference system (see Chapter 12).

A Dominant QR Complex in Standard lead III
If there are QR complexes in all three of the inferior leads but the terminal *R* wave is tallest in Standard lead III, then the diagnosis of complicating right bundle branch block should be entertained (Diagram C of Fig. 25; Electrocardiographic Study 53). The terminal *R* wave vector will, under this circumstance, be directed anteriorly and to the right (see Chapter 9).

C   Evaluation of a Prominent Q Wave in Standard Lead III

A prominent *Q* wave of even a QS deflection may appear in Standard lead III which is not the result of myocardial infarction but which may be an expression of one of the following:

1. a normal phenomenon;
2. acute pulmonary embolism;
3. left axis deviation with left bundle branch block;
4. left posterior hemiblock;
5. a negative delta wave;
6. Vagotonia.

The differential diagnosis is considered below.

THE NORMAL Q WAVE IN STANDARD LEAD III

The normal QRS complex may reflect a prominent initial *Q* wave. This will occur when the complex is *equiphasic* in Standard lead III with an *initial negative* component. This results in an initial *Q* wave which is equal to the height of the ensuing *R* wave. The *Q* wave thus constitutes 100 per cent of the ensuing *R* wave. Since most pathological *Q* waves constitute more than 25 per cent of the ensuing *R*

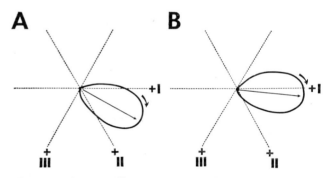

Fig. 27. Diagrams illustrating normal frontal plane vector loops with clockwise rotation. A, the mean axis is directed at +30 degrees. B, the mean axis is directed at +10 degrees. The events depicted in B will result in a larger initial *q* wave than the events depicted in A.

wave, this normal manifestation may lead to erroneous diagnosis. In addition, the associated normal *T* wave is frequently negative, thereby tending to increase even further the simulation of myocardial infarction.

The potential confusion of this manifestation with the pathological *Q* wave of inferior wall myocardial infarction is usually due to a lack of appreciation of the Standard lead III axis relationship to the depolarization process.

The normal frontal plane loop is inscribed around the mean QRS axis and is clockwise in direction in 65 per cent of cases (Fig. 27). It tends to be counter-clockwise when associated with horizontal axes, and clockwise when associated with vertical axes, but this is not invariably so.

Consider now the following examples of normal ventricular activation:

Example 1. The mean manifest frontal plane QRS axis is directed precisely at $+30°$, a normal axis (Diagram A of Fig. 27). The QRS axis is, as a result, perpendicular to the Standard lead III lead axis which will consequently reflect an equiphasic QRS complex, a QR or an RS complex. When this is associated with a clockwise QRS vector loop, the initial forces are directed to the negative pole of Standard lead III and the initial QRS deflection will thus be negative, resulting in a prominent Q wave (Diagram A of Fig. 27). There may be a tiny initial q wave in lead AVF since the initial part of the QRS vector loop may also enter the negative zone of the lead AVF axis.

Example 2. The mean manifest frontal plane QRS axis is directed at $+10°$ (Diagram B of Fig. 27), also a normal QRS axis. The QRS vector loop is again inscribed in a clockwise direction. More of the loop will now be located in the negative zone of Standard lead III axis, and it is only the terminal part of the loop which enters the positive zone of the Standard lead III axis. This will result in a prominent Q wave followed by a tiny terminal r wave, a Qr complex.

The Effects of Respiration

The anatomical axis of the left ventricle is frequently parallel to the lead AVR axis and perpendicular to the Standard III axis. Thus, if the mean QRS axis is directed at $+30°$ (perpendicular to the Standard lead III axis) slight shifts in anatomical position, as affected by respiration, may cause marked changes in the QRS complex in Standard lead III. For example, with the QRS axis at $+30°$ and a clockwise loop, Standard lead III will, as indicated above, reflect a QR complex. Inspiration will tend to depress the anatomical axis of the heart due to downward movement of the diaphragm. Hence, the QRS axis and the QRS loop will also tend to shift inferiorly to a slight extent. Consequently, less of the loop will be situated in the negative zone of Standard lead III. This will result in a diminution of the normal Q wave in Standard lead III. Maximal expiration has the opposite effect, shifting the loop more into the negative zone of Standard lead III, and thereby tending to accentuate the so-called abnormal, prominent, Q wave in Standard lead III.

The differential diagnosis of a normal but prominent Q wave is based on:

(a) the correct vectorial evaluation of the initial 0·04 sec vector with reference to the mean QRS axis (as reflected above).

(b) the absence of other electrocardiographic signs of myocardial infarction.

FURTHER OBSERVATIONS OF THE VECTORIAL EVALUATION OF A PROMINENT Q WAVE IN STANDARD LEAD III

A prominent Q wave in Standard lead III should also be evaluated in terms of its vectorial relationship to the anatomy of the heart, and particularly to a potential infarction site. Thus, the pathological Q wave of myocardial infarction reflects an initial 0·04 sec vector which, as indicated in Chapter 1, is *directed away from the area of infarction*[G31]. The principle is considered with reference to Fig. 28.

Diagram A of Fig. 28 illustrates an initial 0·04 sec QRS vector which is situated within the region of $0-+30°$ on the frontal plane hexaxial reference system. The vector is within the negative zone of the Standard lead III axis, but within the positive zones of the Standard lead II and lead AVF axes. A Q wave will thus appear in Standard lead III but not in Standard lead II or lead AVF. This initial 0·04 sec vector is, however, directed laterally and to the left, i.e. it is not directed away from the inferior wall of the heart, and thus is unlikely to be an expression of inferior-wall myocardial infarction. Diagram B of Fig. 28 illustrates an initial 0·04 sec QRS vector which is situated within the region of $0--30°$ on the frontal plane hexaxial reference system. The vector is within the negative zones of the Standard lead III and lead AVF axes, but within the positive zone of the Standard lead II axis. Q waves will thus appear in Standard lead III and lead AVF but not in Standard lead II. This initial 0·04 sec QRS vectors is also directed laterally and to the left, and *not* away from the inferior wall of the heart. It is therefore unlikely to be significant of inferior wall myocardial infarction.

Diagram C of Fig. 28 illustrates an initial 0·04 sec QRS vector which is situated within the region counter-clockwise from $-30°$ on the frontal plane hexaxial reference system. This vector is situated within the negative zones of the Standard lead III, lead AVF and Standard lead II axes. All these leads will thus reflect initial Q waves. This initial vector is directed superiorly, i.e. away from the inferior wall of the ventricle and may consequently be indicative of inferior wall myocardial infarction.

Thus, a Q wave in Standard lead III is suggestive of inferior wall myocardial infarction when the following criteria are satisfied:

1. The duration of the Q wave must be at least 0·04 sec, i.e. one small square in width.

2. A Q wave of at least 0·02 sec duration must be present in lead AVF.

3. A Q wave of any duration must be present in Standard lead II.

Note: Left posterior hemiblock may be associated with

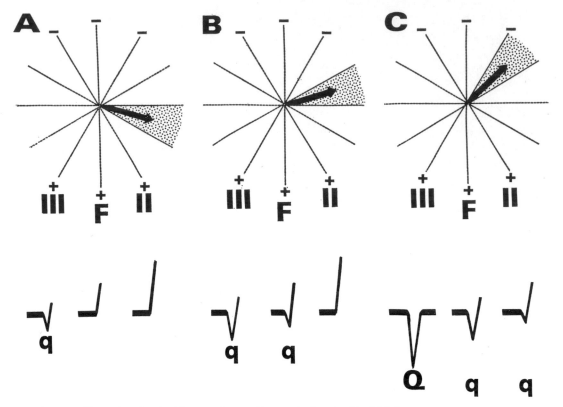

FIG. 28. Diagrams illustrating the significance of a *q* or *Q* wave in Standard lead III. See text.

initial *q* waves in Standard leads II and III and lead AVF. The terminal vector will, however, be directed inferiorly and to the right and will be of large magnitude thereby resulting in a very tall *R* wave in Standard lead III (see Chapter 12).

ACUTE PULMONARY EMBOLISM

The clinical presentation of acute pulmonary embolism, sudden onset of dyspnoea, hypotension, restlessness, collapse, tachycardia and acute chest pain, is similar to that of acute myocardial infarction. Furthermore, the condition is frequently characterized electrocardiographically by the appearance of a prominent *Q* wave and an inverted *T* wave in Standard lead III. It is therefore evident that acute pulmonary embolism simulates acute inferior wall myocardial infarction. In addition, acute pulmonary embolism may be associated with inverted *T* waves and possibly elevated S-T segments in leads V1–V4, and can therefore simulate acute anteroseptal myocardial infarction. Distinction is based on a careful evaluation of both the electrocardiographic parameters and the clinical presentation.

THE ELECTROCARDIOGRAPHIC MANIFESTATIONS OF ACUTE PULMONARY EMBOLISM

Acute pulmonary embolism may manifest with:

(a) electrocardiographic changes which affect the frontal plane leads.

(b) electrocardiographic changes which affect the horizontal plane leads, and

(c) abnormalities of cardiac rhythm: ectopic atrial tachyarrhythmias[C57, D39, D40, L65, M66, M91, O1, P14, R20, S96, S125, W17, W64, W65, W66, Z6].

Electrocardiographic Manifestations Affecting the Frontal Plane Leads

The following electrocardiographic manifestations of acute pulmonary embolism may appear in the frontal-plane leads:

1. The S1 Q3 T3 pattern.
2. S-T segment depression in Standard leads I and II.
3. A 'staircase' ascent of the S-T segment in Standard leads I and II.
4. Right axis deviation.
5. An *R* wave in leads AVR.
6. Transient right bundle branch block.
7. Tall peaked *P* waves in Standard lead II.

The S1 Q3 T3 Pattern

The S1 Q3 T3 pattern is a well-recognized triad consisting of a prominent *S* wave in Standard lead I, a prominent *Q* wave in Standard lead III, and an inverted *T* wave in Standard lead III (Electrocardiographic Study 98).

The prominent S wave in Standard lead I. This is a frequent manifestation of acute pulmonary embolism. The abnormal *S* wave usually undergoes rapid resolution. Immediately after the embolic event, it is usually broad and shallow, but this usually changes within a few hours to a deep and narrow deflection[D39]. The *S* wave ultimately regresses. This may occur early, within 24 hours, or the return to normal may be more gradual, extending over a number of weeks.

The prominent Q wave in Standard lead III. A deep prominent *q* or *Q* wave in Standard lead III is an important component of the electrocardiographic triad of acute pulmonary embolism. The *Q* wave is always followed by an ensuing *R* wave, i.e. it forms part of a qR complex. A QS complex is *not* associated with acute pulmonary embolism. Furthermore, the magnitude and deviation of the *Q* wave does not conform with the criteria of a pathological *Q* wave in acute myocardial infarction, i.e. the *Q* wave is not 0·04 sec in duration or longer, and the magnitude is not, as a rule, 25 per cent or more of the ensuing *R* wave. In addition, a prominent *Q* wave may occasionally appear in lead AVF or even Standard lead II.

The T wave inversion in Standard lead III. The *T* wave inversion in Standard lead III is almost always associated with the S1 Q3 abnormality. It is due to a left axis deviation of the *T* wave, further to the left than + 30° on the frontal plane hexaxial reference system. It is frequently in the region of − 30°, and consequently is usually associated with an inverted *T* wave in lead AVF, and an equiphasic *T* wave in Standard lead II. The *T* wave inversion in Standard lead III and lead AVF adds to the simulation of acute myocardial infarction.

Mechanism: The electrocardiographic manifestation is due to a clockwise loop with a terminal appendage which is directed superiorly and to the right (Fig. 29). The beginning of the loop is situated in the negative zone of Standard lead III, resulting in the prominent initial *Q* wave, and the terminal part of the loop is situated in the negative zone of Standard lead I, resulting in the terminal *S* wave. It will also result in a terminal *r* wave in lead AVR (see below).

Note: The S1 Q3 T3 pattern may also occur in left posterior hemiblock. The distinction is based mainly on a clinical basis. In left posterior hemiblock the *R* wave in Standard lead III is usually much taller than in acute pulmonary embolism.

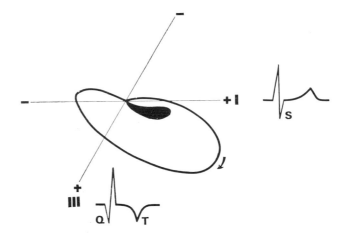

FIG. 29. Frontal plane vectorcardiogram of acute pulmonary embolism illustrating the genesis of the S1 Q3 T3 pattern. See text.

S-T Segment Depression in Standard Leads I and II

Marked depression of the S-T segment in Standard lead II, and to a lesser degree in Standard lead I[L65], may occur in association with acute pulmonary embolism (Electrocardiographic Study 98).

A 'Staircase' Ascent of the S-T Segment in Standard Leads I and II

This unusual pattern, best seen in Standard leads I and II, consists of flattening of the initial part of the S-T segment and *T* wave followed by a more or less sharp rise and then again by flattening of the terminal portion of the *T* wave[M66, M91, Z6].

Right-axis Deviation

Acute pulmonary embolism is usually associated with a rightward deviation of the *mean* frontal plane QRS axis by 20° or more (Electrocardiographic Study 98). The rightward deviation may, in fact, be quite marked, the mean frontal plane QRS axis being deviated to the region of between 90° and 100°, and rarely, even further rightward.

A Prominent R Wave in Lead AVR

Acute pulmonary embolism may be associated with the appearance of a prominent *R* wave in lead AVR (Electrocardiographic Study 98). This empirical observation is a further manifestation of the right axis deviation and the right ventricular dominance. It is due to a terminal appendage of the vectorcardiographic loop which is directed superiorly and to the right (see above and Fig. 29).

Transient Right Bundle Branch Block

Transient right bundle branch block is an important and not infrequent manifestation of acute pulmonary embolism[D39, W65]. The mechanism is probably a compression effect on the right bundle branch secondary to the increased pressure within the right ventricle[S23].

Tall, Peaked P Waves in Standard Lead II

Tall, sharply pointed, peaked P waves may appear in Standard lead II[W65]. Since similar P wave changes may occur with tachycardia *per se*, the significance of altered P waves in acute pulmonary embolism, which is nearly always associated with sinus tachycardia, is uncertain.

Electrocardiographic Manifestations Affecting the Horizontal Plane Leads

The following electrocardiographic manifestations of acute pulmonary embolism may appear in the horizontal plane leads:

1. T-wave inversion in the right precordial leads.
2. S-T segment elevation in the right precordial leads.
3. S-T segment depression in the left precordial leads.
4. Clockwise rotation.
5. An increase in R wave amplitude in the right precordial leads.
6. Diminution in amplitude and slurring of the S wave in the right precordial leads.
7. Transient right bundle branch block: an rSR' or RSR' pattern in the right precordial leads.
8. A prominent S wave in lead V6.

T Wave Inversion in Right Precordial Leads

This is a frequent electrocardiographic manifestation of acute pulmonary embolism[W64]. It almost always involves leads V1–V3, and less commonly lead V4 (Electrocardiographic Study 98). Unlike most of the other electrocardiographic changes occurring in acute pulmonary embolism, the T wave changes are more persistent and may take from 3–6 weeks to become upright again. The manifestation may mimic acute anteroseptal infarction.

S-T Segment Elevation in the Right Precordial Leads

The T-wave inversion which occurs in the right precordial leads in acute pulmonary embolism is, at times, associated with minimal elevation and coving of the S-T segments. This further adds to the simulation of acute anteroseptal infarction.

S-T Segment Depression in the Left Precordial Leads

Acute pulmonary embolism may occasionally be associated with S-T segment depression in the left precordial leads, leads V5 and V6[R20]. The depression is usually not marked, and may reflect horizontality, plane depression, with a sharp-angled ST-T junction (Electrocardiographic Study 98).

Clockwise Rotation

Acute pulmonary embolism may be associated with clockwise rotation around the oblique anatomical axis. The transition zone is displaced to the left, to leads V5 or V6, and may indeed be absent in the precordial leads (Electrocardiographic Study 98). Consequently rS or RS patterns appear in leads V1–V4 (V5 or V6). This is a frequent occurrence. The deviation of such a leftward shift of the transition zone is variable, ranging from a few hours to several weeks.

An Increase in R Wave Amplitude in the Right Precordial Leads

The r wave normally recorded by the right precordial teads is not infrequently increased in amplitude. This is due lo the development of right ventricular dominance. This is associated with a diminution in the associated S wave (see below), thereby resulting in an increase in the rS ratio. The manifestation is particularly marked in leads V2 and V3 (Electrocardiographic Study 98), but may, in the event of marked clockwise rotation, appear in all the precordial leads.

A qR Complex in Lead V1

The tall R wave in lead V1 of right ventricular dominance may occasionally be preceded by a small q wave, resulting in a qR complex. The differential diagnosis of a qR complex in lead V1 is discussed in Chapter 6.

Diminution in Amplitude and Slurring of the S Wave in the Right Precordial Leads[S96]

Early and transient right ventricular enlargement (i.e. dilatation and/or hypertrophy) following acute pulmonary embolism may be reflected electrocardiographically by diminution in the amplitude of the S wave[S96] (Electrocardiographic Study 98) with slurring of the ascending limb, or flattening of the nadir. This is seen particularly in lead V1 and less frequently in leads V4R and V2. These changes may be associated with a diminution of the R/S ratio in right precordial leads (see above). The absence of these abnormalities in control electrocardiographic tracings before the embolic event exclude other causes of right ventricular enlargement. Their appearance soon after a clinical episode suggestive of pulmonary embolism may represent sensitive electrocardiographic alterations of early right ventricular enlargement or hypertrophy of the crista supraventricularis of the right ventricle.

Transient Right Bundle Branch Block[D39, W65]

This will manifest with an rsR' or RSR' pattern in the right precordial leads.

Prominent S Wave in Lead V6
A transient but prominent *S* wave may appear in lead V6 (Electrocardiographic Study 98). This is the expression of a terminal vector which is directed superiorly and to the right.

Paroxysmal, Ectopic, Atrial Tachyarrhythmias
The atrial arrhythmias most frequently seen in acute pulmonary embolism are atrial flutter, atrial fibrillation, atrial tachycardia and atrial extrasystoles. The incidence of these arrhythmias varies considerably in different series. This may be due to their transient nature, as a result of which they may be missed. When atrial tachyarrhythmias occur in acute pulmonary embolism, they are frequently associated with a rapid ventricular response[W17], resulting in significant haemodynamic disturbance.

The most important factors responsible for the genesis of these atrial tachyarrhythmias following acute pulmonary embolism are distension of the right atrium, an increase in circulating catecholamines, and ischaemia of the S-A (sinoatrial) node due to reduced coronary perfusion.

Despite the variable electrocardiographic changes frequently associated with acute pulmonary embolism, it should be stressed that a significant number of patients, 20 per cent or more, may show no gross electrocardiographic abnormality following the embolic event. It should also be emphasized that many of the electrocardiographic manifestations occur very early, within minutes to a few hours, after the onset of the embolic incident, and may consequently be missed.

Furthermore, some of the changes may be very transient, alternating or disappearing with an improvement in the haemodynamic state. Thus, to detect the transient electrocardiographic patterns of acute pulmonary embolism, tracings should be recorded as early as possible (within 1–2 hours) after the onset of symptoms, and followed by frequent serial tracings.

The Mechanism of the Electrocardiographic Manifestations
The exact mechanisms responsible for the QRS changes in acute pulmonary embolism are not known. It has been variously attributed to cardiac rotation[W66], a raised diaphragm[O1], coronary artery insufficiency which could be due to:

1. reflex coronary spasm,
2. poor coronary perfusion secondary to collapse, and sudden dilatation of the right ventricle causing stretching and narrowing of the right coronary artery[O1], and
3. a high right ventricular pressure in association with a low aortic perfusion pressure in coronary blood flow through the right ventricle[D40].

The S-T segment and *T* wave manifestations of acute pulmonary embolism may be related to right ventricular strain[M91], and possibly subendocardial ischaemia due to the poor coronary perfusion resulting from shock and anoxia[K7].

Differential Diagnosis from Acute Myocardial Infarction
The differential diagnosis between acute myocardial infarction and acute pulmonary embolism is based on the following:

1. Sinus tachycardia is invariable with acute pulmonary embolism, and may also occur with acute myocardial infarction. However, acute myocardial infarction may be associated with sinus bradycardia, whereas this does not occur with acute pulmonary embolism.

2. The Q wave which appears in Standard lead III in acute inferior wall myocardial infarction is wide, 0·04 sec or longer, and usually constitutes 25 per cent or more of the ensuing *R* wave. The Q3 of pulmonary embolism, while prominent, does not have these marked characteristics. Furthermore, acute inferior-wall myocardial infarction is usually associated with prominent or significant Q waves in Standard lead II and lead AVF, whereas significant, prominent, Q waves in Standard lead II and lead AVF are very uncommon in acute pulmonary embolism (Electrocardiographic Study 98).

3. Acute inferior wall myocardial infarction is not usually associated with the electrocardiographic features of acute anteroseptal injury and/or ischaemia, whereas this is a common feature in acute pulmonary embolism.

4. Acute inferior wall myocardial infarction is associated with coved and elevated S-T segments in Standard lead II and III and lead AVF. However, in acute pulmonary embolism the S-T segments are usually isoelectric in Standard lead III and lead AVF and may, in fact, be depressed in Standard lead II (Electrocardiographic Study 98).

5. Acute inferior wall myocardial infarction is usually associated with protracted serial changes, whereas the manifestations of acute pulmonary embolism tend to be transient and of short duration.

When the electrocardiographic manifestations of a patient with acute chest pain appear to resemble that of acute inferior infarction in association with acute anteroseptal infarction, the diagnosis of acute pulmonary embolism should always be considered.

LEFT AXIS DEVIATION WITH LEFT BUNDLE BRANCH BLOCK

Left axis deviation with left bundle branch block will

present with a QS deflection in Standard lead III. With significant left axis deviation, an expression of left anterior hemiblock, the mean manifest frontal plane QRS axis will be directed to the region of $-30°$ counter-clockwise to $-90°$. This will result in deep S waves in Standard leads II and III and lead AVF. These leads will, in the absence of left bundle branch block, also have initial r waves, the expression of initial septal activation or, more likely, initial activation of the postero-inferior wall (Diagram A of Fig. 53; see Chapter 12). In other words, these leads will reflect rS complexes. If, in addition, there is incomplete left bundle branch block, the initial r wave will disappear, resulting in a completely negative deflection, a QS complex (Diagram B of Fig. 53). This may mimic the pathological Q wave of myocardial infarction. The differential diagnosis is based on:

(a) the absence of the classical S-T segment and T wave changes of myocardial infarction.

(b) the features of left bundle branch block in other leads, particularly the left lateral leads V5 and V6.

LEFT POSTERIOR HEMIBLOCK

In left posterior hemiblock the initial QRS force, the initial 0·02 sec vector, is directed superiorly and to the left. This will result in rather prominent, but not abnormal, initial q waves in Standard leads II and III and lead AVF. The terminal QRS vector is, however, directed inferiorly and to the right, thereby resulting in a very tall R wave in Standard lead III (Electrocardiographic Studies 46 and 47). The manifestation is also associated with secondary T wave changes. The T wave is directed superiorly and to the left (Diagram C of Fig. 46), thereby resulting in upright T waves in Standard lead I and lead AVL and low to inverted T waves in Standard leads II and III and lead AVF (Electrocardiographic Studies 47 and 48). The phenomenon is considered in greater detail in Chapter 12.

A NEGATIVE DELTA WAVE

When the delta-wave axis is directed superiorly and to the left, for example, at $-60°$ on the frontal plane hexaxial reference system, it will be negative in Standard leads II and III and lead AVF, and may mimic the pathological Q wave of inferior wall myocardial infarction (Electrocardiographic Study 69). The problem and differential diagnosis is considered in greater detail in Chapter 11.

COMPLICATIONS OF INFERIOR WALL MYOCARDIAL INFARCTION

Inferior-wall myocardial infarction may have the following electrocardiographic complications:

1. Extension of the infarction.
2. Right bundle branch block.
3. Left bundle branch block.
4. Diaphragmatic peri-infarction block.
5. Left anterior hemiblock.
6. Complicating A-V conduction disturbances.
7. Complicating ectopic rhythms.

EXTENSION OF THE INFARCTION

Inferior-wall myocardial infarction is frequently associated with an extension of the infarction process to the adjacent regions of the heart. The inferior infarction may, for example, extend to the posterior, lateral (superior), apical or anteroseptal walls (Electrocardiographic Studies 23, 27, 28, 31, 32, 33 and 34).

Posterior Wall Extension

Extension of the infarction to the true posterior wall may involve the parameter of ischaemia only, manifesting with a T wave change only. Or, it may involve all the parameters of the infarction process, those of necrosis, injury and ischaemia.

Extension of the ischaemic process to the posterior wall is a frequent manifestation, and is reflected by tall, symmetrical T waves in the precordial leads (see Diagram C of Fig. 19; Electrocardiographic Study 30).

When all the parameters of infarction extend to the posterior wall, the electrocardiogram will, in addition to the classic features of inferior myocardial infarction, manifest with tall R waves, tall symmetrical T waves, and possibly depressed S-T segments in the right precordial leads (Electrocardiographic Studies 31, 32 and 33; see Chapter 7).

Lateral Wall Extension: Infero-apical Infarction

Lateral extension of an inferior-wall myocardial infarction tends to involve the apical rather than the true left lateral (superior) wall. Lateral extension may involve the parameter of ischaemia only, and this will be reflected by low to inverted T waves in leads V5 and V6 (Electrocardiographic Studies 26, 27, 31, 32, 33 and 34). When lateral extension involves all the parameters of infarction, i.e., necrosis, injury and ischaemia, the fully evolved pattern of infarction—Q wave, coved and elevated S-T segment and inverted, symmetrical T wave—will appear in lead V6 and possibly in lead V5. In addition, the R wave in leads V5 and V6 is always diminished in amplitude (Electrocardiographic Study 28).

If extension of the infarction occurs to the more proximal region of the lateral (superior) wall, the infarction pattern would theoretically also appear in Standard lead I. This is, however, *very rare*. A more common electrocardiographic manifestation of lateral wall extension is the appearance of a QS rather than a QR complex in Standard lead II.

Antero-septal Wall Extension

Inferior-wall myocardial infarction may rarely extend to, or be associated with, anteroseptal infarction or extensive anterior infarction. When this occurs, the parameters of infarction will be seen in the precordial leads as well as the inferior leads (Electrocardiographic Study 2).

COMPLICATING RIGHT BUNDLE BRANCH BLOCK

Inferior-wall myocardial infarction may be complicated by, or superimposed upon, right bundle branch block. When this occurs, the initial vectors are unchanged, and the infarction pattern is recognized from the initial QRS abnormalities in Standard lead II and III, and lead AVF (see Chapter 9 and Electrocardiographic Study 53). With right bundle branch block, however, there is a terminal rightward and anterior QRS force which is reflected by a prominent R wave in Standard lead III. The terminal R wave in Standard lead III is the tallest and most prominent of the terminal R waves in the three conventional leads orientated to the inferior wall (Diagram C of Fig. 25, and Electrocardiographic Study 53). This is in contrast to (a) the manifestations of diaphragmatic peri-infarction block, where the terminal R waves tend to be more or less of equal magnitude or only minimally taller in Standard lead III (Diagram B of Fig. 25), or (b) the manifestations of uncomplicated inferior wall myocardial infarction, where the terminal R wave is of greatest magnitude in Standard lead II (see Diagram A of Fig. 25; see Chapter 12).

ASSOCIATED LEFT BUNDLE BRANCH BLOCK

Inferior-wall myocardial infarction may be associated with left bundle branch block. When this occurs, the diagnosis of myocardial infarction is based on specific modifications of the QRS complex and the presence of primary S-T segment and T wave changes (see Chapter 10). The S-T segments, in contrast to uncomplicated left bundle branch block, are elevated in Standard lead II and III and lead AVF, i.e. they are deviated in the *same* direction as the terminal QRS deflection (see Chapter 10 and Electrocardiographic Study 61).

COMPLICATING DIAPHRAGMATIC, DIVISIONAL, PERI-INFARCTION BLOCK: LEFT POSTERIOR HEMIBLOCK

This is reflected by a wide frontal plane angle, greater than 100°, between the initial and terminal 0·04 sec QRS vectors. The initial 0·04 sec QRS vector, the expression of the myocardial necrosis, is directed superiorly and to the left. The terminal 0·04 sec QRS vector, the expression of the left posterior hemiblock, is directed inferiorly at approximately +90°. This terminal QRS vector is reflected by the inscription of terminal R waves in Standard leads II and III and lead AVF, which are more or less of equal magnitude, or possibly a little taller in Standard lead III (Electrocardiographic Studies 48, 49 and 50). The principles governing peri-infarction block are discussed in greater detail in Chapter 12.

Note that focal peri-infarction block is probably present in uncomplicated inferior wall myocardial infarction, and is reflected by the terminal R wave of the QR complex in Standard lead II (see Chapter 12).

LEFT ANTERIOR HEMIBLOCK

Inferior wall myocardial infarction may be associated with left anterior hemiblock. This may mask or modify both the QRS and T wave manifestations of the inferior wall myocardial infarction.

The Effect on the QRS Complex

In left anterior hemiblock the initial QRS vector is directed inferiorly as a result of initial activation of the postero-inferior wall. The terminal QRS vector is directed superiorly and to the left (Fig. 45, Diagrams C of Figs. 47 and 48, and Diagram A of Fig. 52). If an associated inferior infarction spares the posterior region of the inferior wall (Diagram A of Fig. 51), the initial QRS force of left anterior hemiblock is unaffected. Since this is directed inferiorly, it will inscribe initial positive deflections in Standard leads II and III and lead AVF, and thereby mask the QRS manifestations of inferior-wall myocardial infarction (Electrocardiographic Studies 37, 44 and 45). If the *whole* of the inferior wall is affected, anterior as well as posterior regions (Diagram B of Fig. 51), then the initial forces of the left anterior hemiblock are obliterated and there is no effect on the initial forces of the infarction pattern (Electrocardiographic Study 29). These principles are discussed in greater detail in Chapter 12.

The terminal QRS vector of left anterior hemiblock may also modify the terminal QRS manifestations of inferior-wall myocardial infarction. Since the terminal QRS vector is directed superiorly and to the left, it will be reflected by negative deflections in all three of the inferior leads. Thus, the usual QR complex in Standard lead II of uncomplicated inferior wall myocardial infarction is changed to a QS complex, and all three inferior leads, Standard leads II and III and lead AVF, tend to reflect QS complexes. When this occurs, Standard lead I and particularly lead AVL, will have relatively tall *R* waves, the expression of the marked left axis deviation (Electrocardiographic Study 29).

The Effect on the T Wave

With the advent of left anterior hemiblock, the *T*-wave vector tends to deviate inferiorly to the region of +60° clockwise to +80° on the frontal plane hexaxial reference system (Diagram B of Fig. 46). This will cause the *T* waves to be upright in the inferior leads, Standard leads II and III and lead AVF, and may consequently modify or mask the inverted *T* waves of inferior wall myocardial infarction. The phenomenon is considered in greater detail in Chapter 12.

COMPLICATING A-V CONDUCTION DISTURBANCES

Inferior-wall myocardial infarction is more readily complicated by A-V conduction disturbances than anterior wall infarction. First degree A-V block and particularly the Type I second-degree A-V block, the Wenckebach Phenomenon, is common (see Chapter 17).

COMPLICATING ECTOPIC RHYTHMS

Inferior wall myocardial infarction is not infrequently associated with various forms of enhanced ectopic automaticity, especially *idionodal tachycardia* and *idioventricular tachycardia* (see Chapter 17).

Chapter 6

Anterior Wall Myocardial Infarction

Anterior wall myocardial infarction refers to infarction which involves the anterior wall of the *left ventricle*—the interventricular septum—and *not* the anatomical anterior wall of the heart—the free wall of the right ventricle. The anterior wall of the left ventricle may be arbitrarily divided into an *anteroseptal* region and an *anterolateral* region. The anteroseptal region may be further subdivided into *high-*, *mid-* and *low-*septal regions (Fig. 30). The anterolateral region may be further subdivided into *apical* and *high-lateral* regions (Fig. 30). Anterior wall myocardial infarction may thus be arbitrarily subdivided into one or more of the aforementioned regions. Localization of the infarction is made from the appearance in leads which are orientated to these specific regions of the infarction pattern; *pathological Q wave* or *QS complex*, *elevated S-T segment* and *abnormal T wave*. The localization involves all the three phases of myocardial infarction, the hyperacute phase, the fully evolved phase, and the chronic phase (see Chapter 4).

It must be stressed that localization is based on electrode orientation, and since this orientation, particularly in the case of anterior wall myocardial infarction, may be modified by such factors as body build, accurate electrode placement and heart position, there is of necessity a measure of overlap in the localization.

CLASSIFICATION

CLASSIFICATION OF THE ANTERIOR WALL MYOCARDIAL INFARCTIONS

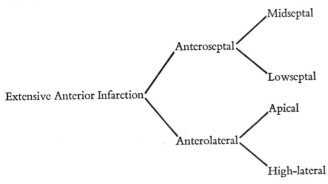

EXTENSIVE ANTERIOR-WALL MYOCARDIAL INFARCTION

Extensive anterior wall myocardial infarction is, in effect, a combination of anteroseptal and anterolateral infarction. The infarction patterns appear in the leads orientated to the anterior and anterolateral wall of the left ventricle, leads V1–V6, Standard lead I, and lead AVL.

THE HYPERACUTE EARLY INJURY PHASE

This is characterized by slope-elevation of the S-T segment and injury block in the anterior orientated leads (Electrocardiographic Studies 2, 3, 5 and 6, and Tracing A of Study 12). Reciprocal S-T segment depression may occur in Standard lead III and lead AVF.

THE FULLY EVOLVED PHASE

This is characterized by pathological Q waves, QS complexes, coved and elevated S-T segments, and inverted arrow-head *T* waves in all the leads orientated to the anterior and anterolateral wall (Electrocardiographic Studies 2, 3, 5, 6, 12B, 13–19). The S-T segment elevation is usually most marked in the mid-precordial leads, V2–V4. Reciprocal S-T segment depression and tall symmetrical *T* waves may appear in Standard lead III and lead AVF. The pathological Q waves or QS complexes are due to loss of (a) the septal vectors of ventricular depolarization (Vectors 1a and b of Fig. 11), (b) the paraseptal vectors of ventricular depolarization, especially the left paraseptal vector (Vector 2a of Fig. 11), and (c) the left free wall vectors of ventricular depolarization (Vectors 3 and 4 of Fig. 11). The initial small *r* wave of the rS complex normally recorded by leads V1–V3 (and possibly lead V4) is lost, thereby resulting in a QS complex. Qr or QR complexes usually appear in the left lateral leads, leads V5 and V6, Standard lead I and lead AVL, thereby reflecting a pathological Q wave with an ensuing *R* or *r* wave. While

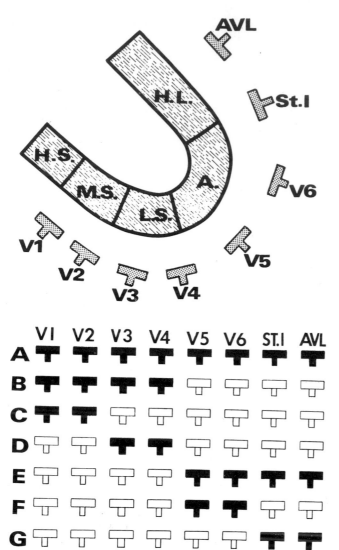

FIG. 30. Diagram illustrating the classification of the anterior wall myocardial infarction. H.S. = High septum. M.S. = Mid septum. L.S. = Low septum. A. = Apical. H.L. = High-lateral.

QS complexes are common in leads V1–V4, and may even be prominent in Standard lead I and lead AVL, they are uncommon in leads V5 and V6, which usually reflect Qr or QR complexes (Electrocardiographic Studies 15, 17 and 18). This is because the apical extension of the infarction tends to be subendocardial, rather than transmural, and is associated with surviving overlying healthy subepicardial tissue. Compare this manifestation with the genesis of the terminal R wave of the QR complex in Standard lead II in cases of inferior wall myocardial infarction (see Chapter 5). Another possible explanation is that leads V5 and V6 may be somewhat inferiorly orientated and consequently reflect late inferior-wall potentials.

Anterior Wall Myocardial Infarction Manifesting with QS Complexes in all the Precordial Leads

Anterior wall myocardial infarction may occasionally manifest with QS complexes in *all* the precordial leads, leads V1–V6, and also in Standard lead I and lead AVL (Electrocardiographic Studies 10, 11 and 12). This may be due to the following:

(a) There is an extensive transmural myocardial infarction of the whole anterior wall, and particularly the anterolateral wall of the left ventricle. When this occurs, a Qr complex may be reflected by lead V7.

(b) There is a marked clockwise rotation of the heart so that leads V5 and V6 constitute the transition zone. In other words, the left lateral leads are not accurately orientated to the apex, but rather to the septal region. When this is the case, leads V7 and V8, in the absence of a very extensive transmural infarction, will definitely reflect Qr or QR complexes.

(c) The infarction is associated with a marked degree of left anterior hemiblock. This tends to diminish the positivity of the QRS deflections in the left lateral leads. Thus, in most cases of uncomplicated left anterior hemiblock, leads V5 and V6 usually reflect an rS complex. The superimposition of myocardial infarction will, in many instances, transform the rS complex into a QS complex.

The Significance of a Precordial Leads QS Complex in Anterior Wall Myocardial Infarction

A QS complex which appears in the left lateral leads, leads V5 and V6, usually connotes a transmural infarction of the left free wall. A QS complex which appears in the right precordial leads, however, does not necessarily connote a transmural infarction of the anterior left ventricular wall, the interventricular septum. It can represent either a transmural infarction of the interventricular septum or a subendocardial infarction of the left (posterior) side of the interventricular septum. This is because a subendocardial infarction of the left side of the interventricular septum, the functional subendocardium of the interventricular septum (see page 76), results in a loss of the first septal vector (Vector 1a of Fig. 11). This results in a loss of the initial r wave of the rS complex normally reflected by the right precordial leads, and which is consequently transformed into a QS complex. Such a QS complex *is not* the expression of transmural infarction. (See Chapter 8 and Fig. 33).

ANTEROSEPTAL MYOCARDIAL INFARCTION

Anteroseptal myocardial infarction is, in effect, a combination of midseptal and lowseptal infarction. The infarction results in the loss of the septal and paraseptal vectors of ventricular depolarization (Vectors 1 and 2 of Fig. 11).

THE CLASSIC ELECTROCARDIOGRAPHIC PRESENTATION

The infarction patterns are present in leads V1–V4 (Diagram B of Fig. 30, and Electrocardiographic Studies 14, 19, 20, 21 and 22).

The fully evolved phase of anteroseptal myocardial infarction is characterized by the following. QS patterns appear in leads V1–V3. A QR pattern is frequently present in lead V4. Leads V5 and V6 reflect the loss of the small initial q wave of the qR complex usually recorded by these leads (see also comment below). This is due to the abolition of the first vector of septal depolarization (Vector 1a of Fig. 11). In addition, the resulting solitary R wave (which is not preceded by a q wave) in the left lateral leads may be, and usually is, diminished in amplitude (Electrocardiographic Studies 14, 19, 20, 21 and 22). This may be due to some lateral subepicardial extension of the infarction. Coved and elevated S-T segments, and sharply pointed arrow-head inverted T waves appear in lead V1–V4. These manifestations are usually more marked with this anteroseptal location than with any other location of the infarction site.

The parameter of myocardial injury, the elevated and coved S-T segment, and especially the parameter of myocardial ischaemia, the inverted arrow-head T wave, tend to extend more laterally, and may thus also be present in leads V5 and V6.

The only electrocardiographic stigmata of myocardial infarction which may manifest in the chronic stabilized phase of anteroseptal infarction are QS complexes in leads V1–V3 or V4. The abnormal S-T segments and T waves of the acute phase will have regressed. The precordial leads, however, still reflect the electrocardiographic parameters of chronic coronary insufficiency, for example, the T waves in the right precordial leads may be taller than the T waves in the left precordial leads (see Chapter 15).

Note that if the classic features of anteroseptal infarction, the QS complexes in leads V1–V4, are associated with what appears to be the normal small initial q wave (of the qR complex) in leads V5 and V6, it *suggests* a lateral subendocardial extension of the infarction. In other words, there is a more extensive anterior-wall infarction even though the characteristic *pathological* Q waves are not present in leads V5 and V6.

OTHER FORMS OF ELECTROCARDIOGRAPHIC PRESENTATION

FAILURE OF THE NORMAL PROGRESSIVE r WAVE INCREASE FROM LEADS V1–V4

At times, the presence of anteroseptal myocardial infarction may be evident from a diminution in the amplitude of the initial r or R wave in leads V3 and V4. There is a failure of the normal progressive increase in the initial r waves from leads V1–V4. These leads may actually show a progressive diminution in R or r wave (Electrocardiographic Study 41).

A progressive diminution in r or R wave may also occur with right ventricular dominance. In this condition, however, there will be clinical evidence for the right ventricular dominance and other electrocardiographic manifestations of right ventricular dominance such as tall R waves in the right precordial leads, right axis deviation, and P pulmonale. A differentiating feature of importance is the associated T-wave pattern. In right ventricular dominance the associated T-wave inversion will be more marked in leads V1 and V2 than in leads V3 and V4, whereas in anteroseptal myocardial infarction the associated T-wave inversion will be more marked in leads V3 and V4 than in leads V1 and V2.

A progressive diminution in r or R wave may also occur with mirror-image dextracardia. In this case, however, the characteristic abnormal rightward QRS and P wave axes in the frontal plane leads will reveal the true diagnosis.

qrS COMPLEXES IN LEADS V1 AND V2: SMALL INITIAL q WAVES IN LEADS V1 AND V2

The presence of a small initial q wave preceding the rS complex in leads V1 and V2 is suggestive of anteroseptal infarction. This diagnostic feature is reinforced if there are QS or Qr complexes in leads V3 and V4. Compare this manifestation with the analogous phenomenon which may affect the inferiorly orientated leads in inferior wall myocardial infarction (see Chapter 12, p. 110; Electrocardiographic Study 37).

FAILURE OF THE NORMAL PROGRESSIVE q WAVE INCREASE FROM LEADS V4–V6

The initial q wave (of a qR complex) is normally deeper in lead V6 than in lead V4. If the reverse appertains, a q wave deeper in lead V4 than in lead V6, it suggests infarction of the lower part of the interventricular septum (see section below in lowseptal infarction, p. 64, and Electrocardiographic Studies 38 and 46).

S-T Segment and *T* Wave Changes Only

Anteroseptal infarction may occasionally present with little or no change of the QRS complexes, the infarction manifesting with the parameters of injury and ischaemia only.

A Qr Complex in the Right Precordial Leads

A Qr complex (pathological Q wave followed by a terminal *r* wave) may be reflected by the right precordial leads in anteroseptal infarction, infarction of the middle and lower thirds of the interventricular septum (Rodriguez and associates)[R29].

Mechanism

A qR pattern will be recorded by a lead (non-conventional) which is orientated to the proximal part of the interventricular septum as, for example, by an electrode situated in the right atrium. This is especially so in cases of right ventricular dominance. The *q* wave is the result of septal activation (Vector 1 of Fig. 11) and possibly activation of the free walls of both ventricles (Vectors 3 and 4 of Fig. 11). The *R* wave is due to late activation of the basal regions of the left ventricle, and particularly the basal region of the interventricular septum, the right ventricular outflow tract or crista supraventricularis. If the lower two-thirds of the interventricular septum is infarcted, the initial *q* wave will be increased in magnitude and duration, i.e. it is transformed into a pathological Q wave. Provided the upper one-third of the interventricular septum is spared, the pathological Q wave is followed by a late *r* wave. The resulting Qr complex will be recorded by leads orientated to the proximal part of the interventricular septum, for example, an intracavity lead. This pattern will be transmitted to the right precordial leads, leads V1 and V2, if, in addition, the right paraseptal region is involved, thereby creating the dead zone window for such transmission. The genesis of this pattern is thus dependent upon:

(a) Infarction of the lower two-thirds of the interventricular septum.

(b) Sparing of the superior one-third of the interventricular septum.

(c) Some degree of right paraseptal infarction.

In addition, the Qr pattern is likely to be of low voltage. This is a distinguishing feature from the qR pattern in the right precordial leads which occurs in cases of right atrial enlargement (see below).

Differential Diagnosis of a qR Pattern in the Right Precordial Leads

A qR, QR, Qr or qr pattern may appear in the right precordial leads in the following conditions:

1. **Anteroseptal myocardial infarction** (see above).
2. **Acute pulmonary embolism** (see p. 54).
3. **Right atrial enlargement.** In the presence of marked right atrial enlargement, the heart frequently undergoes a positional change so that the proximal region of the interventricular septum tends to be orientated to the right precordial leads, particularly lead V1. When this occurs, the qR complex normally recorded by a lead orientated to the proximal part of the interventricular septum will be reflected in lead V1[S106]. The *R* wave tends to be relatively tall, i.e. taller than the *R* wave associated with the QR complexes of septal infarction or acute pulmonary embolism. Such a qR complex may be associated with any form of massive right atrial enlargement, but is especially prone to occur in cases of tricuspid incompetence (Electrocardiographic Study 106).

DIFFERENTIAL DIAGNOSIS OF ANTEROSEPTAL MYOCARDIAL INFARCTION

The following electrocardiographic presentations may simulate anteroseptal myocardial infarction:

1. Left bundle branch block.
2. Left anterior hemiblock.
3. The Type B Wolff-Parkinson-White syndrome.
4. Emphysema, chronic cor pulmonale.
5. The electrocardiographic presentation of acute pulmonary embolism.

The first four conditions listed above may simulate the abnormal QRS complexes, but not the S-T segment and *T* wave manifestations, of anteroseptal infarction. Consequently, they do not present a problem in differential diagnosis during the acute stage of infarction, since the S-T segment and *T* wave abnormalities of myocardial injury and ischaemia make the recognition of the acute infarction pattern evident. These conditions may, however, present some difficulty in the differentiation from the *chronic* stabilized phase of anteroseptal infarction, when only the abnormal QRS changes of the infarction QS complexes in leads V1–V4 may be present. The differential diagnosis is considered in detail below.

It must be emphasized at the outset that the appearance of a single QS complex in the right precordial leads does not constitute evidence of infarction unless there is concomitant electrocardiographic evidence of the infarction such as coved elevated S-T segments and inverted *T* waves. A single QS complex in the absence of such concomitant evidence may be due to faulty electrode placement.

Left Bundle Branch Block

Incomplete or complete left bundle branch block may

present with QS complexes in the right precordial leads. The differential diagnosis from anteroseptal infarction is based on the following:

(a) The characteristic coved and elevated S-T segments of acute myocardial infarction are absent. The S-T segment of uncomplicated left bundle branch block tends to have an upward slope towards a positive T wave. This upward slope is straight or slightly concave-upward. The magnitude of the QRS complex tends to be much larger than the magnitude of the S-T segment elevation, i.e. the QRS/S-T ratio tends to be in the region of 1·5–2 or even greater. If there is a complicating anteroseptal infarction, i.e. if anteroseptal infarction is associated with left bundle branch block, there is a much greater elevation of the S-T segment, and the QRS/S-T ratio tends to diminish and approach unity (see Chapter 10).

(b) In acute myocardial infarction, especially in the fully evolved phase, the T wave in the right precordial leads will be inverted, whereas in uncomplicated incomplete left bundle branch block the T wave will always be upright.

(c) The characteristic manifestations of left bundle branch block will be present in other leads, particularly leads V5 and V6.

(d) A further differentiating features of anteroseptal infarction from left bundle branch block is the appearance of the QRS complexes in the immediately adjacent lateral leads. When, for example, QS complexes appear in leads V1–V3, the form of the QRS complex in lead V4 or the lead constituting the transition zone may afford a clue to the correct diagnosis. If lead V4 reflects a pathological Q wave, i.e. it reflects a Qr complex, then the diagnosis is most likely one of anteroseptal infarction. If the transition from the QS complexes of leads V1–V3 is characterized by a dominant R wave which is not preceded by an initial q wave, the diagnosis is more likely one of left bundle branch block.

LEFT ANTERIOR HEMIBLOCK

Left anterior hemiblock may manifest with QS deflections in the right precordial leads. This is especially prone to occur if the precordial electrodes are placed relatively high on the precordium and/or the heart is relatively low, as occurs in long, thin, slender, asthenic individuals and patients with emphysema. This is discussed in detail in Chapter 12. The differential diagnosis from acute anteroseptal infarction is made by the absence of the classical signs of myocardial injury and ischaemia, the absence of coved and elevated S-T segments, and inverted symmetrical T waves. The differential diagnosis from chronic, old, anteroseptal infarction is made on the following basis.

(a) There is marked left axis deviation in the frontal plane leads. (b) The initial tiny r wave returns when the electrocardiogram is recorded with a slightly lower precordial electrode placement.

Left anterior hemiblock may also mask the QRS manifestations of anteroseptal infarction. Left anterior hemiblock is associated with an initial inferior QRS deflection that may result in the inscription of tiny initial r waves in the right precordial leads (Electrocardiographic Study 60A). This consequently masks the QS complexes of anteroseptal infarction. The true diagnosis may be established by recording the electrocardiogram with the precordial electrodes in a slightly higher precordial electrode placement (see Chapter 12).

THE TYPE B WOLFF–PARKINSON–WHITE SYNDROME

The Type B Wolff–Parkinson–White syndrome results in dominantly negative delta waves and QRS deflections in the right precordial leads. This may mimic anteroseptal myocardial infarction. The diagnosis is made from the recognition of the classical delta waves and shortened P-R intervals in these and other leads, and the absence of the primary S-T segment and T-wave changes of myocardial injury and ischaemia (see Chapter 11).

EMPHYSEMA—CHRONIC COR PULMONALE

QS complexes may appear in the right precordial leads in cases of chronic cor pulmonale, emphysema. This occurs because the heart in emphysema is relatively low in relation to the conventional electrode placement. The precordial electrodes are, as a result, orientated to the proximal regions of the heart, and these regions normally reflect QS complexes. The other electrocardiographic features of emphysema, however, will easily facilitate the differentiation from myocardial infarction. These are:

1. Generalized diminution in amplitude of all the deflections. This affects in particular the QRS complexes in leads V5 and V6 and Standard lead I.

2. The mean frontal plane QRS and P wave axes are usually directed precisely at $+90°$. This, together with the generalized lower voltage, will make a minimal impression of these deflections on Standard lead I.

3. The mean frontal plane T wave axis isa usully directed at $+90°$ or $-90°$.

4. The T waves tend to be low to inverted throughout.

THE ELECTROCARDIOGRAPHIC PRESENTATION OF ACUTE PULMONARY EMBOLISM

Acute pulmonary embolism usually presents with changes

affecting the S–T segment and *T* wave only. It frequently results in *T* wave inversion and, less commonly, S–T segment elevation in the right precordial leads. This may mimic the acute injury and ischaemia of acute anteroseptal myocardial infarction. The diagnosis is discussed on p. 55. Acute pulmonary embolism may at times also present with Qr patterns in leads V1 and V2. This mimics the abnormal QRS complexes of anteroseptal, and particularly midseptal, infarction. However, Qr complexes are unlikely to be present in leads V3 and V4 with acute pulmonary embolism.

MIDSEPTAL MYOCARDIAL INFARCTION

Midseptal infarction is, in effect, a subdivision of anteroseptal infarction, and results in the loss of the midseptal depolarization vectors (vectors 1a and b of Fig. 11). The diagnosis is made from the presence of the infarction pattern in leads V1 and V2 (Diagram C of Fig. 30). QS complexes appear in leads V1 and V2, due to the loss of the small initial *r* wave. The small normal initial *q* wave disappears from leads V5 and V6. In the acute fully evolved phase there will be associated coved and elevated S–T segments and inverted sharply pointed symmetrical *T* waves of acute infarction.

Isolated midseptal infarction is rare. The infarction is usually associated with lowseptal infarction, constituting an anteroseptal infarct.

DIFFERENTIAL DIAGNOSIS

Isolated midseptal infarction may also be simulated by left bundle branch block, the Type B Wolff-Parkinson-White syndrome, the electrocardiographic manifestation of acute pulmonary embolism, and chronic cor pulmonale—emphysema. The differential diagnosis is discussed in the section on anteroseptal infarction (see above).

THE DISTORTING EFFECT OF ATRIAL FIBRILLATION

Atrial fibrillation of recent onset usually manifests with rather coarse, relatively high amplitude 'f' waves which are especially marked in lead V1. If such an 'f' wave is fortuitously superimposed upon the initial part of a pathological QS complex in leads V1 and V2, it may simulate a tiny initial *r* wave and the presence of infarction may consequently be masked (Electrocardiographic Study 43).

LOWSEPTAL MYOCARDIAL INFARCTION

Lowseptal infarction is, in effect, a further subdivision of anteroseptal myocardial infarction. The diagnosis is made from the presence of the infarction pattern in leads V3 and V4 (Diagram D of Fig. 30). Infarction of the lower septum obliterates vectors 2a and b of normal ventricular depolarization, the lower septal and paraseptal forces which are responsible for the initial *r* or *R* waves normally reflected in leads V3 and V4 (see Chapter 2, and Fig. 11). As a result, leads V3 and V4 reflect QS complexes, whereas leads V1 and possibly lead V2 may still reflect the tiny initial septal *r* wave of the normal rS complex. Electrocardiographic Studies 15, 18 and 24, while illustrating relatively extensive anterior infarction, reflect sparing of the midseptal region. In the fully evolved phase, there will be associated coved and elevated S–T segments of myocardial injury and inverted symmetrical *T* waves of myocardial ischaemia. These repolarization manifestations of acute myocardial infarction may extend more widely and may, for example, be present in leads V2–V5.

OTHER FORMS OF ELECTROCARDIOGRAPHIC PRESENTATION

Qr OF QR COMPLEXES IN LEADS V3 AND V4

Lowseptal infarction may present with Qr or QR complexes (instead of QS complexes) in leads V3 and V4 (Electrocardiographic Study 23). This suggests a shift of the transition zone to the right with some epicardial sparing.

LACK OF THE NORMAL INCREASING r WAVE PROGRESSION IN LEAD V3 AND V4

Lowseptal infarction may present with an absence of the normal increasing *r* wave progression in leads V3 and V4 (Electrocardiographic Study 41). This is discussed more fully in the section on anteroseptal infarction (see above).

DISPROPORTIONATE INITIAL q WAVE MAGNITUDE IN LEAD V4

Lowseptal infarction is, for example, also suggested when there is a loss or a failure of the initial *q* wave to increase in depth from leads V3–V6. The initial *q* wave of the qR complex recorded by the left precordial leads normally increases in depth from leads V4 (or lead V3)–lead V6. Failure to do so may indicate the presence of a lowseptal infarction with possible paraseptal involvement. Such failure may manifest as follows:

(a) The initial *q* wave is of abnormal magnitude, and is deeper in leads V3 and/or V4 than in lead V6 (Electrocardiographic Studies 38, 40 and 46).

(b) The initial *q* wave is of normal magnitude, and diminishes progressively from lead V3–V6 (Electrocardiographic Study 13 and 23).

(c) The initial *q* wave is present in leads V3 and V4, and absent in lead V6.

Note that the initial *q* wave referred to above need not be pathological in the sense that it need not be abnormally deep or wide. It is only comparatively out of proportion.

The presence of a prominent Q wave, a Q wave exceeding 3 mm in depth, in the mid-precordial leads, is a pointer to the presence of infarction (Electrocardiographic Studies 38 and 46). If the Q wave is due to infarction, then the amplitude of the ensuing *R* wave will usually be low or relatively low.

qrS COMPLEX IN LEADS V3 AND V4

Mid or lowseptal infarction is suggested when there is a small initial *q* wave, 0·01–0·02 sec in duration, preceding the RS complex of the mid-precordial leads, for example, lead V2 of Electrocardiographic Study 23.

ANTEROLATERAL MYOCARDIAL INFARCTION

Anterolateral myocardial infarction is, in effect, a combination of apical and high-lateral infarction (Fig. 30; see below). The infarction pattern is present in leads V5 and V6, Standard lead I and lead AVL (Electrocardiographic Study 41). The infarction results in the loss of the major vectors of left free wall depolarization (vectors 3a and 4a of Fig. 11). It manifests with pathological Q waves, of QR or Qr complexes, in leads V5 and V6, Standard lead I and lead AVL (see also discussion below on apical and high lateral infarction.

Note that infarction confined to the anterolateral wall does not manifest with QS complexes. QS complexes do not usually manifest in leads V5 and V6 without QS complexes in the right precordial leads as well. When QS complexes do appear in leads V5 and V6, an uncommon occurrence, the manifestation is part of an extensive anterior wall myocardial infarction which will be reflected in all the anteriorly orientated leads. Even anterolateral infarction manifesting with Qr or QR complexes in leads V5 and V6 is rare without involvement of the other precordial leads as well. In other words, it is nearly always part of an extensive anterior infarction. It may also be the expression of an apical extension of an inferior infarction (Electrocardiographic Studies 26 and 28).

The presence of some degree of anterolateral infarction may also be *suspected* even in the absence of pathological Q

waves if the *R* waves of the qR complexes in the left precordial leads tend to be of low amplitude or fail to reflect the normal progression, i.e. fail to become progressively taller from leads V3–V6 (Electrocardiographic Studies 17, 19–25). Other electrocardiographic and clinical confirmation of the infarction must, however, be obtained under these circumstances.

The modification of anterolateral infarction by left anterior and left posterior hemiblock is discussed in Chapter 12.

APICAL INFARCTION

Apical infarction is, in effect, a subdivision of anterolateral myocardial infarction. The diagnosis is based principally on the presence of the infarction pattern in leads V5 and V6 (Diagram F of Fig. 30), since it is these leads which are predominantly orientated to the apex of the heart (Fig. 10). This, however, is an oversimplified approach, since the apex of the heart is a cone shaped structure pointing downward and to the left, and orientated inferiorly and laterally as well as anteriorly. It consequently has surface facing:

(a) laterally–to Standard lead I.
(b) inferiorly–to Standard lead II.
(c) anteriorly–to leads V5 and V6.

Apical infarction may thus be reflected by the infarction pattern in many of these leads (Electrocardiographic Studies 24 and 28). However, the anterior orientation as reflected in Standard lead I and leads V5 and V6 is more common, and apical infarction is not often reflected in Standard lead II, unless the apical infarction occurs as an extension of inferior infarction (Electrocardiographic Study 28). This distributional infarction pattern is due to the loss of the third vector or normal ventricular depolarization (vector 3a of Fig. 11), the principal vector of the left free wall.

ELECTROCARDIOGRAPHIC MANIFESTATIONS

Apical infarction may have the following forms of electrocardiographic presentation:

1. Leads V5 and V6, and possibly Standard leads I and II, reflect QR or Qr complexes. QS complexes are uncommon since adjacent healthy or relatively healthy subepicardial tissue will result in the inscription of late *R* waves, the result of focal peri-infarction block.

2. All of the three Standard leads may reflect *q* or Q waves since the initial 0·04 sec QRS vector, the Q wave vector, is directed superiorly and to the right, i.e. away from the apex.

3. Leads V5 and V6 reflect coved and elevated S-T seg-

ments. The elevation is, however, not as marked as that which occurs in the mid-precordial leads in the case of anteroseptal infarction. Slight coving and elevation of the S–T segment may also be present in Standard lead I, and possibly in Standard lead II.

4. The T waves are inverted and symmetrical in leads V5 and V6, and Standard leads I and II reflect inverted and symmetrical T waves. Since the T wave vector is directed to the right it may be upright in the right precordial leads (Electrocardiographic Studies 24 and 28).

HIGH-LATERAL MYOCARDIAL INFARCTION

High-lateral infarction is, in effect, a subdivision of antero-lateral myocardial infarction, and refers to infarction of the proximal, 'high', or superior region of the left lateral wall (Fig. 10 and Diagram G of Fig. 30). This region is princi-pally orientated to Standard lead I and lead AVL which will reflect the infarction pattern; pathological Q wave, a QR complex, elevated and coved S–T segment and inverted T wave (Electrocardiographic Study 43). This distributional pattern is due to the loss of the fourth vector of normal ventricular depolarization (Vector 4a of Fig. 11). When high-lateral infarction occurs as an isolated or localized phenomenon, it does not present with QS com-plexes. The pathological Q wave is always associated with an ensuing R wave which is not much diminished in amplitude. When QS complexes do appear in Standard lead I and lead AVL, it is always part of a more extensive anterior infarction.

VARIATIONS AND COMPLICATIONS

APICAL EXTENSION

Distal extension to the apex is common. This will be re-flected by the infarction pattern in leads V5 and V6, as well as in Standard lead I and lead AVL, thereby constitut-ing an anterolateral infarction (Electrocardiographic Study 41).

EXTENSION TO THE ANTEROSEPTAL REGION WITHOUT INVOLVEMENT OF THE APICAL REGION—A SEPTOLATERAL INFARCTION (see below)

This is a not infrequent combination. The infarction pattern is then seen in Standard lead I, lead AVL and lead V1–V3 or V4 (Electrocardiographic Studies 20, 22 and 43).

LEFT ANTERIOR HEMIBLOCK

High-lateral infarction is frequently complicated by left anterior hemiblock, thereby resulting in anterolateral peri-infarction block (see below, and Chapter 12).

DIFFERENTIAL DIAGNOSIS OF HIGH-LATERAL INFARCTION

High-lateral myocardial infarction may be simulated by, and must therefore be differentiated electrocardiographic-ally from, (1) uncomplicated left anterior hemiblock, and (2) the Wolff–Parkinson–White syndrome.

UNCOMPLICATED LEFT ANTERIOR HEMIBLOCK

Uncomplicated left anterior hemiblock is characterized by an initial 0·04 sec QRS vector which is directed down-wards, to the right, in the region of +120° on the frontal plane hexaxial reference system. This will result in a promi-nent Q wave in lead AVL which may consequently simu-late high-lateral myocardial infarction (Electrocardio-graphic Study 60A). The differential diagnosis is based on (a) the absence of the classical electrocardiographic features of acute infarction, elevated and coved S–T segments and inverted T waves, and (b) the presence of marked left axis deviation in the frontal plane leads. Thus, the diagnosis of high-lateral myocardial infarction must not be based on the presence of a QR complex in lead AVL alone. There must be, at the very least, evidence of elevated and coved S–T segments and inverted T waves in this lead, and preferably a similar pattern in the adjacent lead, Standard lead I.

The mechanism of this manifestation is analogous to the appearance of a QR complex which occurs in Standard lead III in left posterior hemiblock (see Chapter 12).

THE WOLFF–PARKINSON–WHITE SYNDROME

High-lateral infarction may be simulated by the Wolff–Parkinson–White syndrome when the delta wave is directed at +120° on the frontal plane hexaxial reference system. The delta wave will, under these circumstances, be negative in Standard lead I and lead AVL, and this may simulate the pathological Q waves of high-lateral myo-cardial infarction (Electrocardiographic Study 70; see also Chapter 11). The diagnosis is established by (a) the recog-nition of delta waves as such and the presence of shortened P–R intervals in the other leads, and (b) the absence of the classical coved S–T segments and inverted T waves of myo-cardial injury and ischaemia.

SEPTOLATERAL MYOCARDIAL INFARCTION

A not infrequent presentation or distribution of the myocardial infarction is an anteroseptal infarction in association with a high-lateral infarction. The infarction pattern appears in leads V1–V4, Standard lead I and lead AVL (Electrocardiographic Studies 5, 20, 22 and 43). The apical region is largely spared.

CORRELATIVE ESSAY

THE CAUSES OF PROMINENT Q WAVES OR QS COMPLEXES IN THE LEFT PRECORDIAL LEADS

Prominent, though not necessarily pathological Q waves may appear in the left lateral leads, leads V5 and V6, Standard lead I and lead AVL, in the following conditions:

1. Anterolateral myocardial infarction.
2. Apical fibrosis.
3. Aortic incompetence. ⎫ Expressions of left
4. Ventricular septal defect. ⎬ ventricular diastolic
5. Patent ductus arteriosis. ⎭ overload.
6. Vagotonia.
7. The Duchenne-type of muscular dystrophy.
8. Subaortic stenosis.

ANTEROLATERAL MYOCARDIAL INFARCTION

A prominent Q wave, or, less commonly, a QS complex may appear in the left lateral leads in anterolateral myocardial infarction. When a prominent Q wave in the left lateral leads is due to myocardial infarction, it is always associated with a diminution in the amplitude of the ensuing R wave. This will, in the case of the acute phase of acute myocardial infarction, be associated with the parameters of acute injury and ischaemia, and, in the case of old myocardial infarction, with possible evidence of chronic insufficiency.

APICAL FIBROSIS

Long-standing apical fibrosis resulting, for example, from a cardiomyopathy, may result in prominent Q waves in the left lateral leads, and also in Standard leads I, II and III. There may also be a substantial diminution in the amplitude of the ensuing R wave. The abnormal S-T segment and T wave manifestations of myocardial injury and ischaemia are absent.

AORTIC INCOMPETENCE

A deep, narrow, prominent Q wave may also appear in the left precordial leads in aortic incompetence. This Q wave rarely exceeds 0·04 sec. in duration and is, likewise, associated with a tall ensuing R wave. The T waves are tall and upright. The S-T segment is isoelectric or slightly elevated.

VENTRICULAR SEPTAL DEFECT

A deep, prominent, but relatively narrow Q wave may appear in the left precordial leads, leads V5 and V6, in cases of ventricular septal defect (Electrocardiographic Study 109). This Q wave is not, however, longer than 0·04 sec in duration. It is always associated with a tall, usually very tall ensuing R wave. In other words, the Q wave does not constitute 25 per cent or more of the ensuing R wave. There will be other features of ventricular septal defect such as the Katz-Wachtel phenomenon, viz. tall equiphasic complexes in the mid-precordial leads. Furthermore, the S-T segments and T waves in the left precordial leads do not reflect the features of acute myocardial infarction nor those of coronary insufficiency. The S-T segment is isoelectric or minimally elevated. The T wave is usually tall and upright. Although the chronic stabilized phase of anterolateral myocardial infarction could also manifest with such prominent Q waves in leads V5 and V6, the ensuing R waves would be markedly diminished in amplitude.

PATENT DUCTUS ARTERIOSIS

Patent ductus arteriosis is also associated with the electrocardiographic manifestations of left ventricular diastolic overload. The left lateral precordial leads, leads V5 and V6, reflect rather deep, prominent, but narrow Q waves, which are associated with relatively tall ensuing R waves. The S-T segments are minimally elevated and concave-upwards. The associated T waves are rather tall and symmetrical.

VAGOTONIA

Increased vagotonia, as would occur for example in an athlete, is characterized by the following manifestations in the left lateral leads (Electrocardiographic Studies 100 and 101):

(a) Prominent q waves. The q wave may reach a depth of 3 mm or more, but is narrow.
(b) Rather tall ensuing R waves.
(c) Rather tall and symmetrical T waves.
(d) Slightly elevated and concave-upward S-T segments.
(e) Sinus bradycardia is usual.

Similar electrocardiographic manifestations may appear in the inferiorly orientated leads, Standard leads II and III, and lead AVF (Electrocardiographic Study 100).

THE DUCHENNE TYPE OF MUSCULAR DYSTROPHY

This condition is associated with a relatively characteristic electrocardiographic presentation[P16, S67, W22, Z2]. The right precordial leads reflect tall R waves not unlike that of true posterior infarction or right ventricular dominance. The left lateral precordial leads, as well as the Standard leads, reflect deep prominent, although not necessarily pathological Q waves (Electrocardiographic Study 108). The presentation has been reviewed by Perloff and associates (1967)[P16].

HYPERTROPHIC SUB-AORTIC STENOSIS

Prominent, deep, usually narrow, abnormal Q waves in the left lateral leads is a frequent finding in muscular sub-aortic stenosis[B34, B73, B74, E14, G25, H32, N8, P6, P27, T5, W40, W68]. Similar Q waves may also appear in the inferior orientated leads, Standard leads II and III and lead AVF. This may be associated with tall or relatively tall R waves in the right precordial leads.

Chapter 7

Posterior Wall Myocardial Infarction

The posterior wall of the heart is the posterobasal or dorsal aspect of the left ventricle, and is that part of the left free wall situated between the lateral (superior) and the inferior walls, towards the base of the left ventricular cone (Fig. 10). It is sometimes termed the *true* posterior wall because the inferior wall of the heart was, in old terminology, called the posterior wall. Posterior wall infarction has also been termed *strictly posterior*, *direct posterior*, *posterobasal* and *dorsal* myocardial infarction.

Infarction of the posterior wall is relatively uncommon, and manifests in the conventional electrocardiogram with distinctive features which are manifestly different from the usual presentation of myocardial infarction. The common, classic, electrocardiographic features of acute myocardial infarction—deep, broad *Q* waves, raised and coved S-T segments, and inverted *T* waves—which manifest in leads orientated toward the infarcted area, do not appear in the conventional electrocardiographic leads in true posterior infarction. This is because none of the conventional leads are orientated towards the true posterior surface of the heart (Fig. 10). The diagnosis of true posterior infarction must therefore be made from the *inverse* or *mirror-image* changes in leads which are orientated towards the *un-injured* anterior surface of the heart, viz. the precordial leads, leads V1–V3.

ELECTROCARDIOGRAPHIC MANIFESTATIONS OF TRUE POSTERIOR WALL MYOCARDIAL INFARCTION

Acute Posterior Wall Myocardial Infarction

Acute posterior wall myocardial infarction manifests with the following electrocardiographic features[D38, G36, L47, P15, P33, S38, S112, S114, T15]:

1. Tall and slightly widened *R* waves in the right precordial leads[D38, T15].

2. Tall, upright and symmetrical *T* waves in leads V1–V3.

3. Depressed, concave-upward S-T segments in leads V1 and V2.

These manifestations are reflected in Electrocardiographic Studies 27, 28, 29, 31, 32, 33, 45, 53 and 71, and their genesis is considered below.

TALL AND SLIGHTLY WIDENED R WAVES IN THE RIGHT PRECORDIAL LEADS—LEADS V1–V3

The Mechanism. The posterobasal region of the heart is among the last regions of the heart to be activated, and is equivalent to the basal and sagittal location of vectors 4a and 5a of ventricular depolarization (Fig. 11). Posterior wall myocardial infarction results in a loss of these late posterior wall vectors, and this allows the anterior forces to become dominant since they are then no longer opposed and cancelled by the posterior wall forces. The unopposed anterior wall forces are generated from the free wall of the right ventricle, and possibly the right superior region of the interventricular septum. In simplified representation, depolarization of the normal heart begins in the left side of the interventricular septum and spreads from left to right, i.e. anteriorly, through the septum (Vector 1, Diagram A of Fig. 31). This is followed by more or less simultaneous activation from endocardial to epicardial surfaces of the free walls of the right (anterior) and left (posterior) ventricles (Vector 2, Diagram A of Fig. 31). However, since the left or posterior wall has a larger muscle mass and hence a larger potential electrical force, its activation force will counteract the smaller force of the right (anterior) ventricle which is opposite in direction. The depolarization process is reflected in leads V1 and V2 by a small *r* wave, caused by the septal force moving toward the electrode, followed by a deep *S* wave resulting from the left or posterior wall force being directed away from the electrode

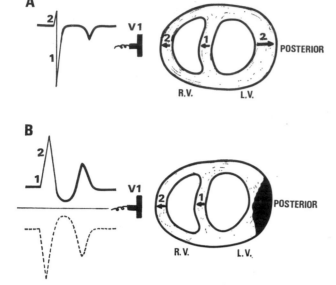

FIG. 31. Diagrams illustrating: A, normal ventricular depolarization, and its effect on lead V1; and B, ventricular depolarization in true posterior wall myocardial infarction, and its effect on lead V1.

(Fig. 31). When the posterior wall is infarcted, the left or posterior wall force is lost (Diagram B of Fig. 31). Thus, activation of the interventricular septum (Vector 1 in Diagram B of Fig. 31) is, in simplified exposition, followed by activation of the free or anterior wall of the right ventricle, and possibly late activation of the right superior region of the interventricular septum (Vector 5a of Fig. 11). Both QRS forces are now orientated towards leads V1, V2 and V3, resulting in tall and widened R waves and diminution of the S waves. This may also be expressed as an increase of the R/S ratio in these leads to greater than 1, the normal being appreciably less than 1.

An annular subvalvular aneurysm of the ventricle may, by pressure on the right coronary artery, give rise to an electrocardiographic presentation of posterior wall myocardial infarction[C24] (Electrocardiographic Study 107).

Levy and associates (1950)[L47] reported 12 cases of myocardial infarction manifesting, *inter alia*, with tall or relatively tall R waves in lead V1. In all these cases the infarct was situated within a relatively small circumscribed area in the free wall of the left ventricle, being dominantly posterior in three cases, posterolateral in eight cases and anterolateral in one case.

There are, however, other conditions which give rise to tall R waves in leads V1–V3, and these must be excluded before the diagnosis of true posterior wall myocardial infarction can be established. The differential diagnosis is considered on p. 71.

TALL AND SYMMETRICAL T WAVES IN LEADS V1–V3

The T wave vector is always directed away from the ischaemic surface of the infarcted area. Thus, in true posterior infarction the T wave is directed anteriorly, away from the posterior surface, resulting in tall symmetrical T waves in leads V1–V3.

The differential diagnosis of tall precordial T waves discussed in Chapter 3.

DEPRESSION OF THE S-T SEGMENT IN LEADS V1–V3

The S-T segment vector is directed toward the injured surface of an infarcted area. Leads orientated to the uninjured surface consequently reflect elevated and coved S-T segments. Thus, in the case of true posterior infarction, the S-T segment vector will be directed towards the posterior surface and away from the conventional leads orientated towards the anterior surface of the heart. This results in *depressed* and *concave-upward* S-T segments in leads V1, V2 and V3 (Electrocardiographic Study 29). The S-T segment depression is not usually marked and may, in fact, be absent, isoelectric, in many cases (Electrocardiographic Studies 27, 31, 32, 33 and 71). This is probably due to the neutralizing or boundary effect of the intervening blood (see Chapter 2).

The electrocardiographic triad of tall R wave, slightly depressed S-T segment and tall, symmetrical T wave in the right precordial leads which occurs in true posterior myocardial infarction is, in effect, the mirror-image of the typical electrocardiographic triad which would be recorded by a lead orientated towards the true posterior wall during the fully evolved phase. The tall R wave is the mirror-image of the pathological Q wave, the depressed S-T segment is the mirror-image of the elevated S-T segment, and the tall symmetrical T wave is the mirror-image of the deeply inverted T wave (dotted line in Diagram B of Fig. 31).

Other Electrocardiographic Manifestations Affecting the QRS Complex

SLURRING OF THE DESCENDING LIMB OF THE R WAVE IN LEAD V1

True posterior myocardial infarction may be associated with a notch in the descending limb of the R wave, giving it a minimimally slurred appearance[G36, P15]. This is due to an abrupt and temporary change in direction of the QRS loop.

DIMINUTION OF THE QRS AMPLITUDE IN THE LIMB LEADS

A reduction of the QRS amplitude to 5 mm or less in the limb leads has been reported in some cases of true posterior myocardial infarction[P15]. This is regarded as a further expression of the anterior shift of electrical forces in true posterior infarction, i.e. away from the frontal plane to the saggital plane.

THE ASSOCIATIONS OF POSTERIOR INFARCTION

EXTENSION OF THE INFARCTION

Posterior myocardial infarction rarely, if ever, occurs as an isolated phenomenon. There is nearly always extension to, and involvement of, the adjacent regions. The extension may involve all the parameters of infarction, necrosis, injury, and ischaemia, or the injury and/or ischaemia only.

The extension may occur:

(a) **inferiorly,** resulting in the association of inferior and posterior infarction[S38] (Electrocardiographic Studies 29, 31, 32 and 33), or

(b) **laterally,** with evidence of high-lateral infarction, or the condition may merely manifest with evidence of lateral ischaemia, low to inverted T waves in leads V5 and V6. (Electrocardiographic Studies 31, 32 and 33).

A-V BLOCK

A-V block of all degrees is a not infrequent complication of posterior wall myocardial infarction. This is because the posterior descending artery is the artery usually involved by the coronary thrombosis. It is a branch of this artery which supplies the A-V node in most cases.

Chronic – Old – Posterior Wall Myocardial Infarction: The Stabilized Phase

The QRS and T wave abnormalities of acute posterior wall myocardial infarction, once present, tend to remain permanently. Thus, acute as well as old posterior wall myocardial infarction are characterized by tall R waves and tall and widened T waves in the right precordial leads. It may consequently be difficult to estimate the age of the infarction solely on the basis of electrocardiographic criteria. Such diagnosis must be based on a correlation of both electrocardiographic and clinical parameters. A possible reason for this is a true loss of the normal, posteriorly directed T wave vector. The normal T wave vector is directed posteriorly and to the left. The reasons for this have already been considered in Chapter 2, p. 14. A true loss of this force, due to loss of viable tissue, would result in a permanent reorientation of the T wave force. With other locations of myocardial infarction the normal, dominantly posterior force would again become dominant with the regression of the infarction pattern.

CORRELATIVE ESSAY

DIFFERENTIAL DIAGNOSIS OF TALL R WAVES IN LEADS V1–V3

Tall R waves in the right precordial leads may be associated with the following conditions:

1 Right ventricular dominance.
2 Certain forms of right bundle branch block.
3 The Type A Wolff-Parkinson-White syndrome.
4 The Duchenne type of muscular dystrophy.
5 Mirror-image dextrocardia.
6 Posterior wall myocardial infarction.
7 Normal variant.

RIGHT VENTRICULAR DOMINANCE

Right ventricular dominance is usually associated with right axis deviation and the P pulmonale of right atrial enlargement. Tall R waves appear in the right precordial leads, leads V1–V3. The associated T waves are usually low to inverted. This is in sharp contrast to the tall and symmetrical T waves which appear in these leads in cases of posterior infarction. There will also be a clinical cause for the right ventricular dominance.

RIGHT BUNDLE BRANCH BLOCK

The initial QRS forces are not altered significantly by the advent of the bundle branch block. This is particularly so in the extremity leads where the initial vectors are virtually or absolutely the same during normal intraventricular conduction as during right bundle branch block conduction. The initial vectors in leads V1 and V2 may, however, be more affected, becoming taller and broader. This has been attributed to the proximity of these precordial electrodes.

The free wall of the right ventricle generates vectors of relatively small magnitude. In right bundle branch block, depolarization of the blocked area begins in the free right wall in close proximity to leads V1 and V2. These forces are directed anteriorly and reflected by the proximity leads V1 and V2, but are too small to be reflected in the more distal leads[G31].

The manifestation of tall and broad R waves in some cases of right bundle branch block means that strictly posteriorly infarction cannot be diagnosed with confidence in the presence of right bundle branch block. Indeed, posterior infarction is the only localization of infarction that cannot be diagnosed with confidence in the presence of right bundle branch block (see Chapter 9). When uncomplicated right bundle branch block manifests with relatively tall initial R waves in the right precordial leads, leads V1–V3, the associated T waves are usually inverted. These manifestations reflect secondary changes to the abnormal intraventricular conduction (see Chapter 9, p. 80). In true posterior myocardial infarction, however, the associated T waves in the right precordial leads are tall and symmetrical. Thus, true posterior infarction may even be suspected in the presence of right bundle branch block if the associated T waves in the right precordial leads tend to be upright and symmetrical (Electrocardiographic Study 53).

THE TYPE A WOLFF-PARKINSON-WHITE SYNDROME

The Type A Wolff-Parkinson-White syndrome is associated with tall R waves in right precordial leads; the manifestation of an anteriorly directed QRS vector (Electrocardiographic Studies 70 and 71). The diagnosis is established by the presence of the typical delta waves and shortened P-R intervals in the right precordial as well as other leads. See also Chapter 11.

THE DUCHENNE TYPE OF MUSCULAR DYSTROPHY

This condition is associated with a relatively characteristic electrocardiographic presentation[P16, S67, W22, Z2]. The right precordial leads reflect tall R waves, not unlike that of true posterior infarction or right ventricular dominance, and the left lateral precordial leads as well as the Standard leads reflect deep, prominent, although not necessarily pathological Q waves (Electrocardiographic Study 108). The presentation has been reviewed by Perloff and associates[P16].

MIRROR-IMAGE DEXTROCARDIA

In mirror-image dextrocardia the R waves will be tall or relatively tall in the right precordial leads. There will also be a progressive diminution in R wave amplitude from lead V1–V6. The characteristic rightward QRS and P wave axes in the frontal plane will reveal the correct diagnosis.

POSTERIOR WALL MYOCARDIAL INFARCTION

This is discussed in detail in this chapter.

NORMAL VARIANT

A rather tall R wave may appear in lead V1 as a normal variant. This is usually associated with an ensuing s or S wave, the resulting Rs ratio being slightly or moderately greater than 1. The associated S-T segment and T wave are normal. When this manifestation appears, electrode placement should be checked.

An *annular subvalvular mitral aneurysm* may also present with tall R waves in the right precordial leads[C24] (Electrocardiographic Study 107). The mechanism, however, is probably pressure upon, and obstruction of, the right coronary artery by the aneurysm.

Chapter 8

Subendocardial Infarction

The accurate diagnosis of pure or dominant subendo-cardial infarction is not as precise nor as clear-cut as that of transmural infarction, or that of dominantly subepicardial infarction and several aspects are controversial. Diagnostic electrocardiographic criteria are not firmly established and are based mainly on S-T segment and T wave changes[C43, L41, L43, P34, Y8]. Such changes may, for example, be simulated by those of transient subendocardial injury and ischaemia of acute coronary insufficiency, as occurs with angina pectoris. The manifestations are at times paradoxical and unpredictable. For example, marked T wave inversion in the precordial leads may occur in a subendocardial in-farction, whereas such T wave inversion would theoretic-ally only be expected from the fully evolved phase of dominantly subepicardial infarction, since the T wave vector is directed away from the surface of ischaemia. The difficulty of establishing a confident diagnosis of myo-cardial infarction on the basis of S-T segment and T wave changes only, and in the absence of QRS change is well recognized[F2, L38, W53]. Furthermore, Cook and associates (1958)[C42] reported six large *non*-transmural infarcts which extended from one-half–three-quarters of the distance from the endocardium to the epicardium, and which were associated with the QRS, S-T segment and T wave changes commonly seen with transmural infarction.

The following aspects of myocardial physiology and electropathology contribute to this difficulty in electro-cardiographic diagnosis:

THE HYPOTHETICAL 'SILENT' SUBENDO-CARDIAL RIND

It has been postulated that a narrow subendocardial rind of tissue *may* be electrocardiographically 'silent' because of (a) rapid instantaneous activation within the subendocardial rind, or (b) the formation and merging of multiple excita-tion fronts resulting in both local and remote cancellation with a resultant zero or near-zero residual[K18, M28, S108]. Activation of and within the rind may consequently not be

reflected electrocardiographically by the QRS complex (Diagram B of Fig. 3). This is considered in greater detail in Chapter 2. *Theoretically*, therefore, an infarct which occurs within or is confined to this hypothetical electro-cardiographically 'silent' region may not present with manifest or marked QRS changes (Diagram B of Fig. 3). It has been observed, for example, that only minor QRS changes result from extensive mechanically induced sub-endocardial trauma (Pruitt and associates, 1945)[P32]. Cook and associates (1958)[C42], in a study of acute subendocardial infarction, showed that the necrosis must involve more than the inner half of the left free wall before significant QRS changes of infarction appear. The electrocardio-graphic diagnosis of such infarction may consequently have to be based on the manifestations of injury and ischaemia only, viz. S-T segment and T wave changes. Since S-T segment and T wave changes of myocardial injury and ischaemia can occur with acute coronary in-sufficiency which is not necessarily associated with in-farction, the diagnosis must of necessity be based on a correlation of clinical, biochemical (enzyme) and electro-cardiographic parameters.

It must, however, be emphasized that the question of the very existence of the so-called 'silent' region has been strongly challenged (see Chapter 2). Studies of ventricular activation by Durrer and associates (1964)[D51] and (1965)[D43] demonstrated that Q waves were recorded by leads orien-tated to the epicardium of dogs with subendocardial in-farction. The magnitude, width and depth, of the Q waves varied with the size and extent of the subendocardial infarct, the larger the infarct, the wider and deeper the pathological Q wave. They consequently concluded that subendocardial infarction was not 'silent' and could be reflected by epicardial orientated leads.

Boineau and associates (1968)[B67] arrived at similar con-clusions from body surface mapping in humans, viz. that (a) subendocardial and non-transmural infarction could produce diagnostic Q waves on the body surface, (b) the subendocardium is not uniquely 'silent', and the presentation of the infarct on the body surface is related to the volume of the infarcted tissue, and (c) that mid and terminal force charges are related to disturbances of intramural conduction within tissue overlying the subendocardial infarct.

Furthermore, the monophasic record obtained by the pressure of an intracardiac electrode on the subendocardium constitutes further corroborative evidence of the normal electrical reaction of the subendocardium[K40].

THE BOUNDARY INTERFACE EFFECT

As a result of the relatively low resistance, high conductivity, of blood (see Chapter 2), the electrical currents generated on the interface of the blood and myocardium tend to be short circuited. Consequently, the S-T segment deviations towards the endocardial surface in the case of subendocardial infarction will not be as marked as in the case of S-T segment deviation towards the epicardial surface in the case of subepicardial infarction.

THE DIFFERENT DEVIATIONS AND MAGNITUDES OF SUBENDOCARDIAL AND SUBEPICARDIAL INJURY

It has been shown experimentally in dogs that subendocardial injury manifests with a significantly shorter duration of electrocardiographic effect than a similar injury to the epicardium[B43, P32]. Moreover, injury to the subepicardium produces a greater electrocardiographic injury effect than an equivalent injury to the subendocardium.

THE ELECTROCARDIOGRAPHIC DIAGNOSIS OF SUBENDOCARDIAL INFARCTION

In the clinical context, there appears to be two distinct electrocardiographic syndromes of acute subendocardial infarction:

1. The electrocardiographic syndrome of **hyperacute subendocardial injury.**
2. The electrocardiographic syndrome of **subendocardial necrosis.**

The Syndrome of Hyperacute Subendocardial Injury

This electrocardiographic syndrome of subendocardial infarction presents with dominant S-T segment and *T* wave changes. There are no significant changes of the QRS complex. The syndrome is, in effect, the mirror-image of the electrocardiographic manifestation of the hyperacute

early injury phase of transmural or dominantly subepicardial infarction.

The syndrome is not, at present, a definitive or pure electrocardiographic diagnosis, but rather a clinical-electrocardiographic correlation. The diagnosis may be entertained when (a) the clinical presentation and biochemical presentation (enzyme studies) justify such a diagnosis, and (b) the electrocardiographic presentation reflects the S-T segment and *T* wave parameters of hyperacute subendocardial injury and ischaemia which tend to last for a relatively long time, longer than would be expected with acute coronary insufficiency, angina pectoris.

THE S-T SEGMENT MANIFESTATION

The hyperacute injury syndrome of acute subendocardial infarction affects both the direction and the shape of the S-T segment (Electrocardiographic Studies 16, 73, 74, 75 and 76).

THE DIRECTION OF THE S-T SEGMENT

The hyperacute injury syndrome of acute subendocardial infarction affects predominantly the anterolateral aspect of the left free wall. Since the S-T segment vector deviates towards the surface of the injury, it will be directed away from the epicardial apex of the heart, i.e. to the *right, anteriorly* and somewhat *superiorly*, at about −150° on the frontal plane hexaxial reference system (Diagrams A and B of Fig. 32). The S-T segment will therefore be:

(a) *depressed in the left lateral precordial leads, leads V4–V6, and Standard leads I and II, and possibly in lead AVL,* (b) elevated in the right precordial leads and particularly lead

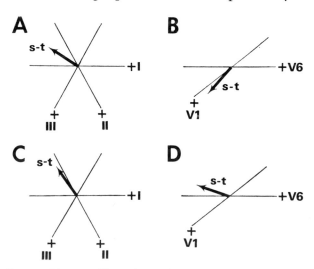

FIG. 32. Diagrams illustrating various S-T segment vectors in subendocardial infarction. See text.

AVR, and (c) equiphasic or isoelectric in Standard lead III (Electrocardiographic Study 76).

When the subendocardial infarction is very extensive, it may result in an S-T segment vector that is directed even more superiorly and to the right in the region of −120° on the frontal plane hexaxial reference system (Diagrams C and D of Fig. 32). The horizontal plane S-T segment axis may, under this circumstance, have a slight posterior deviation (Diagram D of Fig. 32). The S-T segment will then only be elevated in lead V1 and lead AVR, and depressed in leads V2–V6, Standard leads I, II and III, and lead AVF; it will be equiphasic, isoelectric, in lead AVL (Electrocardiographic Study 75). Minor variations in these vectorial directions may occur (Electrocardiographic Studies 73 and 74).

Theoretically, subendocardial infarction of the posterior, left free wall should cause a deviation of the S-T segment vector towards the subendocardial surface of the posterior wall. In other words, there should be an anterior deviation of the S-T segment vector, and this should be reflected by elevated S-T segments in the precordial leads. Although this has been produced experimentally[P35], it is doubtful whether this occurs clinically. This could conceivably be due to (a) a neutralizing anterior wall subendocardial injury, (b) the relatively long distance of the posterior wall from the precordial electrodes, and (c) the modification resulting from boundary conditions[P35] (see above). In this respect it is of interest to compare the minimal S-T segment deviation in the precordial leads which is associated with true posterior infarction (see Chapter 7).

THE SHAPE OF THE S-T SEGMENT

The S-T segment of the hyperacute injury syndrome of acute subendocardial infarction tends to manifest with *slope-depression*; a straight downward slope, or a downward slope that is minimally convex-upward (Electrocardiographic Studies 73–75). It merges smoothly and imperceptibly with the proximal limb of the widened and deepened *T* wave (see below).

THE T WAVE MANIFESTATION

The S-T segment deviation is always associated with some abnormality of the *T* wave. The *T* wave vector is usually directed posteriorly, superiorly and to the right. This is reflected by inversion of the *T* waves in all the conventional leads with the exception of lead AVR and possibly lead AVL, where it may be positive (Electrocardiographic Studies 73 and 75). The inverted *T* waves are, in addition, *increased in magnitude*, i.e. they are very deep. They also tend to be symmetrical and widened, particularly in the mid-precordial leads (Electrocardiographic Studies 73 and 75).

It is apparent that the aforementioned S-T segment and *T* wave changes are, in effect, the mirror-image of those associated with the hyperacute early injury phase of transmural or dominantly subepicardial infarction (see Chapter 4), or the mirror-image of the electrocardiographic manifestations of the variant form of angina pectoris (see Chapter 15). There is little or no alteration of the QRS complex.

The subsequent evolution is a gradual return to normal, usually within several days. The equivalent mirror-image presentation of the fully evolved phase of acute transmural or dominantly subepicardial infarction does not usually occur, although this may occasionally appear to be the case (Electrocardiographic Study 76).

At times, this syndrome of acute subendocardial infarction presents with what appears to be *T* wave changes only, the most striking feature being deeply inverted, symmetrical, sharply pointed and arrow-head *T* waves which are most marked in the mid-precordial leads and Standard lead II. In some of these cases the preceding S-T segment may be minimally depressed, but is frequently normal. Papp and Smith (1951)[P5] described this presentation as 'slight coronary attack' since the clinical and electrocardiographic abnormalities usually disappeared within a short time. Pruitt and associates (1955)[P34] noted similar electrocardiographic presentation with coronary artery disease, constrictive pericarditis, and in valvular heart disease. The pattern may also herald the development of a more extensive transmural infarction (Kossman 1956)[K37].

DIFFERENTIAL DIAGNOSIS

The differential diagnosis of depressed S-T segments in the precordial leads is discussed in a Correlative Essay in Chapter 3, p. 34.

The possible mechanism of these S-T segment and *T* wave changes is discussed in Chapter 2.

The Syndrome of Subendocardial Necrosis

Subendocardial infarction may result in necrosis of myocardial tissue. This manifests with pathological Q waves, the expression of the necrosis, and ensuing r or R waves, the expression of the overlying healthy or relatively healthy tissue. (Diagram C of Fig. 3. Compare also Diagrams C and D of Fig. 22). Since the amount of thickness of overlying healthy tissue must *ipso facto* be diminished, the height of the ensuing R wave is also diminished, the height of the ensuing R wave is also diminished.

This form of subendocardial infarction frequently occurs

as a lateral subendocardial extension of a transmural infarction. The transmural infarction is reflected by QS complexes, and the subendocardial extension by Qr or QR complexes in adjacent leads (see Electrocardiographic Studies 17, 18, 28, 31 and 32).

The Sites of Subendocardial Necrosis

Subendocardial infarction manifesting with subendocardial necrosis may occur in two specific locations:

1. the subendocardium of the left side of the interventricular septum, the physiological subendocardium of the interventricular septum (see Chapter 2). This is anterior wall subendocardial infarction; and

2. the subendocardium of the free wall of the left ventricle.

SUBENDOCARDIAL INFARCTION OF THE LEFT SIDE OF THE INTERVENTRICULAR SEPTUM: ANTERIOR WALL SUBENDOCARDIAL INFARCTION

Subendocardial infarction involving the left side of the interventricular septum may manifest with QS complexes typical of transmural infarction, despite the fact that the infarction is not transmural and only involves the left side of the interventricular septum. This is because of the bilateral endocardial to centre-septal form of septal depolarization as compared with the single endocardial-to-epicardial form of left free wall depolarization. Activation begins within the subendocardial regions of both sides of the interventricular septum, each activation front being directed medially, i.e. towards each other (Fig. 33). The activation front from the left side of the interventricular septum dominates that arising from the right side, and the resultant initial QRS vector is thus directed anteriorly and from left to right (Vector 1 in Diagram A of Fig. 33). This is reflected by a small initial r wave in leads V1 and V2. Thus, the r wave of the rS complex normally recorded by the leads orientated to the anterior wall of the interventricular septum reflects dominant activation of the left side of the septum, the electrophysiological subendocardial surface. Infarction confined to this left or posterior subendocardial region of the interventricular septum (the anterior wall of the left ventricle) would thus result in the disappearance of the small initial r wave of the rS complex. This complex is consequently changed into a QS complex (Diagram B of Fig. 33). It is abundantly clear, however, that this *does not necessarily* reflect transmural infarction. Infarction of the interventricular septum may indeed be transmural when QS complexes manifest in the right precordial leads, but this phenomenon could equally well

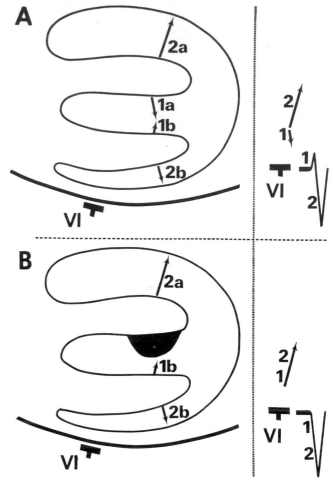

FIG. 33. Diagrams illustrating the effect of subendocardial infarction involving the left side of the interventricular septum on the precordial electrocardiogram. See text.

be the expression of a subendocardial infarct confined to the left side of the septum, the true subendocardial region.

Notched or slurred QS complexes resembling those associated with transmural infarction were found in cases where the infarct was localized to the subendocardial one-half of the myocardium[M92].

Thus, while a QS complex in the *left lateral* precordial leads usually represents a transmural infarction, a QS complex in the right precordial leads does not necessarily do so. A QS complex in leads V1–V3 may reflect transmural anteroseptal infarction, but could also represent subendocardial infarction of the left side of the interventricular septum.

It is important also to appreciate that in an electrocardiographic sense the left subendocardial surface of the interventricular septum acts physiologically as the true subendocardial surface of the left ventricles, whereas the right subendocardial surface behaves electrophysiologically as the subepicardial surface (for further discussion of this aspect see Chapter 2). It is interesting to note that QS complexes in the left lateral leads (leads V5 and V6, Standard lead I and lead AVL), are not very common with infarction of the left free wall, the apex, the high-lateral or superior regions of the left ventricle. These leads will in most cases reflect QR or Qr complexes (Electrocardiographic Studies 17, 18, 28, 31, and 32). In other words, most infarctions of the free wall of the left ventricle tend to be associated with some epicardial sparing.

SUBENDOCARDIAL INFARCTION OF THE LEFT FREE WALL

There is little doubt that pathological Q waves can and do occur with subendocardial infarctions or with infarctions which are dominantly subendocardial[B67, D51]. *Theoretically* this would occur when the necrotic subendocardial infarct is greater than the thickness of the hypothetical 'silent' subendocardial rind. It must, however, be emphasized that even the extent, the thickness, of this hypothetical subendocardial rind is uncertain. Estimates vary from one-third or less to two-thirds of the myocardial thickness. When the infarct is theoretically greater than the thickness of the rind, it *will* manifest with changes of the QRS complex, and pathological Q waves followed by an R or r wave, a QR or Qr complex, will be recorded. The latter, i.e. the r or R wave, represents activation of the overlying surviving myocardial tissue, probably by focal peri-infarction block (see Chapter 12). The R or r wave is to some extent proportional to the degree of surviving *epi*cardial tissue,

and is always reduced in amplitude. It is thus evident that pathological Q waves can then be associated with some forms of subendocardial infarctions. Even if the postulated subendocardial 'silent' rind does not exist, the Q wave would be proportional to the degree of subendocardial involvement (Diagrams C and D of Fig. 22). The electrocardiogram would manifest with Qr or QR complexes. The Q wave represents the pathological Q wave of the necrosis, and the r or R wave represents the late activation of the overlying healthy or relatively healthy subepicardial tissue by focal or peri-infarction block. This will be associated with *elevated* and *coved S-T segments* and *inverted T waves* due to the overlying injured and ischaemic tissues. Whereas the region of necrosis in such cases is dominantly subendocardial, the regions of myocardial injury and/or myocardial ischaemia are probably transmural or nearly so. The reason for the anterior rather than the posterior deviation of the S-T segment in such cases is probably the combination of boundary and electrical image effect.

These subendocardial infarctions usually occur as subendocardial extensions of a transmural infarction. This may occur as a lateral extension of an anterior infarction (Electrocardiographic Studies 17 and 18), or as a lateral-apical-extension of an inferior infarction (Electrocardiographic Studies 28, 31 and 32).

It should again be emphasized that while QS complexes usually connote transmural infarction, this only applies to the free wall of the left ventricle. Non-transmural and dominantly subendocardial infarction of the *left side of the interventricular septum* can also present with QS complexes (see above).

Chapter 9

Myocardial Infarction Associated with Right Bundle Branch Block

Myocardial infarction may result in right bundle branch block. It may also be superimposed upon a pre-existing right bundle branch block. The accurate electrocardiographic diagnosis of acute myocardial infarction in the presence of right bundle branch block is based primarily on an appreciation of the genesis, mechanism and electrocardiographic manifestations of ventricular activation in cases of uncomplicated right bundle branch block. This will be considered first.

UNCOMPLICATED RIGHT BUNDLE BRANCH BLOCK

VENTRICULAR ACTIVATION: THE QRS COMPLEX

In right bundle branch block, conduction down the left bundle branch is impeded, and activation of the lower one-third of the interventricular septum therefore proceeds normally, proceeding from left to right[B49, M76, S105, S118] (Vector 1 of Fig. 34). This is reflected by a small initial r wave in leads orientated to the right ventricle and right side of the interventricular septum, and a small initial q wave in leads orientated to the left ventricle and left side of the interventricular septum. This is followed by endocardial-epicardial activation of the free wall of the left ventricle (Vector 2 of Fig. 34). This vector is directed to the left, inferiorly and somewhat to the right[S107]. It is also a little smaller than normal, for it tends to be overlapped and thus somewhat neutralized by the ensuing and oppositely directed activation front of right septal depolarization[S109, S112, S118] (Vector 3 of Fig. 34). This activation of the right side of the interventricular septum is effected by the activation front which arises in the left side of the interventricular septum[H29]. This right-sided activation is *slow* and *anomalous* in character, tending to be longitudinal or tangential rather than transverse (endocardial-epicardial). It would seem that the Purkinje system is programmed for the rapid transmission of the activation process from a central distributing point which is normally in the subendocardium. Activation entering the system from another direction, i.e. within the myocardium, is also transmitted but is a bizarre, relatively slow and ineffective manner[W3] (see also discussion on the physiological intraseptal barrier in Chapter 2). The deflection resulting from this form of anomalous activation is relatively *increased in magnitude* and *delayed*. This right septal and paraseptal activation is followed by activation of the free wall of the right ventricle which is also anomalous in character, for the reasons mentioned above. The slow, abnormal, anomalous form of activation is responsible for the marked notchings and slurrings of the terminal bizarre and widened deflection[M35, M73, M74, M75, M76]. The mean vector representing these terminal deflections, the summation of Vectors 3 and 4, is directed anteriorly and to the right. The QRS complex is, as a result, prolonged to 0.11 sec or longer.

Leads orientated to the right ventricle, for example, lead V1, reflect the following:

(a) An initial small r wave due to left septal depolarization (Vector 1 of Fig. 34).

(b) A relatively deep S wave—due mainly to depolarization of the left free wall (Vector 2 of Fig. 34).

(c) A terminal bizarre and slurred R wave—due to late and anomalous right septal and right free wall depolarization (Vectors 3 and 4 of Fig. 34)[B6, E13, K22, W48].

Leads orientated to the left ventricle, leads V5 and V6, and Standard lead I, reflect the following:

(a) An initial small q wave, due to left septal depolarization (Vector 1 of Fig. 34).

(b) A relatively tall R wave, due mainly to depolarization of the left free wall (Vector 2 of Fig. 34).

(c) A terminal bizarre and slurred S wave, due to late and anomalous right septal and right free wall activation (Vectors 3 and 4 of Fig. 34).

Leads orientated to the mid-precordium, leads V2–V3 (V4), tend to reflect a rR's or RR's complex (Fig. 34).

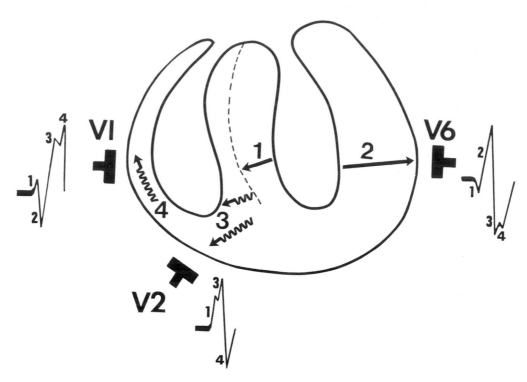

FIG. 34. Diagrammatic representation of ventricular depolarization in right bundle branch block. See text.

THE SECONDARY S-T SEGMENT AND T WAVE CHANGES

The abnormal intraventricular conduction is associated with secondary S-T segment and *T* wave changes. These secondary changes of repolarization are the direct result of the abnormal intraventricular conduction due to the right bundle branch block, and do not connote any primary disorder of the ventricular myocardium. The principles governing these secondary changes are the same as those associated with other forms of abnormal intraventricular conduction, such as left bundle branch block, ectopic ventricular beats, and the Wolff-Parkinson-White syndrome (discussed in Chapters 10, 11, 12 and 13).

The S-T segment and *T* wave vectors are directed *away from the terminal QRS vector*. In other words, if the terminal QRS deflection is positive, the S-T segment and *T* waves will be negative (depressed), and vice versa. The relationship may be expressed vectorially as a spread or angle between the S-T segment and *T* wave vectors and the terminal QRS vector greater than 140°. The S-T segment, when depressed, slopes downward and is usually straight with a slight, at times barely perceptible, upward convexity. It blends with the proximal limb of the *T* wave which cannot be accurately separated from the S-T segment (see Diagram A of Fig. 67).

THE DIAGNOSIS OF MYOCARDIAL INFARCTION IN THE PRESENCE OF RIGHT BUNDLE BRANCH BLOCK

MANIFESTATIONS AFFECTING THE QRS COMPLEX

It is clear that initial ventricular activation (Vectors 1 and 2 of Fig. 34) during right bundle branch block does not differ materially from that recorded during normal activation, i.e. during activation uncomplicated by right bundle branch block. This is in contrast to the situation in left bundle branch block, where the initial vectors are markedly different from that recorded during normal activation. Right bundle branch block, in effect, merely results in the addition of a terminal vector which is directed anteriorly and to the right. This has several important implications:

1. The diagnosis of any abnormality affecting the initial QRS deflections such as myocardial infarction, ventricular hypertrophy, etc., is *not affected by the advent of the right bundle branch block*.

2. Since the initial vectors of right bundle branch block are unchanged, and phasic aberrant ventricular conduction is usually of the right bundle branch block type (Chapter 17), the recognition of aberrantly conducted beats is

facilitated by the comparison of the initial vectors during both normal and anomalous conduction .

Since the basic QRS deflections are not changed by the advent of the right bundle branch block, any abnormality affecting these initial forces will still be evident after the advent of the block. This principle is illustrated in Fig. 35. Diagram A shows the basic deflections in leads V2 and V6 as recorded during normal intraventricular activation. Diagram B illustrates the advent of right bundle branch block. The initial QRS forces are essentially unchanged, there merely being the addition of a terminal R′ wave in lead V2 and a terminal S wave in lead V6. Diagram C illustrates anterior myocardial infarction which is *not* complicated by right bundle branch block. Lead V2

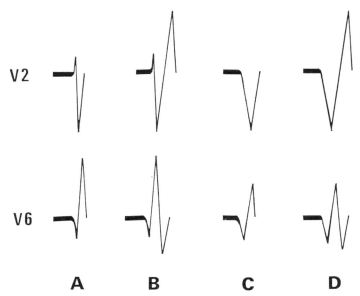

V2

V6

A   B   C   D

FIG. 35. Diagrams illustrating: A, normal QRS complexes in leads V2 and V6; B, the effect of right bundle branch block; C, the effect of anteroseptal myocardial infarction on normal intraventricular conduction; and D, the effect of anteroseptal myocardial infarction in the presence of right bundle branch block. See text.

reflects a QS complex of transmural infarction. Lead V6 reflects a QR complex of dominant subendocardial infarction. Diagram D illustrates the superimposition of the pattern of right bundle branch block on the pattern of the anterior wall myocardial infarction. This again results in a terminal R deflection in lead V2 and a terminal S wave in lead V6. The parameters of the infarction are clearly discernible and are not in any way masked by the advent of the right bundle branch block.

The principle is evident in Electrocardiographic Study 52, a tracing of lead V2 showing acute anteroseptal myocardial infarction with intermittent right bundle branch block, which was dependent upon critical rate. The first

two complexes represent acute myocardial infarction with right bundle branch block. The ensuing four complexes show the acute myocardial infarction without the right bundle branch block. It is clear that the initial QRS forces, the QS deflections of acute myocardial infarction, are essentially unchanged during right bundle branch block conduction.

MANIFESTATIONS AFFECTING THE S-T SEGMENT AND T WAVE: PRIMARY S-T SEGMENT AND T WAVE CHANGES

As indicated above, uncomplicated right bundle branch block is associated with secondary S-T segment and T wave changes which are secondary to the abnormal intraventricular conduction. When right bundle branch block is complicated by acute myocardial infarction, the S-T segments and T waves reflect marked changes which are primary in character, and the direct result of the acute myocardial infarction. These changes are as follows:

1. *The S-T segment is displaced in the* **same direction** *as the terminal,* **positive** *QRS deflection of the right precordial leads.* The S-T segment in acute anterior wall myocardial infarction is elevated in leads V1–V3 despite the terminal R′ deflection of the bundle branch block. In other words, the S-T segment is deviated in the *same* direction as the terminal positive R′ deflection in these leads. Indeed, in extensive anterior wall myocardial infarction it is usually elevated in *all* the precordial leads (Electrocardiographic Studies 51, 54 and 60B). In cases of inferior wall myocardial infarction, the S-T segment will be elevated in Standard leads II and III and lead AVF (Electrocardiographic Study 53).

2. *The S-T segment becomes coved, convex-upward* (Electrocardiographic Studies 51, 52, 53, 54 and 60B).

3. *The T wave becomes symmetrical, inverted and arrow-head in configuration* (Electrocardiographic Studies 51–54).

In other words, the S-T segment and T wave develop the same characteristics as when they occur in association with acute myocardial infarction that is not complicated by the bundle branch block.

Further Observations

1. At times, however, the initial r wave of the rsR′ pattern in the right precordial leads may be taller than normal, resulting in an RsR′ pattern (Electrocardiographic Study 53). This may be partly due to a lack of the normal opposition of the left to right septal force; Vector 1a of the normal depolarization in Fig. 11 is no longer chronologically opposed by Vector 1b. The relatively tall initial R

wave in the right precordial leads may consequently make it difficult to diagnose the presence of true posterior infarction, which is the only infarction that cannot be diagnosed with confidence in the presence of right bundle branch block (Grant 1957)[G31]. The condition may, nevertheless, still be suspected electrocardiographically if there is an associated tall symmetrical T wave, a primary T wave change.

2. With rate-dependent right bundle branch block, or with atrial extrasystoles conducted with phasic aberrant ventricular conduction having a right bundle branch block pattern, a Q wave may appear in leads V_1–V_3, indicative of septal infarction. This is in contrast to the manifestation during non-aberrant ventricular conduction, when these leads reflect an rS complex. This has been attributed to an additional complicating septal focal block, a transient rate-dependent block of the septal fibres of the left bundle branch[G2].

3. The advent of complete right bundle branch block during the course of acute myocardial infarction increases the mortality[B15, D8, G15, H42, N16].

Chapter 10

Myocardial Infarction Associated with Left Bundle Branch Block

Myocardial infarction may cause left bundle branch block, or it may be superimposed upon a pre-existing left bundle branch block. Reports of the combination are relatively infrequent[B10, B11, C19, E15, F16, M39, M87, P3, R8, R38, S61, S99, S113, S116, S117, W33, W42, W44, W46, W53, W54, W55]. The association has been reported with an incidence of 8 per cent[M39]. Since left bundle branch block radically alters the sequences of ventricular activation, the manifestations of acute myocardial infarction are also significantly changed in the presence of left bundle branch block, and may present considerable diagnostic difficulty. Indeed, Wilson and associates (1945)[W55] observed that 'in the presence of left bundle branch block it is seldom possible to make a diagnosis of myocardial infarction on the basis of electrocardiographic findings alone'. Others, too, have stressed the difficulty of recognizing the electrocardiographic features of myocardial infarction in the presence of left bundle branch block[B10, B11, M39, W33, W42]. Nevertheless, the manifestations of myocardial infarction in the presence of left bundle branch block may, at times, be clearly evident and even characteristic. The understanding of these manifestations is based on the original experimental work by Wilson and associates[W44, W46, W53, W54, W55, R38, S99], which was subsequently developed by others[C1, K21], particularly Dressler and associates (1950)[D33], Pantridge (1951)[P3], Sodi-Pallares and associates[S113, S116, S117] and Chapman and Pearce (1957)[C19].

The accurate diagnosis of acute myocardial infarction in the presence of left bundle branch block is based primarily on an appreciation of the genesis, mechanism and electrocardiographic manifestations of ventricular activation in cases of uncomplicated left bundle branch block. This will be considered first.

UNCOMPLICATED LEFT BUNDLE BRANCH BLOCK

VENTRICULAR ACTIVATION: THE QRS COMPLEX

In uncomplicated left bundle branch block activation of the left side of the interventricular septum, the left septal mass, and the free wall of the left ventricle is *delayed* and *anomalous* in character[B83]. The anomalous activation process is an expression of slow, abnormal intramyocardial conduction[B83]. It has been shown that the Purkinje system is in fact used in this anomalous form of left bundle branch block activation[A10, B68, W3], but the activation process tends to be longitudinal, tangential or oblique, rather than centrifugal (an endocardial to epicardial spread). It would seem that the Purkinje system is programmed for the rapid transmission of the activation process from a central distributing point which is normally the left ventricular subendocardium. Activation entering the system from another direction, i.e. from *within* the myocardium, is also transmitted, but not in a very effective manner[W3].

There are three major ventricular activation processes in left bundle branch block. These, in chronological order, are:

1. Right septal activation.
2. Delayed and anomalous left septal activation.
3. Delayed and anomalous activation of the free left ventricular wall.

RIGHT SEPTAL ACTIVATION

The First Component of Left Bundle Branch Block Activation
In contrast to normal intraventricular conduction (see Chapter 2 and Fig. 11), ventricular activation in left bundle branch block begins in the subendocardial regions of the *right* side of the interventricular septum, in the region of the anterior papillary muscle, i.e. in the inferior subendocardial region of the right septal mass[B49, M76, S118]. The activation process then proceeds from *right to left* through the septum (Vector 1A of Fig. 36), resulting in a vector of relatively small magnitude which is directed *anteriorly*, *inferiorly* and to the *left*[S107]. This represents the normal right septal force which, unlike normal intraventricular conduction, is not opposed by a concomitant and greater

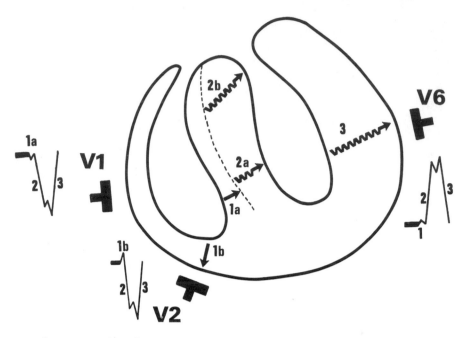

FIG. 36. Diagrammatic representation of ventricular depolarization in left bundle branch block. See text.

left to right force of the left septal mass. The unopposed right septal force then becomes manifest electrocardiographically, and is reflected as (a) a small initial positive deflection in leads orientated to the left side of the interventricular septum, and (b) as a small negative deflection in leads orientated to the right side of the interventricular septum (Fig. 36). This right septal activation process will be termed the first component of left bundle branch block activation. It is reflected in leads V5 and V6 as a small initial positive deflection which is but a tiny, at times imperceptible, initial positive incident preceding the bizarre and dominantly positive QRS complex (Figs. 36, 37 and 38). This tiny initial positive incident will be labelled *r1*. This first component is of very small magnitude and may not be seen unless sensitive recording apparatus is used[H12, K22, W53, W54]. It may, nevertheless, still be evident in electrocardiograms recorded by the conventional electrocardiograph. Leads orientated to the right ventricle, particularly lead V1, may show a small initial negative deflection (Figs. 36 and 38).

This right septal activation process may be complemented or reinforced by some activation of the free right ventricular wall in the paraseptal region[B6, H12]. This produces a force which is directed anteriorly and to the right of Vector 1A, and is labelled Vector 1B in Fig. 36. The right precordial leads, particularly leads V2 and V3, may reflect this initial paraseptal force as a small positive deflection (Fig 36). In some cases, however, these initial right ventricular forces are not manifest, since they occur

synchronously with, and hence are opposed by, the stronger and anomalous right to left activation force of the left septal mass (see below).

The slightly inferior direction of the right septal force may, at times, be directed somewhat inferiorly, and is consequently reflected by an initial negativity in left atrial leads or leads orientated to the base of the left heart, particularly lead AVL. Lead AVL may thus reflect a tiny initial Q wave[S113], although it may also manifest without an initial *q* wave. However, all other leads orientated to the left side of the heart, e.g. leads V5 and V6 and Standard lead I, will reflect *initial positivity*.

DELAYED AND ANOMALOUS LEFT SEPTAL ACTIVATION

The Second Component of Left Bundle Branch Block Activation
Following activation of the right septal mass, the activation process continues through the septum from right to left to activating the lower left septal mass (illustrated as Vector 2a of Fig. 36)[B49, B83, H29, M74, M75, M76, S107, S112]. It has been postulated that this activation process has to 'jump' a physiological barrier of delay between the right and left sides of the septum[S109, S112, S118]. This concept has, however, been questioned[D43, E13, W3]. Activation of the left septal mass is anomalous in character, and it is conceivable that this delayed anomalous activation, which is most probably due to ectopic and abnormal entry of the activation process into the septal Purkinje system (as described

on page 79) may be responsible, in part, for the effect of the so-called septal barrier. This results in a force of large magnitude directed posteriorly and to the left (illustrated as Vector 2a of Fig. 36). This will be termed the second component of left bundle branch block activation, and is reflected by a tall R wave in leads orientated to the left side of the interventricular septum. This tall R wave will be labelled R2. Leads orientated to the right side of the interventricular septum will reflect a deep negative deflection, which will be termed the primary S wave. Further delay in the activation of the superior regions of the interventricular septum (Vector 2B of Fig. 36) may result in slurring or delay, a plateau, of the apex of the bizarre QRS complex recorded by leads orientated to the left ventricle[S107].

DELAYED AND ANOMALOUS ACTIVATION OF THE FREE LEFT VENTRICULAR WALL

The Third Component of Left Bundle Branch Block Activation
Septal activation is followed by delayed activation of the left ventricular wall. This is also anomalous in character (see above) and results in a force of large magnitude which is directed *posteriorly*, *superiorly* and to the *left* (illustrated by Vector 3 of Fig. 36). This will be termed the third component of left bundle branch block activation. This force is responsible for the large terminal positive deflection recorded by leads orientated to the left ventricle, and which will be labelled R3 (Fig. 36). Right precordial leads (leads V1–V3) will reflect a large terminal S wave, which will be termed the secondary S wave.

Comment

It is clear that in cases of left bundle branch block the left precordial leads, leads V5 and V6, and also Standard lead I, *cannot reflect an initial Q wave or a terminal S wave*.

THE LEFT CAVITY POTENTIAL

A lead sited *within* the left ventricular cavity and orientated to the left side of the interventricular septum will reflect an RS or rRS complex. The small r wave of the rRS complex represents the first component of left bundle branch block activation. The R wave of the rRS complex or RS complex represents the second component of ventricular activation. The S wave of the rRS or RS complex represents the third component of ventricular activation, the activation of the left free wall, which is directed *away* from the left ventricular cavity.

SUMMARY

TABLE 3   Left bundle branch block as manifest in the left precordial leads

		LEADS V5 AND V6
Right septal activation	First component	r1
Left septal activation	Second component	R2
Left ventricular activation	Third component	R3

The Electrocardiographic Manifestations of Uncomplicated Left Bundle Branch Block

THE QRS CHANGES OF UNCOMPLICATED LEFT BUNDLE BRANCH BLOCK

Complete left bundle branch block manifests empirically with the following QRS manifestations (Electrocardiographic Study 59A):

PROLONGED QRS DURATION

The QRS complex is prolonged to 0·12 sec or more, and may be as long as 0·20 sec. This is due to the delayed and anomalous activation of the left septal mass and the free wall of the left ventricle.

BIZARRE QRS MORPHOLOGY IN LEADS V5 AND V6

Leads orientated to the left ventricle reflect a wide notched 'M' or plateau-shaped QRS complex. This may be preceded by a very small r wave, thus resulting in an rRR complex consisting of the r1, R2 and R3 deflections.

DELAYED INTRINSICOID DEFLECTION IN LEADS V5 AND V6

The ventricular activation time is prolonged, the intrinsicoid deflection being delayed to 0·09 or 0·10 sec.

THE QRS MORPHOLOGY OF LEAD AVL

Lead AVL may reflect the following:

(a) an RsR complex (the s representing the notched plateau).

(b) an RR complex (an unnotched plateau).

(c) a qRsR or a qRR complex. This reflects the additional manifestation of the first component of left bundle branch block activation (Vector 1a of Fig. 36) or, more likely, the vector of the right paraseptal mass (Vector 1b of Fig. 36) as a tiny q wave. The first tall R wave represents the R2 deflection (the second component of ventricular activation), and the second tall R wave represents the R3 deflection (the third component of ventricular activation). The first component may be isoelectric and thus not manifest, and lead AVL will consequently reflect a notched, wide, dominantly positive R wave.

THE QRS MORPHOLOGY IN LEADS V1 AND V2

Leads V1 and V2 usually reflect a widened notched QS complex or a dominantly widened and notched negative deflection which may be preceded by a small r wave. The r wave represents Vector 1b of the first component of left bundle branch block activation. The deep negative deflection consists of the primary and secondary S waves; the second and third components of left bundle branch block activation.

THE S-T SEGMENT AND T WAVE MORPHOLOGY IN UNCOMPLICATED LEFT BUNDLE BRANCH BLOCK

In uncomplicated left bundle branch block the S-T segment and T wave are *normally* displaced in a direction *opposite to that of the main QRS deflection* (Electrocardiographic Study 59A). Thus, if the main QRS deflection is positive, the S-T segment will be depressed and the T wave inverted (Diagram B of Fig. 37). If the main QRS deflection is negative, the S-T segment will be elevated and the T wave upright (Diagram A of Fig. 37). The principle may be expressed with greater accuracy in terms of the vectorial relationship between the main QRS vector and the S-T segment and T wave vectors. In uncomplicated left bundle branch block, the S-T segment and T wave vectors are normally directed away from the main QRS vector, the angle between them being between 150° and 180°[G31]. These changes are, in fact, a normal physiological or secondary response to the abnormal anomalous intraventricular conduction. They do not reflect primary abnormality or disease, and hence are termed secondary S-T segment and T wave changes.

If the S-T segment and/or T wave vectors are deviated in the *same direction* as the main QRS deflection, i.e. the angle between them is narrowed, a primary disturbance affecting the S-T segment and/or T wave is present (Diagram F of Fig. 37). This may be expressed vectorially as follows. If the angle between the mean manifest frontal plane T wave axis and the mean manifest frontal plane axis of the *terminal* QRS deflection is less than 110°, primary myocardial disease is probably present.

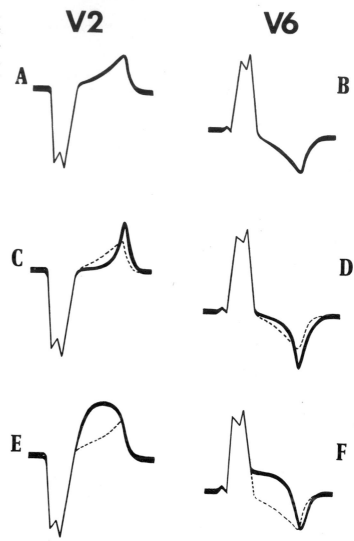

FIG. 37. Diagrams A and B illustrate the normal QRST configuration in left bundle branch block. Diagrams C and D illustrate the effect of myocardial ischaemia on the S-T segment and T wave in left bundle branch block. Diagrams E and F illustrate the effect of anterior wall myocardial infarction on the S-T segment and T wave in left bundle branch block. See text.

THE MORPHOLOGY OF THE S-T SEGMENT AND T WAVE IN LEADS ORIENTATED TO THE LEFT VENTRICLE

In uncomplicated left bundle branch block, leads which are orientated to the left ventricle, leads V5 and V6, Standard lead I and lead AVL, will reflect a dominantly positive QRS deflection. They will therefore be associated with depressed (negative) *secondary* S-T segment and T wave. The depressed S-T segment will usually have a straight downward slope, or a slope that is minimally convex-upwards (Diagram B of Fig. 37). The T wave is *inverted* and *asymmetrical* with a relatively *blunt apex* (Electrocardiographic Study 59A).

THE S-T SEGMENT AND *T* WAVE IN LEADS ORIENTATED TO THE RIGHT VENTRICLE

In uncomplicated left bundle branch block, leads which are orientated to the right ventricle, leads V1–V3, will reflect a dominantly negative QRS deflection. They will therefore be associated with an elevated (positive) *secondary* S-T segment and *T* wave changes. The *elevated* S-T segment has a straight upward slope, or an upward slope that is minimally concave-upwards. The *T* wave is *upright*, *asymmetrical* with a relatively *blunt* apex (Diagram A of Fig. 37, Diagram A of Fig. 39; Electrocardiographic Study 59A). This is, in effect, the mirror-image of the electrocardiographic manifestation in the left precordial leads.

THE QRS : S-T SEGMENT RATIO IN LEAD V2

The ratio of the QRS amplitude to the S-T segment amplitude in lead V2 is normally always greater than one, and is frequently 2:1 or even 3:1 (Electrocardiographic Studies 57, 59, 61B and 63)[S17].

THE ELECTROCARDIOGRAPHIC MANIFESTATIONS OF MYOCARDIAL INFARCTION ASSOCIATED WITH LEFT BUNDLE BRANCH BLOCK

The electrocardiographic manifestations of myocardial infarction in the presence of left bundle branch block will first be described empirically. Their genesis and significance are considered thereafter.

Anterior Wall Infarctions

The manifestations of anterior wall infarctions may be evident in all the precordial leads, but are usually best seen in the left precordial leads.

MANIFESTATIONS IN THE LEFT PRECORDIAL LEADS—LEADS V5 AND V6—AND STANDARD LEAD I

The normal uncomplicated left bundle branch block pattern in lead V6 has, as indicated above, *no* initial Q wave or terminal *S* wave, and the two dominant deflections, the R2 and R3 deflections described above, are of appreciable magnitude (Diagram B of Fig. 37), Electrocardiographic Study 59A). With the advent of myocardial infarction, leads orientated to the left ventricle may reflect the following modifications of this left bundle branch block pattern:

1. The wide and bizarre QRS complex reflects an initial small *q* wave (Diagram H of Fig. 38; Standard lead I of Electrocardiographic Studies 63 and 64; leads V5 and V6, and Standard lead I of Electrocardiographic Study 65).

2. The initial *tall R* wave (the R2 deflection or second component of left bundle branch activation, as described above) becomes diminished in amplitude (Diagrams I and K of Fig. 38; Electrocardiographic Study 59). This deflection may also become slurred, rounded or dome shaped. (Diagrams J, L, M, N of Fig. 38; Electrocardiographic Studies 59, 60 and 62). The appearance, when fully developed, is quite characteristic, giving rise to a slope which ends in a rather sharp spike, the R3 of the third component of ventricular activation. The appearance may be likened to a dome-and-dart configuration analogous to the dome-and-dart configuration of a left atrial *P* wave[M83]; (Electrocardiographic Studies 60, 62 and 65).

3. The wide and bizarre QRS complex may develop a terminal *S* wave (Diagrams K, L, M, N and O of Fig. 38; Electrocardiographic Studies 60 and 62).

4. The terminal tall *R* wave of the left bundle branch block pattern (the R3 deflection or the third component of left bundle branch block activation, as described above) becomes diminished in amplitude and may disappear completely, to be replaced by an *S* wave. The bizarre QRS complex then takes the form of an initial *r* or *R* wave, or a qr complex, which is followed by an *S* wave, i.e. an rS, RS or qrS complex (Diagrams L, M and N of Fig. 38).

5. There is a **general diminution in the amplitude of all the components of the QRS deflection**[C19, K19] (Diagrams I to O of Fig. 38; Electrocardiographic Studies 59–63).

6. All the left precordial leads may reflect QS complexes (Diagram O of Fig. 38). This may be associated with absent initial *r* waves in the right precordial leads so that all the precordial leads reflect QS complexes[W43]. This is particularly prone to occur with extensive and massive infarction involving the free left ventricular wall, the interventricular septum and the right paraseptal areas[W43].

MANIFESTATIONS IN THE LEAD IMMEDIATELY TO THE LEFT OF THE TRANSITION ZONE—LEAD V4 (OR LEAD V5)

Lead V4 (at times lead V5) usually represents the lead immediately to the left of the transition zone, and in uncomplicated left bundle branch block usually reflects a dominantly upright QRS complex. The complex is broad, notched or slurred, and at times associated with a terminal *S* wave (Diagram D of Fig. 38; Electrocardiographic Study 59)[C19]. In cases of complicating myocardial infarction this lead may become dominantly negative (Diagrams E and F of Fig. 38; Electrocardiographic Study 60). The

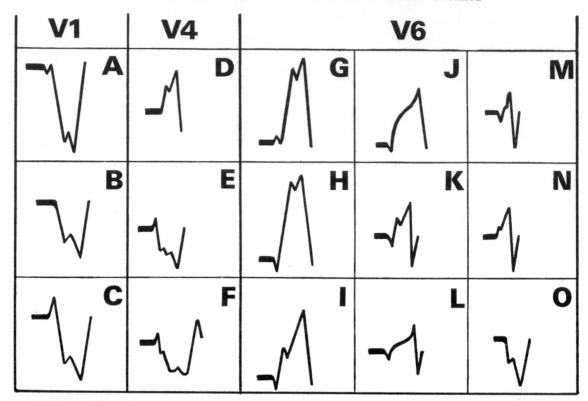

FIG. 38. Diagrams illustrating the various QRS patterns associated with anterior wall myocardial infarction complicated by left bundle branch block. See text.

negativity may be preceded by an initial small *r* wave, the ensuing *S* wave being bizarre and notched (Electrocardiographic Study 61A)[C19]. The notch is usually on the proximal limb of the *S* wave. There may also be a terminal small *r* or larger *R* wave. This lead may thus manifest with:

    (a) a notched QS complex[C19].

    (b) an rS complex with the *S* wave notched and bizarre (Diagram E of Fig. 38).

    (c) an rSr complex, with the *S* wave notched and markedly bizarre (Diagram F of Fig. 38).

MANIFESTATIONS IN THE RIGHT PRECORDIAL LEADS—LEADS V1–V3

With the advent of anterior wall myocardial infarction, leads orientated to the right ventricle may reflect the following modifications of the normal left bundle branch block pattern: 1. The QRS complex is diminished in amplitude, i.e. there is a diminution in the depth of the dominantly negative QRS complex (Diagram B and C of Fig. 38; Diagram B of Fig. 39; Electrocardiographic Studies 59, 60, 64 and 65).

    2. A prominent initial *r* wave develops in leads V1–V3 (Electrocardiographic Studies 59, 60, 62 and 65). The

dominantly negative QRS complex may be associated with the development of a small initial *r* wave, if this was not previously present.

Note: an initial *r* wave in the right precordial leads may be a normal manifestation of uncomplicated left bundle branch block, but if pre- and postinfarction tracings are available, the development of a small initial *r* wave, if previously absent, may constitute corroborative, though not definitive, evidence of infarction. For this manifestation to be meaningful, the electrode placement must be very accurate. Furthermore, the masking or unmasking effect of left anterior hemiblock must not be present (see Chapter 12). If an initial *r* wave was present before the infarction, it may become taller, at times considerably taller, with the advent of the infarction (Diagram C of Fig. 38; Diagram B of Fig. 39; Electrocardiographic Studies 59 and 62). This may be associated with a diminution of the QRS amplitude in the left precordial leads. In other words, the 'centre of electrical gravity' is deviated towards the right (Electrocardiographic Study 62).

    3. There may be a progressive diminution in the height of the initial *r* wave from leads V1–V4[C19, P3]. In uncomplicated left bundle branch block the initial *r* waves usually increase from V1–V4 (Electrocardiographic Study 61D).

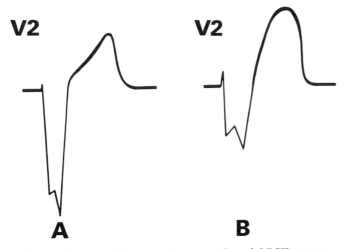

FIG. 39. Diagram A illustrates the uncomplicated QRST pattern in lead V2 of left bundle branch block. Diagram B illustrates the QRST pattern in lead V2 of left bundle branch block complicated by anterior wall myocardial infarction.

4. All the precordial leads, right as well as left, may reflect QS deflections[W43].

Inferior Wall Myocardial Infarction with Left Bundle Branch Block

The modifications of the left bundle branch block QRS pattern with the advent of inferior wall myocardial infarction have not been well documented. The manifestations are reflected in Standard leads II and III and lead AVF, and are essentially the same, or analogous to, those of the left precordial leads in left bundle branch block with anterior wall myocardial infarction.

1. There may be a reduction in the amplitude of the QRS complex, the amplitude being reduced to 5 mm or less (Electrocardiographic Studies 61 and 62). This reduction in amplitude may not be as apparent as that which occurs in the left precordial leads with anterior wall myocardial infarction, since the amplitude in uncomplicated left bundle branch block is not particularly large. The manifestation may be obvious if serial tracings are recorded.

2. If the QRS complex is dominantly positive, there may be a small initial q wave. Note that, as with the precordial leads, a dominantly positive QRS complex in uncomplicated left bundle branch block cannot be preceded by any initial negativity.

3. If the QRS complex is dominantly positive, the advent of myocardial infarction may be associated with the development of a terminal S wave. As with the precordial leads, a dominantly positive QRS complex in uncomplicated left bundle branch block cannot have a terminal S wave. This terminal S wave may be notched.

4. The notch in the M-shaped complex of left bundle branch block may become particularly marked, i.e. there is a relatively deep S wave to the RSR' complex (Electrocardiographic Study 61).

The aforementioned manifestations of anterior and inferior wall myocardial infarction reflect the modifications of the three basic components of left bundle branch block activation, and may be due to infarction of the interventricular septum and/or the free wall of the left ventricle[P17, S104, S110]. Their genesis is considered below.

THE GENESIS OF THE QRS MANIFESTATIONS, AND THE LOCALIZATION OF MYOCARDIAL INFARCTION IN THE PRESENCE OF LEFT BUNDLE BRANCH BLOCK

Infarction of the Right Lower Interventricular Septum

MODIFICATION OF THE FIRST COMPONENT OF LEFT BUNDLE BRANCH BLOCK ACTIVATION

When the infarct involves predominantly the right lower third of the interventricular septum (Diagram A of Fig. 40), the first component, the small right to left right-septal force (Vector 1a of Fig. 36) is abolished. The r1 deflection is consequently not recorded by the left precordial leads or leads orientated to the inferior left wall. The initial ventricular activation process is then right paraseptal depolarization (Vector 1b of Fig. 36), or depolarization of even more remote regions of the free right ventricular wall (Diagram A of Fig. 40). These small forces are directed *away* from the left precordial leads and Standard lead I, thereby resulting in a small initial q wave, i.e. a qRR' complex (Diagram A of Fig. 40; Electrocardiographic Studies 63, 64 and 65). The tiny initial r wave which may normally be present in right precordial leads in cases of uncomplicated left bundle branch block may become a little more prominent, or a tiny r wave may appear in the right precordial leads, if previously absent. The second component of left bundle branch block activation may not be appreciably affected and the R2 wave is not necessarily much changed. There may be a slight diminution in the height of the R2 wave depending upon the degree of encroachment of the infarction on the left septal mass (see next section). Thus, infarction of the right lower third of the interventricular septum is reflected by a small initial q wave in the left precordial leads, leads V5 and V6, and perhaps in Standard lead II. A small initial q wave may also appear in lead AVL but, in this case, it does not

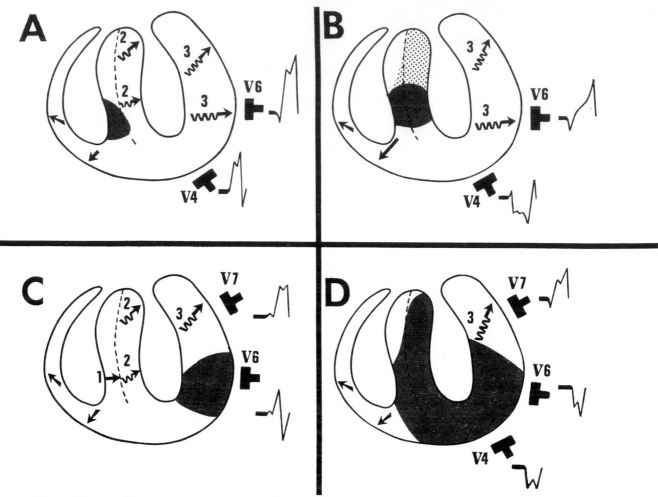

FIG. 40. Diagrams illustrating the effect of various sites of anterior wall myocardial infarction on the depolarization associated with left bundle branch block. See text.

necessarily have the same significance, since a small initial *q* wave may appear in lead AVL in cases of uncomplicated left bundle branch block (see p. 85). If, however, pre- and postinfarction tracings are available, a normal initial *q* wave in lead AVL may become more marked (deeper) with the advent of the infarction (Electrocardiographic Study 63).

Differential Diagnosis

Anterolateral Peri-infarction Block

A qR complex may appear in the left precordial leads in anterolateral peri-infarction block (see Chapter 12)[G4, G31].

(a) Anterolateral peri-infarction block is associated with a *wide angle* between the initial 0·04 sec QRS vector and the terminal 0·04 sec QRS vector—an angle that exceeds 100°. A wide angle is uncommon in uncomplicated left bundle branch block.

(b) Anterolateral peri-infarction block rarely reflects a diminution in the amplitude of the first tall R wave, the

R2 deflection or the second component of left bundle branch block activation, whereas left bundle branch block with myocardial infarction frequently does. In other words, if the initial *q* wave is followed by a tall or relatively tall and unslurred *R* wave, and there is a left axis deviation with a wide angle between the initial and terminal QRS deflections, the presentation is likely to be anterolateral peri-infarction block. If, on the other hand, the initial *q* wave is followed by a relatively small, slurred and rounded *r* or *R* wave, it is likely to be left bundle branch block with myocardial infarction.

Trans-septal Infarction

MODIFICATION OF THE FIRST AND SECOND COMPONENTS OF LEFT BUNDLE BRANCH BLOCK ACTIVATION

When the infarct is trans-septal and involves the full

thickness of the interventricular septum, both the first and second components of left bundle branch block activation are modified (Diagram B of Fig. 40). Loss of the first component is reflected by the appearance of a tiny initial q wave in leads V5 and V6, and a relatively prominent r wave in leads V1 and V2 (as described above). The second component of left bundle branch block activation is diminished or lost, and results in the *abolition or a reduction in magnitude of the large right to left anomalous left septal mass activation force*. The R2 wave of the left ventricular leads, leads V5 and V6, is diminished in size and may become slurred and deformed, forming a possible dome-and-dart appearance (Diagram B of Fig. 40; Electrocardiographic Studies 59, 60 and 65). The reduction in size of the R2 deflection is probably proportional to the degree of the involvement of the left septal mass. Furthermore, the right paraseptal forces (Vector 1b of Fig. 36) and perhaps even the forces of the more remote regions of the right ventricle are no longer opposed by the stronger anomalous right to left force of the left septal mass, as occurs in uncomplicated left bundle branch block. They consequently become manifest, thereby contributing to the magnitude of the R wave in the right precordial leads. This R wave may become increasingly taller concomitant with greater involvement of the interventricular septum (Electrocardiographic Study 62). If the right parseptal regions are spared, but the lower interventricular septum involved, the electrocardiogram may manifest with a diminishing amplitude of the initial r wave from lead V1–V4 (Electrocardiographic Study 65). The initial tiny r wave represents the right paraseptal forces which becomes lost in the electrode orientated to the inferior regions of the interventricular septum (Electrocardiographic Study 65). QS complexes (reflecting a loss of the initial r wave) may appear even further to the left, for example, in leads V2 or V3.

If the infarct is very extensive, and the right paraseptal regions as well as the interventricular septum and the left free wall are involved, then the left to right paraseptal force is also lost. The electrocardiogram may then manifest without the initial r wave and all the precordial leads will then reflect QS deflections, the proximal limb of the S wave being, in addition, frequently notched.

Infarction of the Left Free Wall

MODIFICATION OF THE THIRD COMPONENT OF LEFT BUNDLE BRANCH BLOCK ACTIVATION

When the infarct involves the free wall of the left ventricle, the third component of ventricular activation in left bundle branch block, the R3 deflection, is abolished or reduced in magnitude. A lead orientated to the left ventricle, for example, lead V5 or lead V6, is, in effect, orientated through the electrophysiological hole of the necrotic and electrically inert infarcted area situated in the free wall of the left ventricle, and is orientated towards the left side of the interventricular septum. The effect is thus similar to the effect on a lead sited within the left ventricular cavity, as described on p. 85 (Diagram C of Fig. 40). Leads V5 and V6 will consequently record an RS or rRS complex. These positive deflections are an expression of the first (r1) and second (R2) components of left bundle branch block activation, and the negative deflection is the result of the delayed forces which depolarize the unaffected regions of the left ventricle being directed away from the electrode orientated over the hole. This is an expression of the third component which, in this instance, is directed away from the electrode. Leads which are orientated to the higher, more remote, unaffected regions of the left ventricle—Standard lead I and lead AVL, or leads V7 and V8—may reflect the typical left bundle branch block configuration, and this must be sought for (Diagram D of Fig. 40). Leads V5 and V6 may also present with a *diminution* in the amplitude of the third component of ventricular activation, thereby resulting in a reduction of the R3 deflection (Electrocardiographic Study 61). This may also be associated with a terminal S wave (Electrocardiographic Studies 60 and 62). The reduction of the second and third components of left bundle branch block activation may also be reflected by a diminution in the negative components, the primary and secondary S waves, of the right precordial leads.

Trans-septal Infarction Associated with Infarction of the Free Left Ventricular Wall

The following electrocardiographic manifestations may occur with extensive infarction, involving the interventricular septum as well as the free wall of the left ventricle (Diagram D of Fig. 40).

1. A small initial q wave is recorded by leads V5, V6 and Standard lead I, representing the loss or modification of the first component of left bundle branch block activation.

2. There is a generalized reduction in voltage, due to modification of the second and third components of left bundle branch block activation. The first normal major QRS deflection may be completely lost, so that the lead reflects a dominantly negative deflection. This is particularly prone to occur in the lead immediately to the left of the transition zone, lead V4, or occasionally lead V5 (Electrocardiographic Studies 60 and 65).

3. A terminal S wave, the expression of transmural left ventricular infarction, may appear in the left precordial leads (Electrocardiographic Studies 60 and 62).

4. Right precordial leads may reflect an initial *r* or *R* wave (Electrocardiographic Studies 60 and 62).

When myocardial infarction complicates left bundle branch block, there is in most cases a loss of QRS voltage which affects, in particular, the complexes of the precordial leads, leads V1–V6. This loss of voltage is far more marked than the potential analogous reduction in voltage which may affect the QRS complexes of the frontal plane leads. With normal intraventricular conduction the QRS complexes of the precordial leads are nearly always larger than the QRS complexes of the frontal plane leads.

Similarly, in uncomplicated left bundle branch block, the QRS complexes of the horizontal plane leads, the precordial leads, are larger than those of the frontal plane leads. Thus, if the QRS complexes of the precordial leads are of *smaller* magnitude than those of the frontal plane leads, it is corroborative evidence or a pointer to the presence of infarction or some other pathological process, for example fibrosis, which may affect the ventricles (Electrocardiographic Studies 59 and 60).

With massive infarction involving the interventricular septum, the left free wall and right paraseptal regions, the electrocardiogram may manifest with dominant QS complexes in the left precordial leads, or throughout the conventional precordial leads[W43]. When this occurs, the characteristic or minimally modified left bundle branch block pattern may still be evident in leads V7 and V8, or in lead AVL (Diagram D of Fig. 40).

The aforementioned principles governing the electrocardiographic diagnosis of myocardial infarction in the presence of left bundle branch block have received experimental support[M71].

The S-T Segment and T Wave Manifestations of Myocardial Infarction Associated with Left Bundle Branch Block

The S-T segment and *T* wave manifestations in acute myocardial infarction complicating left bundle branch block reflect acute injury and ischaemia respectively. Their interpretation and significance are, with some modification, governed by the same principles as when they occur with acute myocardial infarction uncomplicated by left bundle branch block.

THE T WAVE MANIFESTATIONS

In uncomplicated left bundle branch block the *T* wave has asymmetrical limbs with a relatively blunt apex (Diagrams A and B of Fig. 37; Diagram A of Fig. 39). This manifestation is modified by the advent of acute myocardial infarction.

The *T* wave becomes inverted in the right precordial leads in anterior wall myocardial infarction. The *T* wave is usually inverted in all the precordial leads, but the inversion in the right precordial leads constitutes a primary change since the *T* wave is normally upright in these leads in uncomplicated left bundle branch block (Electrocardiographic Studies 58, 59, 60 and 65). The *T* wave inversion is minimal and is not as marked as that associated with anterior myocardial infarction in the presence of normal intraventricular conduction. The inverted *T* waves in the right precordial leads as well as those in the left precordial leads also tend to become more symmetrical.

The same primary *T* wave changes may occur in the inferiorly orientated leads, Standard leads II and III, and lead AVF, in inferior wall myocardial infarction (Electrocardiographic Study 61).

THE S-T SEGMENT MANIFESTATIONS

In uncomplicated left bundle branch block the S-T segment is displaced in a direction opposite to that of the main QRS deflection, the vectorial angle between them being between 150° and 180°. Furthermore, the S-T segment in leads orientated to the left ventricle has a straight or relatively straight downward slope, or a slope that is minimally convex-upwards. The S-T segment in leads orientated to the right ventricle has a straight upward slope or a slope that is minimally concave-upwards.

The advent of acute myocardial injury, as occurs for example in acute myocardial infarction, may alter these manifestations by effecting a *change in the deviation of the S-T segment* and a *change in the shape of the S-T segment*.

1. The S-T segment is deviated or displaced in the *same direction as the dominant QRS deflection* in the left precordial leads in anterior myocardial infarction, and in the inferiorly orientated leads in inferior wall myocardial infarction.

2. The S-T segment elevation is exaggerated in the right precordial leads.

3. The S-T segment becomes *coved*, convex-upward.

MANIFESTATIONS OF ACUTE MYOCARDIAL INJURY AFFECTING THE S-T SEGMENT

(a) There is an upward displacement, an elevation of the S-T segment, in leads V5 and V6 (Diagram F of Fig. 37, Standard lead I and lead AVL of Electrocardiographic Studies 63 and 64; Electrocardiographic Studies 59B, 64 and 65). This constitutes a primary change since the S-T segment is normally depressed in these leads in cases of uncomplicated left bundle branch block. This is also evident in the inferiorly orientated leads, Standard leads II and III, and lead AVF, in inferior wall myocardial infarction (Electrocardiographic Study 61).

In extensive anterior wall myocardial infarction complicated by left bundle branch block, the S-T segment is elevated in all the precordial leads, V1–V6 (Electrocardiographic Studies 59, 64 and 65), or dominantly in the right precordial leads (Electrocardiographic Study 58). The elevation is particularly marked in the right precordial leads (Electrocardiographic Study 64). This is because the *injury* of acute myocardial infarction is extensive and usually involves the greater part of the anterior wall of the heart, including the interventricular septum and the right paraseptal regions. Thus, Leads V1–V3 are *also* orientated to the injured surface and will also reflect the injury pattern; the coved and elevated S-T segments (Diagrams E and F of Fig. 37).

The elevation in the right precordial leads constitutes an exaggeration of the secondary S-T segment change, since the S-T segment in uncomplicated left bundle branch block is also elevated in these leads. However, the associated coving of the S-T segment, the large magnitude of the S-T segment elevation, and the diminution of the QRS:S-T ratio (see below) are pointers to the presence of the infarction.

(b) The S-T segment becomes symmetrically curved and convex-upward, blending imperceptibly with the proximal limb of the *T* wave (Electrocardiographic Studies 58, 59, 60, 61, 64 and 65)[C19, D33, K19, S116, S117]. The associated *T* wave is usually inverted with pointed arrow-head configuration (see below). The significance of the elevated S-T segment is essentially the same, whether followed by an upright *T* wave (leads V5 and V6 of Electrocardiographic Study 63) or an inverted *T* wave.

THE QRS/S-T RATIO

In uncomplicated left bundle branch block, the ratio of the QRS magnitude to the S-T segment magnitude in leads V1 and V2 is always greater than unity, and is commonly about 2:1 (Diagram A of Fig. 39)[S17]. In other words, the QRS deflection is always of larger magnitude than the associated S-T segment elevation. The elevation of the S-T segment and reduction in the QRS magnitude which occurs with the advent of acute myocardial infarction results in a diminution of the QRS/S-T ratio (Diagram B of Fig. 39). The S-T segment amplitude approximates that of the QRS amplitude, and the ratio may become unity or even less than one (compare Diagrams A and B of Fig. 39, Electrocardiographic Studies 58, 59, 60, 64 and 65).

FURTHER COMMENTS

1. If there are complicating ventricular extrasystoles, the infarction pattern may be more evident in the ventricular extrasystoles than in the conducted left bundle branch block pattern[D33, S116] (see Chapter 13). The infarction pattern may also become evident in the relatively normal conduction which sometimes follows the long or relatively long compensatory pause of the ventricular extrasystole.

2. The diagnosis of coronary insufficiency in the presence of left bundle branch block is considered in Chapter 15 and 16.

3. The advent of complete left bundle branch block during the course of acute myocardial infarction increases the mortality[B15, D8, G15, H42, N16].

Chapter 11

The Wolff-Parkinson-White Syndrome and Myocardial Infarction

The Wolff-Parkinson-White (WPW) syndrome may occasionally be associated with acute myocardial infarction. The association is entirely fortuitous, and merely reflects the occurrence of myocardial infarction in an individual with a pre-existing WPW syndrome. The WPW syndrome may, however, significantly modify the electrocardiographic presentation of acute myocardial infarction. Moreover, the WPW syndrome in itself can mimic the electrocardiographic effects of myocardial infarction and coronary artery disease. The recognition of these manifestations and their inter-relationship is thus important to the cardiologist.

The basic features of the uncomplicated WPW syndrome will be presented first, and then their significance in relationship to coronary artery disease, and myocardial infarction in particular, will be considered.

THE BASIC MANIFESTATIONS OF THE WOLFF-PARKINSON-WHITE SYNDROME

The WPW syndrome is due to the presence of a congenital anomalous A-V pathway which enables the sinus or supraventricular impulse to bypass the impedence, conduction delay, of the main A-V nodal pathway, and activate or pre-excite part of the ventricular myocardium anomalously. The syndrome has three basic characteristics (Fig. 41):

1. **A shortened P-R interval.**
2. **A widened QRS complex.**
3. **A delta wave – a slurred and thickened proximal limb of the QRS complex.**

There are associated secondary S-T segment and *T* wave changes which are secondary to the abnormal intraventricular conduction (discussed below on p. 98). These classic features are evident in Electrocardiographic Studies 69 and 70.

The WPW syndrome is also associated with a tendency to reciprocating tachyarrhythmias.

The activation front of the sinus or other supraventricular impulse is conducted down both the normal and anomalous pathways concomitantly. The impulse is, however, conducted more quickly through the anomalous pathway and consequently reaches the ventricles earlier than the impulse travelling through the normal A-V pathway, hence the shortened P-R interval. Part of the ventricular myocardium is then activated or pre-excited by the early impulse. This form of ventricular activation is *slow* and *abnormal* since it occurs through ordinary myocardial tissue and not the specialized conducting tissue. It is represented by the delta wave (Fig. 41). The region of ventricular myocardium so pre-excited is known as the *pre-excitation area*. The concomitant conduction through the normal A-V conduction pathway proceeds at the normal but relatively slower rate. Once this excitation front reaches the ventricles, however, further onward transmission proceeds through the rapid and efficiently transmitting specialized conducting system, the bundle of His, bundle branches and Purkinje network. Consequently, this excitation front is rapidly transmitted through the ventricles, activating the ventricular myocardium and recording the normal QRS complex. It is evident, therefore, that the normal excitation front eventually overtakes the pre-excitation front to

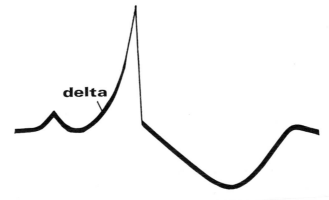

FIG. 41. Diagrammatic representation of the classic fusion complex of the Wolff-Parkinson-White syndrome.

activate the remaining responsive ventricular myocardium. The typical QRS complex of the WPW syndrome is thus a *fusion complex*; the initial part, the delta wave, is recorded by the impulse conducted through the anomalous pathway. The normal remainder of the QRS complex is recorded by the impulse conducted through the normal A-V nodal pathway.

It is thus evident that the anomalous activation produces an abnormal vector, the delta wave vector, which is superimposed upon the beginning of the QRS complex and hence may mask or modify the initial QRS vector of conventional, normal, ventricular activation. Since it is the initial QRS forces which are affected by the necrosis of myocardial infarction, it is these forces in particular which may be affected. In addition, the remainder or non-delta wave part of the QRS deflection, which represents ventricular activation by the impulse conducted through the normal A-V pathway, may be altered. This alteration, which may also modify the manifestations of myocardial infarction, is reflected by a *change in direction of the QRS force*, the mean manifest frontal and horizontal plane QRS axes. Thus, there may be right or left axis deviation of the frontal plane QRS axes. This is usually associated with the Type *A* WPW syndrome[S18]. In the horizontal plane, the QRS axis may become more anteriorly orientated, the Type *A* WPW syndrome, or more posteriorly orientated, the Type *B* WPW syndrome (see below).

The Mode of Pre-excitation

In contrast to the normal endocardial-epicardial form of ventricular activation, pre-excitation results in an epicardial-endocardial form of activation[S16]. Since a part of the subendocardial region may be electrocardiographically 'silent' (see Chapter 2), activation beginning in the epicardium will theoretically have a greater potential electrocardiographic effect than a similar degree of activation beginning in the endocardium. This is because early epicardial activation is not balanced or opposed by a manifest subendocardial vector. Thus, subepicardial pre-excitation usually has a significant effect electrocardiographically.

The Types of Wolff-Parkinson-White Syndrome

The WPW syndrome has been classified into two types[R39].

Type A is characterized by dominantly positive QRS complexes and delta waves in the right precordial leads (Electrocardiographic Study 70), and is due to pre-excitation of the basal region of the left ventricle.

Type B is characterized by dominantly negative QRS complexes and delta waves in the right precordial leads,

and is due to pre-excitation of the basal region of the right ventricle.

THE SIGNIFICANCE OF THE WOLFF-PARKINSON-WHITE SYNDROME IN RELATIONSHIP TO MYOCARDIAL INFARCTION

When the WPW syndrome occurs in association with myocardial infarction, it may give rise to various and diverse problems in diagnosis (Electrocardiographic Studies 71 and 72). The first report was made by Fischer in 1938[F16], and the problems surrounding the association has since evoked much interest[A11, B1, D32, E5, F16, G9, G16, G20, G24, G40, K6, K28, L1, L2, L3, L40, L63, P22, R12, R37, S36, S113, S127, S132, T4, V8, W13, W60, W61, Z4]. The syndrome is of significance in three important respects:

1. The uncomplicated WPW syndrome may simulate the electrocardiographic manifestations of myocardial infarction.

2. The WPW syndrome may mask the electrocardiographic manifestations of co-existing myocardial infarction.

3. The WPW syndrome may augment or exaggerate the electrocardiographic manifestations of co-existing myocardial infarction.

Simulation of the Electrocardiographic Manifestations of Myocardial Infarction by the Wolff-Parkinson-White Syndrome

The WPW syndrome may simulate almost any form of electrocardiographic presentation, and is particularly prone to mimic myocardial infarction[E5, K6, K47, L63, W14]. The delta wave axis of the WPW syndrome may have a mean manifest frontal plane axis which is directed within a range of $-70°$ to $+120°$ (Zao, 1958[Z1], Grant, 1957[G31], Schamroth 1973[S18]; shaded area of Fig. 42).

If the delta wave axes are located at the two extremes of this range (Vectors D1 and D2 of Fig. 42), they will be reflected by negative deflections in certain of the conventional leads and may thus simulate the pathological Q waves of inferior wall myocardial infarction (Electrocardiographic Study 69)[E5, W13], or anterolateral wall myocardial infarction (Electrocardiographic Study 70)[K6]. The delta wave axes of the Type *A* WPW syndrome in particular tend to be concentrated in two regions on the frontal plane hexaxial reference system (Schamroth, 1973)[S18]:

1. In the region of $-10°$ to $-70°$.
2. In the region of $+60°$ to $+120°$.

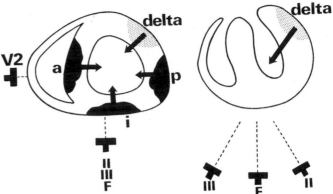

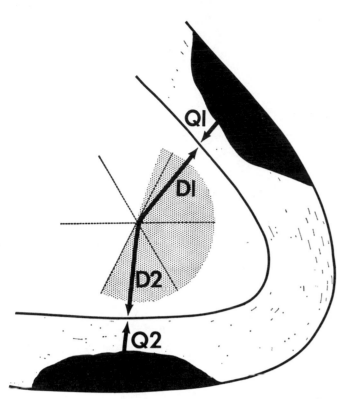

FIG. 42. Diagram illustrating the effect of a superiorly directed delta wave vector (D1) on the Q wave of high-lateral myocardial infarction (Q1), and the effect of an inferiorly directed delta wave vector (D2) on the Q wave of an inferior wall myocardial infarction (Q2), The shaded area on the hexaxial reference system indicates the range of the delta wave vectors.

FIG. 43. Diagrams illustrating the effect of an anterior and inferior directed delta wave vector on anterior wall myocardial infarction (a), inferior wall myocardial infarction (i), and true posterior wall myocardial infarction (p). See text.

Furthermore, if the delta wave and QRS vectors are directed posteriorly, as usually occurs in the Type B WPW syndrome, it will be reflected by initial negative deflections in the right precordial leads and may simulate anteroseptal myocardial infarction[K47, L63]. If the delta wave and QRS vectors are directed anteriorly, as occurs in the Type A WPW syndrome, the resulting dominantly positive deflections in the right precordial leads, leads V1–V3, may simulate true posterior wall infarction (Fig. 43).

SIMULATION OF INFERIOR WALL MYOCARDIAL INFARCTION

If there is a left axis deviation of the delta wave vector further to the left than −30°, for example an axis of −70°, the delta wave vector will be directed away from the positive poles of Standard leads II and III and lead AVF[5, L2] and will consequently be reflected by initial negative deflections in these leads, which may simulate the pathological Q wave of inferior wall myocardial infarction (Vector D1 of Fig. 43)[K6, S36, W13]. This is evident in Electrocardiographic Study 69.

SIMULATION OF ANTEROLATERAL WALL MYOCARDIAL INFARCTION

If there is a right axis deviation of the delta wave vector, for example an axis of +100°, the delta wave vector will be directed away from the positive poles of lead AVL and Standard lead I (Vector D2 of Fig. 42), and would consequently be reflected by initial negative deflections in these leads, which may simulate the pathological Q waves of anterolateral wall myocardial infarction (Electrocardiographic Study 70).

SIMULATION OF ANTEROSEPTAL WALL MYOCARDIAL INFARCTION

When the pre-excitation affects the anterior wall of the heart, the right ventricle, the epicardial-endocardial activation results in a delta wave vector which is directed posteriorly. This is usually associated with the Type B WPW syndrome. The posteriorly directed delta wave force will be reflected by negative deflections in leads V1–V3 or V4, and may thus simulate the pathological Q waves of anteroseptal myocardial infarction[K47, L63].

SIMULATION OF TRUE POSTERIOR WALL MYOCARDIAL INFARCTION

Pre-excitation may affect the posterior wall of the heart, the posterior wall of the left ventricle. This is usually associated with the Type A WPW syndrome. When this occurs, the resulting epicardial-endocardial form of activation will result in an anteriorly directed delta wave vector which is reflected by initial positive deflections in the right precordial leads, leads V1–V3 or V4. Moreover, the associated intraventricular activation effected by the normally conducted impulses, the non-delta wave excitation, usually results in an anterior directed QRS vector which will further contribute to the positivity of the QRS deflections in the right precordial leads. These dominantly positive QRS deflections in the right precordial leads can simulate true posterior wall myocardial infarction (Electrocardiographic Study 71; see Chapter 7).

THE DIFFERENTIAL DIAGNOSIS

The distinction of the aforementioned manifestations of the WPW syndrome which can mimic myocardial infarction from true myocardial infarction, is made on the following basis:

  1. The presence of the characteristic manifestations of the WPW syndrome, positive delta wave, widened QRS complex, shortened P-R interval, secondary S-T segment and T wave changes in leads other than those showing the apparent infarction pattern.

  2. The absence of the manifestations of coronary insufficiency or myocardial infarction in the other components of the electrocardiographic deflections, the S-T segment and T wave.

  3. Normalization of the WPW syndrome either spontaneously or, for example, by the administration of atropine or Rauwolfia alkaloids[G9, L63, P38] will result in the loss of the delta waves and reveal the normality of the basic uncomplicated pattern (see Electrocardiographic Study 71).

The Masking of the Electrocardiographic Manifestations of Myocardial Infarction by the Wolff-Parkinson-White Syndrome

The delta wave vector modifies the initial QRS complex and hence may mask or modify the initial abnormal QRS forces of myocardial infarction.

THE MASKING OF INFERIOR WALL MYOCARDIAL INFARCTION

If the delta wave vector is directed downwards and to the right in the region of $+90°$ to $+100°$ on the frontal plane hexaxial reference system (Vector D2 of Fig. 42), it will be reflected by positive initial deflections in Standard leads II, III and lead AVF, and hence will mask or counteract initial abnormal, pathological Q wave forces of inferior wall myocardial infarction, whose vector is directed upwards and to the left (Vector Q2 of Fig. 42), away from the inferior wall necrosis (Electrocardiographic Study 71).

THE MASKING OF ANTEROLATERAL WALL MYOCARDIAL INFARCTION

If the delta wave is directed upwards and to the left in the region of $-30°$ to $-70°$ on the frontal plane hexaxial reference system (Vector D1 of Fig. 42), it will counteract the forces of anterolateral myocardial infarction whose initial pathological, Q wave, vector is directed downwards and to the right (Vector Q2 of Fig. 42), away from the lateral wall necrosis and away from Standard lead I and lead AVL.

THE MASKING OF ANTEROSEPTAL WALL MYOCARDIAL INFARCTION

If the delta wave is directed anteriorly (an expression of posterior wall pre-excitation, usually the Type A WPW syndrome (see Fig. 43), it will result in positive deflections in the right precordial leads, leads V1–V4. This may mask the pathological Q waves of anteroseptal myocardial infarction in these leads (Electrocardiographic Study 71). The diagnosis may, at times, be suspected when the initial r or R waves are seen to diminish in amplitude from leads V1 or V2 to leads V3 or V4[L35], and when there are primary S-T segment and T wave changes (see below).

The Significance of Changes in the Associated S-T Segments and T Wave

The presence of acute myocardial infarction may also be suspected under the aforementioned circumstances when there are associated primary S-T segment and T wave changes of injury or ischaemia and/or changes in the morphology of the T wave.

PRIMARY S-T SEGMENT AND T WAVE CHANGES

When intraventricular conduction is abnormal, as in bundle branch block, pre-excitation, or with ventricular ectopic beats, there are concomitant S-T segment and T wave changes which are secondary to the abnormal intraventricular conduction, and, as such, have no primary significance. These secondary changes usually constitute a deviation of the S-T segment and sometimes the T wave in a direction opposite to that of the terminal QRS deflection. Thus, if the terminal deflection of the QRS complex is upright, the S-T segment will be depressed and vice versa. In the case of the WPW syndrome, the greater the degree of pre-excitation, the greater the degree of the secondary S-T segment and T wave changes (Tamagna and associates, 1948)[T4]. In other words, the secondary S-T segment and T wave changes bear a close causal relationship to the delta wave. This relationship may be more important than the relationship to the QRS complex, but requires further study. With the advent of ischaemia, injury or other primary myocardial disease, the S-T segments may be primarily affected. These primary S-T segment changes are characterized by an S-T segment shift in the *same direction* as that of the dominant QRS deflection, a change that is not due to the WPW syndrome alone. This is particularly so with dominantly upright QRS complexes when the associated S-T segment is elevated. This is reflected in Electrocardiographic Study 71, where the presence of acute anterior wall myocardial infarction in association with the Type *A* WPW syndrome may be suspected from the elevation of the S-T segments and the *T* waves in the precordial leads, i.e. a displacement of the S-T segments in the *same direction* as the dominant QRS deflection.

PRIMARY MORPHOLOGICAL CHANGE OF THE S-T SEGMENT AND T WAVE

The diagnosis of myocardial ischaemia due to acute coronary insufficiency or myocardial infarction in the presence of the WPW syndrome may be entertained when the S-T segment and *T* wave have the characteristics of the injury type manifestations, i.e. when the *T* wave is sharply pointed, symmetrical and arrow-head in appearance and when the S-T segment is elevated and upwardly coved (Electrocardiographic Study 72). These may be the only electrocardiographic signs which reflect the presence of infarction or acute insufficiency[F16, G16, G20, S113, W61, Z1].

It is thus evident that it may be difficult to establish a confident electrocardiographic diagnosis of myocardial infarction in the presence of the WPW syndrome. Such diagnosis can at times be based on the appearance of electrocardiographic signs of injury and ischaemia, i.e. primary S-T segment and *T* wave changes, together with a clinical picture suggestive of myocardial infarction. This has been emphasized by others[F16, G16, G20, S113, W61]. A diligent search should always be made for complexes which do not show pre-excitation so that accurate diagnosis can be made.

The diagnosis of the infarction becomes clearly evident from the normal beats when the WPW syndrome is intermittent[B1, D32, S36, S127, S132, V8, W61, Z4].

See Chapter 16 for interpretation of the exercise test in the presence of the WPW syndrome.

Augmentation of the Electrocardiographic Effects of Myocardial Infarction by the Wolff-Parkinson-White Syndrome

The delta wave and QRS forces associated with the WPW syndrome may augment co-existing pathological QRS forces of myocardial infarction if they are orientated in the *same direction*[S36].

When the pre-excitation involves the posterior wall of the left ventricle, the Type *A* WPW syndrome, the anteriorly directed delta and QRS forces will be reflected by dominantly positive QRS deflections in the right precordial leads. This will thus augment a co-existing true posterior wall infarction (Fig. 43)[S36]; (Electrocardiographic Study 71).

The electrocardiographic effects of myocardial infarction could theoretically also be augmented under the following circumstances:

(a) A left axis deviation of the delta wave force could augment the electrocardiographic effects of inferior wall myocardial infarction.

(b) A right axis deviation of the delta wave force could augment the electrocardiographic effects of anterolateral wall myocardial infarction.

(c) Posteriorly directed delta wave and QRS forces could augment the electrocardiographic effects of anteroseptal myocardial infarction.

These phenomena have not, as yet, been reported.

Chapter 12

Myocardial Infarction Associated with the Hemiblocks and Other Disturbances of Intraventricular Conduction

Acute myocardial infarction may be associated with various forms of intraventricular conduction disturbance. These are:

1. Acute injury block.
2. Infarction block. This may be subdivided into:
    (a) Intra-infarction block.
    (b) Peri-infarction block. This may be further subdivided into:
        (i) Focal peri-infarction block.
        (ii) Divisional peri-infarction block.
3. Bundle branch block.
4. The 'S1 S2 S3' syndrome.

ACUTE INJURY BLOCK

Acutely injured myocardial tissue is associated with a delay in conduction, a delay in the process of depolarization, *through* the injured zone. The delayed conduction is known as *acute injury block*[B91], and has the following characteristics (Diagram C of Fig. 23):

1. The delay is reflected by a relatively slow inscription of the R wave, resulting in a **delay of the intrinsicoid deflection** to 0·045 sec or longer, an **increased ventricular activation time.**
2. There may be an **increase in the duration of the QRS complex** which may be prolonged to 0·12 sec.
3. There is frequently an **increase in the amplitude of the QRS complex.** This is because the delayed activation front is no longer balanced or neutralized by the earlier activation of distant healthy regions of the ventricular myocardium.
4. The manifestations appear *early* in the evolution of acute myocardial infarction, i.e. during the hyperacute phase, i.e.:

(a) before the development of the abnormal, pathological, Q waves,

(b) during the phase of hyperacute injury as reflected by marked slope-elevation of the S-T segments,
(c) before the inversion of the *T* waves.
5. The manifestations are usually of short duration, and disappear when the manifestations of necrosis (the pathological Q waves) and ischaemia (the deeply inverted *T* waves) appear.

Injury block is a *constant feature* during the early, hyperacute, injury phase of myocardial infarction[C40, P1]. It may be missed, however, because it occurs transiently. The features of injury block are evident in Electrocardiographic Studies 1 (Standard leads II and III, and lead AVF), 2 (Standard leads II and III and leads AVF, V5 and V6), 4 (Standard leads II and III, and lead AVF), and 7 (Standard leads II and III and lead AVF).

INFARCTION BLOCK

Infarction block is a conduction defect which may occur during the fully developed stage of acute myocardial infarction. The block is the direct result of the infarction process. Consequently, in order to establish the diagnosis of infarction block, it must be clearly evident, both chronologically and from the concomitant electrocardiographic manifestations of infarction, that the block is the direct result of the infarction.

There are two principal forms:

1. Intra-infarction block.
This is an expression of the activation of some surviving myocardial fibres *within* the necrotic tissue.
2. Peri-infarction block.
This is an expression of a delay in conduction through, and activation of, the tissue *surrounding* the myocardial infarction. It constitutes an epiphenomenon of the infarction.

INTRA-INFARCTION BLOCK

If the necrotic tissue of a myocardial infarction is homogeneously necrotic, i.e. there are no surviving islets of living tissue within the necrotic zone, then the pathological Q wave or QS complex recorded by an electrode orientated to the surface of the necrotic zone will be smooth and regular without any notch or slur. In other words, the electrocardiogram will reflect the perfect Q wave or QS complex, the expression of a perfect, unobstructed window effect, for example leads V2–V4 of Electrocardiographic Study 19.

If, however, there are surviving islets of viable tissue within the necrotic zone, then delayed activation of these surviving islets will result in minor, small, positive deflections within the pathological Q wave or QS complex, thereby resulting in irregularities such as notching and slurring. This is known as intra-infarction block. Examples are depicted in leads V4–V6 of Electrocardiographic Study 24, and Electrocardiographic Studies 38 and 52.

These views were propounded by Wilson *et al.* (1935)[W50], and Barker and Wallace (1952)[B7]. The condition was termed intra-infarction block by Cabrera and associates in 1959[C2]. Such islets if viable tissue within a necrotic zone were described by Burch *et al.* (1958)[B88] in necropsy studies, and by Durrer and associates (1961[D42] and 1964[D51]) in physiological studies.

PERI-INFARCTION BLOCK

Peri-infarction block is a delay in conduction through the tissues *surrounding* the infarcted area. The phenomenon is reflected in leads orientated to the surface of the infarcted area by a *late positive deflection*, an R wave, which is inscribed after the pathological Q wave of the myocardial necrosis, and thereby resulting in a Qr or QR complex.

HISTORICAL BACKGROUND

The term 'peri-infarction block' was introduced by First and associates in 1950[F14], who postulated a conduction delay around the necrotic area to explain in the phenomenon. They further postulated that the activation of healthy or relatively healthy tissue overlying an infarction which is dominantly subendocardial, cannot occur in the normal endocardial-epicardial direction. Rather, the activation front arising from neighbouring healthy subendocardial tissue has to circumnavigate the necrotic area by a circuitous route and activate the overlying healthy or relatively healthy subepicardial tissue in a tangential or oblique manner. The tangential activation front would thus be orientated to the epicardial surface overlying the necrotic area, and leads orientated to this area will consequently reflect a late R wave. No reference was made to initial disturbance of the QRS complex.

It is clear, however, that F. N. Wilson and his associates (1935[W50], 1944[W53]) previously recognized the existence of intraventricular conduction defects which occurred in association with myocardial infarction, and which were not necessarily of a bundle branch block.

The concept of peri-infarction block was given further impetus by the studies of Grant (1954[G36], 1956[G30], 1957[G31], 1959[G33]). He postulated that the basic cause was a block in one of the divisions of the left branch by the infarcted tissue; the initial QRS deformity, the pathological Q wave, being due to the loss of forces resulting from the necrosis itself, and the terminal QRS deformity, the delayed, late R wave, being due to a left bundle branch *divisional* block. He further considered that QRS prolongation need not be present, although it did occur in about 10 per cent of cases.

Cabrera and associates (1959)[C2] considered that both the initial and the potential terminal QRS deformities in myocardial infarction could be the expression of late, delayed activation of islets of viable tissue *within* the necrotic zone. In other words, they postulated that *intra*-infarction block was responsible for both deformities.

The term 'post-infarction block' has been used to describe both intra- and peri-infarction blocks (Burchell and Pruitt, 1951[B91], Durrer and associates, 1964[D51]). The prefix 'post' would, however, appear to be semantically redundant, as was pointed out by Rosenbaum and associates (1970)[R48].

The Basic Forms of Peri-infarction Block

There are two basic forms of peri-infarction block:

1. FOCAL PERI-INFARCTION BLOCK

This is a *focal* conduction abnormality complicating myocardial infarction, and is presented in detail on p. 118.

2. DIVISIONAL PERI-INFARCTION BLOCK

This is a peripheral conduction abnormality, a hemiblock, complicating myocardial infarction.

The concepts governing the hemiblocks are fundamental to the understanding of divisional peri-infarction block. They are also pertinent to the diagnosis of coronary insufficiency and myocardial infarction in general. The principles governing the hemiblocks and their significance in relation to coronary artery disease will thus be considered first. Consideration will then be given to their role and application in divisional peri-infarction block.

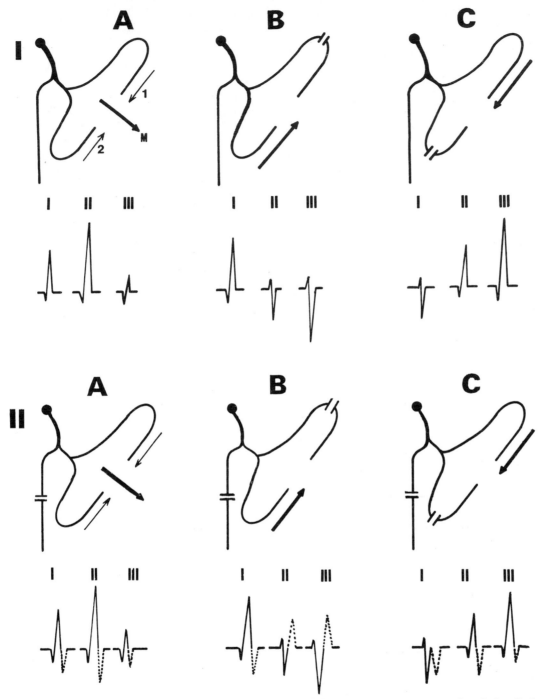

FIG. 44. Diagrams illustrating: I, the genesis of the hemiblocks; and II, the hemiblocks associated with right bundle branch block. See text.

THE HEMIBLOCKS

Basic Anatomy and Physiology

Shortly after leaving the main bundle of His, the left bundle branch divides into a number of rootlets which then proceed in two major sweeps of radiations. These constitute the two major divisions or fascicles of the left bundle branch (Diagram 1A of Fig. 44):

The **anterosuperior division** which spreads anteriorly and superiorly over the subendocardium of the lateral wall of the left ventricle.

The postero-inferior division which spreads inferiorly

and posteriorly over the diaphragmatic surface of the left ventricle.

The fibres of the two divisions meet and anastomose peripherally, forming a closed conduction network, a syncitium with rapid conduction properties.

Recent elegant work by Demoulin and Kulbertus (1972)[D13] showed that the left bundle branch has, in effect, more than two fascicles. Nevertheless, the left bundle branch appears to behave electrophysiologically as if there were only two major fascicles. This anatomical revelation does not, therefore, appear to detract materially from the electrophysiological principles governing the hemiblocks.

The anterosuperior division is relatively long and thin, whereas the posteroinferior division is relatively short and thick[R43]. Furthermore, the posteroinferior division has a double blood supply in contrast to a single blood supply for the anterosuperior division[R45]. The anterosuperior division is closer to the aortic valve, and is therefore more likely to be involved in disease processes affecting the aortic valve[R43]. All these factors contribute to the greater vulnerability of the anterosuperior division.

Conduction Within the Left Bundle Branch System
Conduction through the anterosuperior division results in an activation front directed *inferiorly and, to the right* (illustrated by Vector 1 in Diagram 1A of Fig. 44). Conduction through the posteroinferior division results in an activation front directed *superiorly and to the left* (illustrated by Vector 2 in Diagram 1A of Fig. 44). Since normal activation occurs concomitantly through both divisions, the two vectorial forces summate both complementing and modifying each other's direction, and thereby resulting in a mean QRS force or vector which is directed downward and to the left (illustrated in Vector M in Diagram 1A of Fig. 44). This normal QRS axis is, therefore, commonly directed in the region of $+60°$ on the frontal plane hexaxial reference system.

Hemiblock

When conduction is delayed or interrupted in one of the divisions of the left bundle branch, it is termed a 'hemiblock'[R48]. Perhaps a more appropriate term would be a 'left divisional block'.* When conduction is interrupted

---

* Mild exception could be taken to the use of the prefix 'hemi' in terms of block. It is semantically unsatisfactory to refer to an anatomical location of a block as a hemiblock, particularly so since 'complete block' refers to a pathological entity. Furthermore, it has recently been shown that the left bundle branch has, in effect, more than two divisions, although the pathological effect of interruption is dominantly based on two functional divisions[D13]. The term has, however, through repeated usage in recent years become an accepted entity. Thus, hemiblock will be retained in this text.

in the anterosuperior division of the left bundle branch, it is termed 'left anterior hemiblock'[R48]. The interruption may be due to *fibrosis* (as a result, for example, of coronary insufficiency) or *infarction*. When this occurs, activation will proceed predominantly or solely through the posteroinferior division of the left bundle branch, resulting in a mean frontal plane QRS axis that is directed upwards and to the left, a left axis deviation (Diagram 1B of Fig. 44).

When conduction is interrupted in the posteroinferior division of the left bundle branch, a left posterior hemiblock, activation will occur predominantly or solely through the anterosuperior division, resulting in a mean frontal plane QRS axis that is directed downward and to the right, a *right axis deviation* (Diagram 1C of Fig. 44).

The electrocardiographic characteristics of the left hemiblocks have recently received emphasis by the elegant studies of Rosenbaum and his associates[R48, R49, R50, R51, R52, R53].

Left Anterior Hemiblock

ELECTROCARDIOGRAPHIC CHARACTERISTICS
(Electrocardiographic Studies 42 and 43)

The QRS Complex

1. **The mean frontal plane QRS axis is deviated superiorly and to the left** (Diagram 1B of Fig. 44). The mean QRS axis may be located within a range extending from $-45°$ (an arbitrary lower limit set by Rosenbaum and his associates) counterclockwise to $-80°$ on the frontal plane hexaxial reference system (Vector 4 in Fig. 49). It seems likely, however, that the lower limit may well be $-30°$, since axes between $-30°$ and $-45°$ are usually pathological and, in all probability, also reflect a left anterior hemiblock. Indeed, axes between $0°$ and $-30°$ may also reflect minor degrees of left anterior hemiblock, but this requires further substantiation.

The left axis deviation will be reflected by **deep terminal S waves in Standard leads II and III, and lead AVF, and a tall R wave in lead AVL.**

The other causes of left axis deviation are considered on p. 121.

The Effect on Standard Lead II
Since the frontal plane vector loop in left anterior hemiblock is inscribed in a *counterclockwise* direction (see below), its terminal part will be located in the negative zone of Standard lead II (Fig. 45 and Diagram C of Fig. 47). Consequently, Standard lead II will *not* reflect a terminal R wave. This is an important differentiating feature from the left axis deviation of uncomplicated inferior wall infarction,

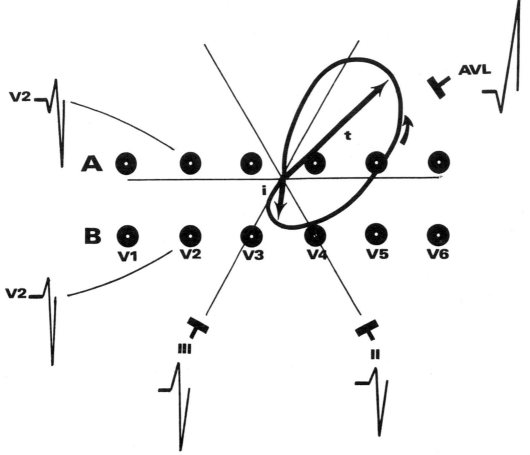

FIG. 45. Diagrammatic illustration of the frontal plane vectorcardiographic loop in left anterior hemiblock, and the initial (i) and terminal (t) QRS vectors. A reflects a relatively high precordial electrode placement. B reflects a relatively low electrode placement. See text.

which is reflected by a clockwise frontal plane vector loop. As a result, the terminal part of this loop will be located in the positive zone of Standard lead II, which will consequently reflect a terminal R wave, i.e. a QR complex (Diagram A of Fig. 47 and Diagram A1 of Fig. 26).

2. The leftwardly directed QRS forces are frequently *increased in magnitude* due to lack of opposing forces from the blocked anterosuperior division.

3. There is a *delay in the inscription of the intrinsicoid deflection* in leads orientated to the high lateral or superior aspect of the left ventricle, particularly AVL[M69, M72]. The delay may also be evident in lead AVR and, with very horizontal hearts, may indeed only be seen in lead AVR[M69, M72].

4. There may be *slurring or notching* of the R wave in lead AVR, and the descending limb of the R wave in lead AVL, and also of the S waves in leads V5 and V6[M69, M72].

5. The *initial 0·02 sec QRS vector is directed inferiorly and to the right* in the region of $+90°$ to $+120°$ on the frontal plane hexaxial reference system[R53, R61]. This will result in the following:

(a) Prominent initial q waves appear in Standard lead I and especially lead AVL. In other words, the normal initial small q waves in these leads become more prominent.

(b) Prominent initial r waves appear in Standard leads II and III and lead AVF.

The rightward deviation of the initial QRS forces may not be apparent unless pre- and post-block tracings are compared (Rosenbaum and associates, 1969)[R53]. If the pre-block tracing reflects a rightward initial force, there may merely be an inferior deviation with the onset of the left anterior hemiblock[R48]. This deviation represents a change from the normal initial midseptal activation, since the first region to be activated in left anterior hemiblock is the postero-inferior region of the left ventricle.

6. Comparison of the pre- and post-block tracings indicate that there is usually *no significant widening of the QRS complex*. If widening does occur, the increase is usually not greater than 0·02 sec.

7. *Prominent S waves appear in the left precordial leads, leads V5 and V6*[M69, M72, R48]. This is the expression of the superiorly directed main QRS force which is directed *away* from the left precordial electrodes. Consequently, an *RS or rS complex is a common finding in leads V5 and V6*. Furthermore, the *S* wave may be slurred.

8. The initial small q waves, normally present in the left precordial leads, leads V5 and V6, tend to disappear. This reflects the change from the normal initial left to right septal activation (see above).

9. The initial inferior and rightward 0·02 sec vector may result in the inscription of small initial *r* waves in the right precordial leads, leads V1–V3 (Electrodes B of Fig. 45). Thus, although the right precordial leads usually reflect the same rS complex as is inscribed during uncomplicated normal intraventricular activation, the genesis of the initial *r* wave is probably different. The initial *r* wave may also be accentuated (Electrocardiographic Study 41). The relationship of the precordial electrodes to the electrical centre of the heart may vary at times due to their being positioned a little above the conventional level and/or a slight lowering of the heart position due, for example, to a long slender physique or emphysema (as illustrated by Electrodes A in Fig. 45). When this occurs, the initial 0·02 sec vector tends to be directed away from the lead V1–V3 electrodes, thereby resulting in obliteration of the initial *r* waves, and the inscription of small initial *q* waves. These small initial *q* waves may be mistaken for an old anteroseptal infarction.

THE T WAVE

Normally, the QRS and *T* wave vectors tend to be similarly directed on the frontal plane hexaxial reference system, the QRS-T angle being narrow and rarely exceeding 60° (Diagram A of Fig. 46). The *T* wave vector in the frontal plane is usually in the region of +8° to +78° (Cerqueira Gomes and associates 1972)[C16]. With the advent

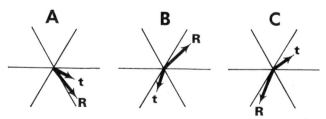

FIG. 46. Diagrams illustrating the relationship between the frontal plane QRS and *T* wave vectors with: A, normal intraventricular conduction; B, left anterior hemiblock; and C left posterior hemiblock.

of left anterior hemiblock, as with the other forms of intraventricular conduction disturbance, there are usually associated secondary abnormalities of repolarization, particularly *T* wave changes. These *T* wave changes manifest as a *T* wave vector which is *opposite in direction to the dominant, and particularly the terminal, QRS deflection*, a phenomenon similar to that which occurs with bundle branch block and ectopic ventricular beats (discussed in Chapters 9, 10 and 13). Thus, with left anterior hemiblock, the *T* wave vector tends to deviate inferiorly, more posteriorly, and at times somewhat to the right (Diagram B of Fig. 46), (Cerqueira Gomes 1972)[C16]. As a result, leads which reflect a dominantly positive QRS complex, such as Standard lead I and lead AVL, tend to have inverted *T* waves; whereas leads with a dominantly negative QRS complex, such as Standard leads II and III, and lead AVF, tend to have upright *T* waves. In other words, there is a *tendency to develop a wide frontal plane QRS-T angle*.

This secondary *T* wave change may simulate or mask the primary *T* wave changes of myocardial ischaemia and/or myocardial infarction. For example, the inverted *T* waves in Standard lead I and lead AVL may mimic the anterolateral myocardial ischaemia of coronary insufficiency or myocardial infarction. The *T* wave vector may also become more aligned with lead V5 (V6). Hence, the *T* wave may become a little taller in lead V5 (V6) and thereby tend to mask the *T* wave inversion of anterolateral left ventricular epicardial ischaemia (Cerqueira Gomes 1972)[C16]. The upright *T* waves in Standard leads II and III, and lead AVF may mask or correct the inverted *T* waves of inferior myocardial infarction[C7, C16] (Electrocardiographic Study 42).

VECTORCARDIOGRAPHIC CHARACTERISTICS
[C8, C9, C11, C15, F9, F11, F12, K48, O3, P36, R53, R61, S5, T6].

The frontal plane vector loop is inscribed in a *counterclockwise* direction. It is *wide* and *open*, with initial forces directed inferiorly and to the right, and the mean or dominant force directed superiorly and to the left (Fig. 45, Diagrams C of Figs. 47 and 48, and Diagram A of Fig. 52). The loop is frequently *increased in magnitude* due to the lack of balancing forces from the blocked anterosuperior division.

The *intermediate and terminal parts of the loop may be slurred*, reflecting slow activation of the basal part of the left ventricle[M69]. This may imply the presence of a concomitant left anterior parietal block.

COMMENTS

1. The initial inferior and rightward forces resulting from

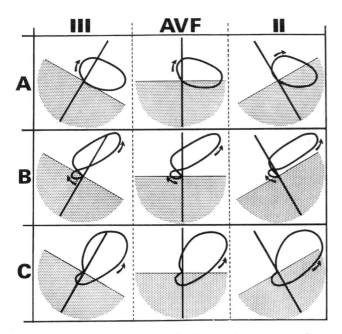

FIG. 47. Diagrams illustrating the frontal plane vectorcardiographic loop and its relationship to the Standard lead III, lead AVF, and Standard lead II lead axes in: A, inferior wall myocardial infarction; B, inferior wall myocardial infarction associated with left anterior hemiblock; and C, uncomplicated left anterior hemiblock.

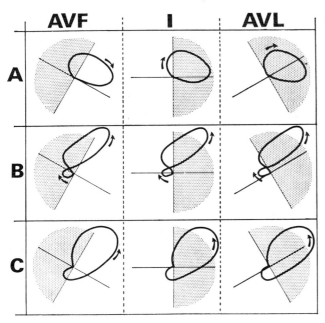

FIG. 48. Diagrams illustrating the frontal plane vectorcardiographic loop and its relationship to the lead AVR, Standard lead I, and lead AVL lead axes in: A, inferior wall myocardial infarction; B, inferior wall myocardial infarction associated with left anterior hemiblock; and C, uncomplicated left anterior hemiblock.

the initial activation of the postero-inferior wall may obliterate or mask the pathological Q wave of inferior wall myocardial infarction, an infarction which involves predominantly the anterior region of the inferior wall (see p. 110).

2. The tiny initial q waves which may appear in leads V1–V3. (see section 9 above) may simulate old anteroseptal infarction.

3. If the initial inferior and rightward 0·02 sec QRS vector results in small initial r waves in leads V1–V3 (see section 9 above) it may mask or modify an anteroseptal infarction, since the QS complexes of the infarction will be transformed into rS complexes (see p. 111, and Electrocardiographic Study 60A). See also Electrocardiographic Study 41.

Left anterior hemiblock was found to be the commonest intraventricular conduction defect in a general hospital population (Cerqueira Gomes and associates, 1970)[C17], constituting 2·6 per cent of 13,061 electrocardiograms recorded over a 10-year period. The significance of left anterior hemiblock in relationship to coronary artery disease is discussed on p. 109.

Note: The causes of left axis deviation are considered in a Correlative Essay on p. 121.

Left Posterior Hemiblock

ELECTROCARDIOGRAPHIC CHARACTERISTICS
(Electrocardiographic Studies 46 and 47)

THE QRS COMPLEX

1. The mean manifest frontal plane QRS axis is rightwardly directed to the region of +90° to +120° on the hexaxial reference system (Vectar 1 in Fig. 49). This results in prominent S waves in Standard lead I and lead AVL, and a tall R wave (of a qR complex) in Standard leads II, III and lead AVF. The R wave is particularly tall in Standard lead III. Other causes of right axis deviation, such as right ventricular dominance, must be excluded on both clinical *and* electrocardiographic grounds before the diagnosis of right posterior hemiblock can be established. Left posterior hemiblock is consequently not a pure electrocardiographic diagnosis, but always a clinical-electrocardiographic correlation.

2. The *mean QRS axis may be increased in magnitude* due to the lack of balancing forces from the posterior division.

3. The QRS complex is not necessarily increased in duration. If widening of the QRS complex does occur, such widening is usually not more than 0·02 sec in duration.

4. The initial 0·02 sec forces are directed superiorly and

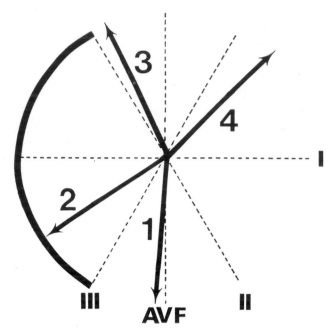

FIG. 49. Diagram illustrating the location of various terminal QRS vectors. See text.

to the left in the region of $-50°$ on the frontal plane hexaxial reference system. These forces are due to early activation of the posterolateral wall of the left ventricle, and result in a small initial r wave in Standard lead I and a small, but prominent, initial q wave in Standard leads II, III and lead AVF. The normal small q wave in these leads is increased in magnitude.

5. There is a *delay in the onset of the intrinsicoid deflection* in lead AVF, to 0·45 sec or longer[B76].

6. The distal limb of the R wave in Standard lead III and lead AVF is frequently notched or slurred[B76].

THE T WAVE

As with other forms of intraventricular conduction disturbances, left posterior hemiblock is usually associated with secondary abnormalities of repolarization, particularly T wave changes. The T wave vectors tend to be opposite in direction to the dominant QRS deflection. Thus, the T wave vector is directed to $-30°$ on the frontal plane hexaxial reference system, i.e. opposite to that of the main QRS axis (Diagram C of Fig. 46). As a result, leads with a dominantly positive QRS complex, Standard leads II and III and lead AVF, tend to have inverted T waves. Leads with a dominantly negative QRS complex, Standard lead I tend to have upright T waves. In other words, there is a tendency to develop a wide frontal plane QRS-T angle.

These secondary T wave changes may simulate or mask the primary T wave changes of ischaemia and/or infarction.

For example, the inverted T waves in Standard leads II and III and lead AVF may mimic the inferior ischaemia of coronary insufficiency or inferior wall myocardial infarction. The upright T waves in Standard lead I and lead AVL may mask or correct the inverted T waves of anterolateral myocardial infarction (Electrocardiographic Study 48).

VECTORCARDIOGRAPHIC CHARACTERISTICS

The frontal plane vector loop is inscribed in a *clockwise direction*[F9, F11, F12]. The initial forces are inscribed superiorly and to the left, and the mean or dominant force is inscribed inferiorly and to the right (Diagram B of Fig. 50). The loop is frequently *increased in magnitude* due to the lack of balancing forces from the blocked posteroinferior division.

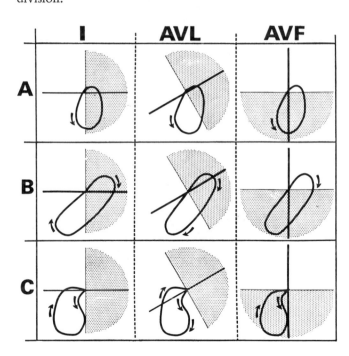

FIG. 50. Diagrams illustrating the frontal plane vectorcardiographic loop and its relationship to the Standard lead I, lead AVL and lead AVF lead axes in: A, uncomplicated anterolateral myocardial infarction; B, uncomplicated left posterior hemiblock; and C, anterolateral myocardial infarction associated with left posterior hemiblock. Compare with Fig. 55.

Left posterior hemiblock, occurring as an isolated phenomenon, is very rare. It occurred in 0·01 per cent of 13,061 electrocardiograms recorded over a 10-year period in a general hospital population (Cerqueira Gomes and associates 1970)[C17]. The significance of left posterior hemiblock in relationship to coronary artery disease is discussed on p. 112.

THE SIGNIFICANCE OF THE LEFT HEMIBLOCKS IN RELATION TO CORONARY ARTERY DISEASE

The left hemiblocks have an important bearing on the electrocardiographic diagnosis of coronary artery disease:

1. They may simulate the electrocardiographic manifestations of myocardial infarction.

2. They may modify or mask the electrocardiographic manifestations of myocardial infarction.

3. They may complicate myocardial infarction, forming an integral part of divisional peri-infarction block.

4. Left anterior hemiblock (a left axis deviation) and left posterior hemiblock may reflect the presence of coronary insufficiency. (See Chapter 15).

5. The hemiblocks may herald the development of complete bilateral bundle branch block.

The first three of these categories are considered in detail below.

1 Simulation of the Electrocardiographic Manifestations of Myocardial Infarction by the Left Hemiblocks

Left anterior hemiblock may, at times, simulate high-lateral myocardial infarction or anteroseptal myocardial infarction.

SIMULATION OF HIGH-LATERAL MYOCARDIAL INFARCTION

THE EFFECT ON THE QRS COMPLEX

In left anterior hemiblock, the initial 0·02 sec vector is directed inferiorly and to the right. This is reflected by a prominent q wave of the qR complex in Standard lead I and lead AVL. The q wave, particularly in lead AVL, may at times be, or appear to be, significantly large, thereby simulating a high-anterolateral myocardial infarction, especially an old high-lateral myocardial infarction, since there are usually no S-T segment or T wave signs of acute myocardial infarction. The distinction from true infarction is based on the following:

(a) The q wave does not reach the pathological duration of 0·04 sec.

(b) There is no marked reciprocal widening of the initial r waves (of the rS complexes) in Standard leads II and III and lead AVF to 0·04 sec, as would be expected in high-lateral myocardial infarction complicated by left anterior hemiblock.

(c) There are no S-T segment changes of acute myocardial infarction.

THE EFFECT ON THE T WAVE

Anterolateral myocardial infarction may be further simulated by the secondary T wave changes of left anterior hemiblock (see above, p. 106). This causes inverted T waves in Standard lead I and lead AVL which may simulate the anterolateral ischaemia of coronary insufficiency or anterolateral myocardial infarction.

SIMULATION OF ANTEROSEPTAL MYOCARDIAL INFARCTION

The inferior and rightward direction of the initial 0·02 sec vector in left anterior hemiblock may result in the inscription of small initial q waves in leads V1–V3. This will then be reflected by qrS complexes, which may simulate anteroseptal infarction. This manifestation is especially likely if the electrodes are incorrectly placed slightly above the conventional level, namely relatively high to the electrical centre of the heart and/or associated with the downward displacement of the heart, as would occur in individuals with a slender physique or emphysema (Electrodes A of Fig. 45). The differentiation from infarction is based on the following:

(a) The q waves do not reach the pathological duration of 0·04 sec.

(b) There are no S-T segment and T wave changes of infarction.

(c) The small initial q waves will disappear when the electrodes are placed at a slightly lower level, whereas they will persist or become accentuated in the case of true anteroseptal myocardial infarction.

2 The Modification or Masking of the Electrocardiographic Manifestations of Myocardial Infarction by Left Hemiblock

Left anterior hemiblock may mask or modify the electrocardiographic manifestations of myocardial infarction, anteroseptal myocardial infarction and anterolateral myocardial infarction.

MODIFICATION OF THE ELECTROCARDIOGRAPHIC EFFECTS OF INFERIOR MYOCARDIAL INFARCTION BY LEFT ANTERIOR HEMIBLOCK

THE EFFECTS ON THE QRS COMPLEX

The inferior and rightward initial 0·02 sec vectors may

mask or modify the pathological Q waves of inferior myocardial infarction.

The pathological Q wave of inferior myocardial infarction is the expression of a superiorly directed initial 0·04 sec vector (see Chapter 5). The initial inferior and rightward vector of left anterior hemiblock will therefore tend to oppose the superiorly directed initial 0·04 sec QRS vector of the inferior infarction, and will consequently obliterate or modify the pathological Q waves of the infarction[A8, C7, R48].

The principle may, prima facie, appear a little paradoxical, for if the infarction obliterates the normal activation process of the inferior wall, it should also obliterate the initial 0·02 sec vector of the left anterior hemiblock, since this also reflects early activation of the inferior wall.

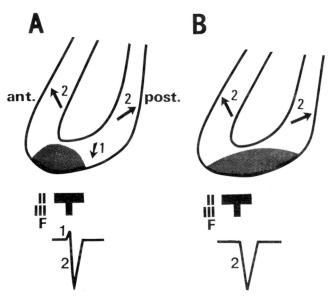

FIG. 51. Diagrams illustrating: A, infarction involving the anterior region of the inferior wall; and B, extensive inferior wall myocardial infarction. See text.

Rosenbaum and associates (1970)[R48] suggest the following hypothesis to explain the so-called paradox: Left anterior hemiblock results in early activation of the *posterior region of the inferior wall*, the area around the posterior papillary muscle. Thus, if the infarction involves the whole inferior wall, anterior as well as posterior regions, the initial vectors of both normal activation and that resulting from left anterior hemiblock will be obliterated (Diagram B of Fig. 51). If, however, the infarction involves predominantly the anterior region of the inferior wall, the unaffected posterior region of the inferior wall will, as a result of a complicating left anterior hemiblock, generate an inferior force which will tend to oppose, and hence obliterate or modify, the initial pathological Q waves (Diagram A of

Fig. 51). The modification of the inferior infarction may take one of the following forms:

(a) The signs of infarction may be obliterated. The QS complexes or the pathological Q waves of the QR complexes in Standard leads II and III and lead AVF of uncomplicated inferior wall myocardial infarction may be changed to rS complexes (Electrocardiographic Studies 44 and 45). When this occurs, however, the initial r wave (of the rS complex) is often tallest in Standard lead III, less tall in lead AVF, and minimal or absent in Standard lead II which usually reflects a QS complex (Diagram F of Fig. 25; Electrocardiographic Study 44). This contrasts with uncomplicated left anterior hemiblock where the initial r waves are usually of equal amplitude in Standard leads II and III and lead AVF (Diagram E of Fig. 25; Electrocardiographic Study 41). In the case of old, chronic, inferior wall myocardial infarction, however, it may be necessary to have pre- and post-block tracings to establish the diagnosis. An example of this is published by Rosenbaum and associates (1970)[R48], their Figs. 7 and 8 in Chapter X.

(b) All the inferior orientated leads, Standard leads II and III and lead AVF, reflect *initial incidents* (Electrocardiographic Study 37). Standard lead III may reflect a small initial ledge or step followed by the major smooth negative deflection of the dominant negative QS deflection. Lead AVF may be similarly, though not so conspicuously, modified. The initial negativity has a slight forward slope. The ledge is small, in most cases merely constituting an angulation in the proximal limb of the QRS deflection.

(c) The initial negative incident described above may be preceded by a very small, at times barely perceptible, r wave which will be most prominent in Standard lead III, least prominent in lead AVF, and absent in Standard lead II which may show a small initial q wave, a qrS complex (Diagram G of Fig. 25; Electrocardiographic Study 37). An example of this manifestation was published by Grant (1959, his Fig. 4)[G33]. Since the inscription of the initial incident is a little slower than the rest of the QRS deflection, it is a little thicker and hence slightly more conspicuous than the rest of the QRS complex. This is evident in Fig. 11, Chapter X of Rosenbaum and associates (1970)[R48].

(d) The dominantly negative deflections in Standard leads II and III and lead AVF may reflect very small initial rs complexes. The entire inscription thus presents as an rsr 'S' complex (Diagram H of Fig. 25; Electrocardiographic Studies 18 and 25).

As indicated by Castellanos and associates (1971)[C7], Standard lead II is probably the most useful indicator for distinguishing between the left axis deviation of uncomplicated inferior wall myocardial infarction and inferior wall myocardial infarction complicated by left anterior hemiblock.

A terminal r or R wave (of a Qr of QR complex) would indicate uncomplicated inferior wall myocardial infarction, since a terminal positivity does not occur with left anterior hemiblock.

A QS complex with initial slurring or deformity would indicate inferior wall myocardial infarction with left anterior hemiblock.

These aspects are considered further in the Correlative Essay on The Differential Diagnosis of the Terminal and Initial QRS Vectors in Inferior Wall Myocardial Infarction (p. 119).

When acute inferior wall myocardial infarction is complicated by left anterior hemiblock, the presence of infarction may also be diagnosed from the concomitant signs of myocardial injury and ischaemia, the raised S-T segments and inverted T waves (Electrocardiographic Study 45).

THE EFFECTS ON THE T WAVE

Left anterior hemiblock is frequently associated with secondary T wave changes which are upright in Standard leads II and III and lead AVF (discussed in greater detail earlier in this Chapter, p. 106 and 108). This may consequently modify or correct the inverted T waves of inferior wall myocardial infarction (Cerqueira Gomes, 1972[C7, C16]; Electrocardiographic Studies 44 and 45).

MODIFICATION OF THE ELECTROCARDIO-GRAPHIC EFFECTS OF ANTEROSEPTAL MYOCARDIAL INFARCTION BY LEFT ANTERIOR HEMIBLOCK

The initial inferior and rightward 0·02 sec vector of left anterior hemiblock may result in the inscription of small initial r waves in the right precordial leads, leads V1–V3 (Electrocardiographic Study 60A). This may consequently mask anteroseptal infarction[A8, R48]. It is particularly likely to occur if the electrodes are placed a little low relative to the heart position, i.e. just below the conventional placements (Electrodes B of Fig. 45). The diagnosis of incorrect placement is further substantiated if all the QRS complexes of the precordial leads tend to resemble lead AVF (Electrocardiographic Study 60A). The manifestation may, however, cause some difficulty in the case of old, chronic, anteroseptal infarction when the characteristic S-T segment and T wave abnormalities of the acute incident are not present. The diagnosis can be established by recording the electrocardiogram with the electrodes in a slightly (mini-

mally) higher position. This will usually obliterate these initial r waves[R48].

MODIFICATION OF THE ELECTROCARDIO-GRAPHIC EFFECTS OF ANTEROLATERAL MYOCARDIAL INFARCTION BY THE LEFT HEMIBLOCKS

The electrocardiographic manifestations of anterolateral infarction may be modified by both left anterior and left posterior hemiblock.

MODIFICATION OF ANTEROLATERAL INFARCTION BY LEFT ANTERIOR HEMIBLOCK

The frontal plane vectorcardiographic loop with a large anterolateral transmural infarction is inscribed in a counter-clockwise direction. See next section, p. 112, for greater detail.

In uncomplicated left anterior hemiblock, the initial vector is directed inferiorly and to the right, resulting in prominent initial r waves in Standard leads II and III and lead AVF, and prominent initial q waves in Standard lead I and lead AVL. The terminal vector is directed upwards and to the left, resulting in prominent R waves in Standard lead I and lead AVL, and deep S waves in Standard leads II and III and lead AVF (Diagram A of Fig. 52; see Fig. 45, Diagrams C of Fig. 47 and 48, and Fig. 53A). The loop is inscribed in a counter-clockwise direction.

When left anterior hemiblock is associated with a large anterolateral infarction, the loop is still inscribed in a counter-clockwise direction, and the initial forces are also directed inferiorly (Diagram B of Fig. 52). The terminal or dominant forces, however, are now deviated superiorly *and to the right*. This dominant force now occurs within the negative zone of Standard lead I as well as Standard leads II and III. This results in a deep negative pathological Q wave in Standard lead I (since both the initial and terminal vectors occur within the negative zone of this lead). The terminal or dominant force, however, still occurs within the positive zone of lead AVL, which will consequently still reflect a dominantly positive terminal R wave, although this will not be as tall as in uncomplicated left anterior hemiblock. The inscription of this terminal R wave will be somewhat delayed, the ventricular activation time will be increased, and it will be preceded by a prominent Q wave. Standard lead II and III will still reflect rS complexes as with uncomplicated left anterior hemiblock. Note that **all three Standard leads now reflect dominantly negative QRS complexes**[B93, G19, L46].

Occasionally, the dominant loop may still be partly in the positive zone of Standard lead I, in which case this lead

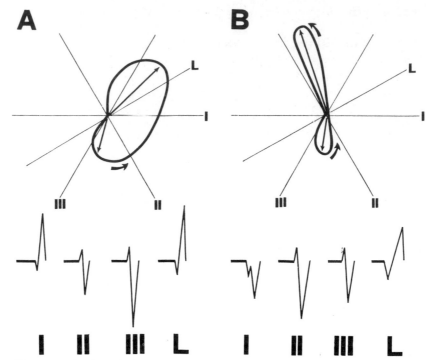

FIG. 52. Diagram illustrating the frontal plane vector and electrocardiograms in: A, uncomplicated left anterior hemiblock; and B, left anterior hemiblock associated with anterolateral myocardial infarction.

will reflect a terminal r or R wave (of a Qr or QR complex). This terminal r or R wave will, under this circumstance, be smaller than the terminal R wave in lead AVL (Electrocardiographic Study 41).

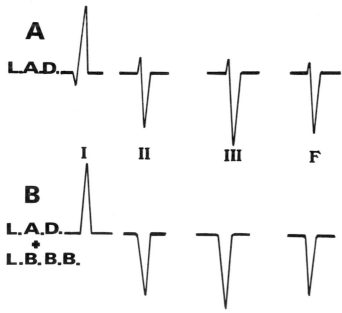

FIG. 53. Diagrams illustrating: A, uncomplicated left axis deviation; and B, left axis deviation associated with incomplete left bundle branch block.

MODIFICATION OF ANTEROLATERAL INFARCTION BY LEFT POSTERIOR HEMIBLOCK

The vector and electrocardiographic features of uncomplicated anterolateral infarction, and uncomplicated left posterior hemiblock will be presented first. Consideration will then be given to the two in combination.

Uncomplicated Anterolateral Myocardial Infarction

A large transmural anterolateral myocardial infarction, or its subdivision of high-lateral myocardial infarction, manifesting with QS complexes in Standard lead I and lead AVL, results in a *rightward deviation of the frontal plane QRS forces* (Fig. 54). This may also occur with a septolateral infarction—an anteroseptal infarction associated with high-lateral infarction. This is because the QRS forces normally generated by this region are directed superiorly and somewhat to the left. Hence, loss of these forces will result in the dominant QRS forces being directed away from the infarction, viz. the lateral and superior surface of the left ventricle, and thus inferiorly and towards the right (Electrocardiographic Studies 11 and 12). Since left posterior hemiblock also presents with a right axis deviation, the association of the two phenomena in the same tracing presents some difficulty in diagnosis. This is considered further below.

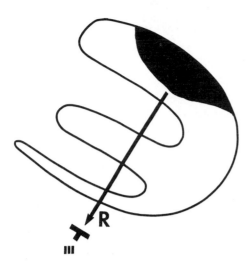

FIG. 54. Diagram illustrating the mean QRS axis in high-lateral myocardial infarction. See text.

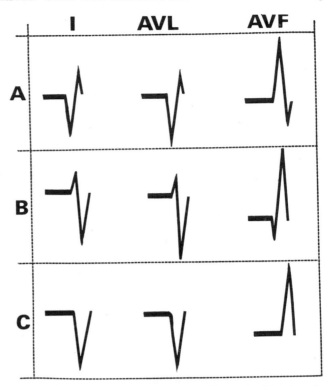

FIG. 55. QRS configurations in Standard lead I, lead AVL, and lead AVF in: A, uncomplicated anterolateral myocardial infarction; B, uncomplicated left posterior hemiblock; and C, anterolateral myocardial infarction associated with left posterior hemiblock. Compare with Fig. 50.

Uncomplicated anterolateral myocardial infarction is usually associated with a terminal r wave in Standard lead I, and less commonly in lead AVL. In other words, the pathological Q wave in these leads is followed by a terminal r wave resulting in a Qr complex. This, as stated, is invariably so in Standard lead I (Electrocardiographic Study 5B).

The dominantly positive R wave in lead AVF is at times followed by a terminal s wave in lead AVF.

The aforementioned manifestations are due to the counter-clockwise rotation of the frontal plane loop which is directed inferiorly, and with extensive lateral infarction somewhat to the right (Diagram A of Fig. 50). The initial part of this loop is located in the negative zones of Standard lead I and lead AVL, hence the pathological Q waves in these leads. The terminal part of the loop is located in the positive zones of Standard lead I and possibly lead AVL, resulting with the terminal r wave in these leads (Diagram A of Fig. 55).

The dominant part of the loop is located almost entirely within the positive zone of lead AVF (Diagram A of Fig. 50); hence the dominantly positive QRS complex in this lead (Diagram A of Fig. 55). Moreover, since the loop is inscribed in a counter-clockwise direction, it enters the positive zone of lead AVF immediately, so that there is no initial q wave. The terminal part of the loop may enter the negative zone of lead AVF (Diagram A of Fig. 50), resulting in a small terminal s wave in this lead (Diagram A of Fig. 55). This lead frequently reflects an R wave only (Electrocardiographic Study 5B).

Uncomplicated Left Posterior Hemiblock

Contrast the aforementioned events with those associated with left posterior hemiblock (Diagram B of Fig. 50), where the loop is inscribed in a clockwise direction and is also directed inferiorly and to the right. This means that its initial part enters the negative zone of lead AVF first, thereby resulting in a prominent initial q wave (Diagram B of Fig. 55). The main part of the loop is also located within the positive zone of lead AVF, hence the tall R wave in this lead. These features are reflected in Electrocardiographic Studies 46 and 47. Due to the clockwise rotation of the frontal plane loop, the initial part of the loop is situated within the positive zones of Standard lead I and lead AVL (Diagram B of Fig. 50), which consequently reflect initial r waves. The dominant and terminal parts of the loop are situated in the negative zones of Standard lead I and lead AVL, which consequently reflect deep terminal S waves (Diagram B of Fig. 55).

Anterolateral Myocardial Infarction Associated with Left Posterior Hemiblock

When anterolateral myocardial infarction is associated with left posterior hemiblock, the electrocardiogram manifests with the following features:

(a) Standard lead I and lead AVL reflect pure QS complexes, i.e. there are *no* terminal *r* waves in these leads.

(b) Lead AVF presents with a pure *R* wave, i.e. there is *no* terminal *s* wave.

These features are reflected in Diagram C of Fig. 55 and Electrocardiographic Studies 11 and 12B.

The mechanism of these electrocardiographic manifestations is evident from the frontal plane vector loop (Diagram C of Fig. 50). The initial part of the loop is inscribed inferiorly and to the right in a *counter-clockwise* direction (as with uncomplicated anterolateral myocardial infarction). It is then inscribed inferiorly and to the right in a *clockwise* direction[F9]. This means that the entire loop is situated within the negative zones of Standard lead I and lead AVL, hence the pure QS complexes in these leads, and entirely within the positive zone of lead AVF, resulting with the pure *R* wave in this lead.

3 Left Hemiblock as Complications of Myocardial Infarction

Left anterior hemiblock is a relatively common complication of myocardial infarction. It is especially prone to occur with anterolateral and anteroseptal infarction[C17]. When it occurs in association with inferior wall myocardial infarction, the diagnosis may occasion some difficulty since both conditions result in a left axis deviation. The differential diagnosis is considered on p. 120.

Left posterior divisional hemiblock is a rare complication of myocardial infarction, and only a few cases have been reported [D11, R48, V4, W1]. It may occur in association with right bundle branch block[B64, D11, R48, V4], and may even occur as a transient phenomenon[B64, D11, R48, W1] (Electrocardiographic Study 48). When it occurs in association with anterolateral myocardial infarction, it may cause some difficulty in diagnosis, since both conditions are associated with a dominant right axis deviation. The differential diagnosis is considered on p. 113.

Masquerading Bundle Branch Block

'Masquerading' bundle branch block is basically a right bundle branch block with a left anterior hemiblock which appear, at first glance, to resemble the pattern of left bundle branch block in the frontal plane leads. The principles governing this manifestation are illustrated with reference to the Standard leads (Fig. 56). There are four principal phases which do not necessarily occur in the chronological sequence depicted below:

1. Left anterior hemiblock.

2. Left anterior hemiblock with right bundle branch block.

3. Left anterior hemiblock with right bundle branch block and diminution of the terminal vectors.

4. Left anterior hemiblock with right bundle branch block, diminution of the terminal vectors, and diminution of the initial vectors.

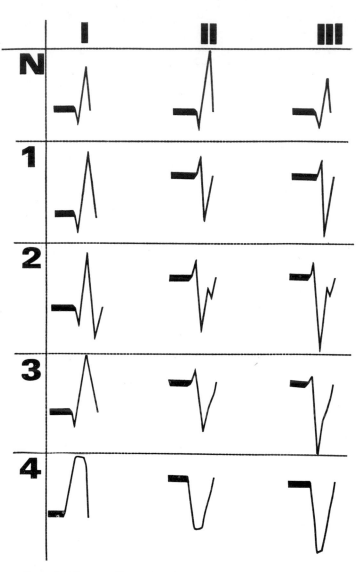

FIG. 56. Diagrams illustrating the genesis of the QRS pattern in 'masquerading' bundle branch block. See text.

Diagram 1 of Fig. 56 illustrates uncomplicated left anterior hemiblock. Standard lead I reflects a prominent initial *q* wave with a relatively tall *R* wave. Standard leads II and III reflect prominent initial *r* waves and deep terminal *S* waves.

Diagram 2 of Fig. 56 illustrates the left anterior hemiblock in association with right bundle branch block. This results in the addition of terminal QRS vectors, a terminal slurred S wave in Standard lead I and terminal R' waves in Standard leads II and III. Note that the initial vectors are unchanged by the advent of the right bundle branch block. It is of interest to note that the depth of the S wave in Standard lead I is inversely proportional to the magnitude of the S waves in Standard leads II and III. In other words, the greater the degree of left anterior hemiblock or the greater the degree of the left axis deviation, the smaller the terminal S wave in Standard lead I.

Diagram 3 of Fig. 56 illustrates the total diminution, i.e. disappearance of the terminal S wave in Standard lead I and the terminal R' waves in Standard leads II and III. The terminal deflection is, so to speak, absorbed into the QRS complex which is widened. This may be due to:

(a) the presence of concomitant left anterior parietal block,

(b) the presence of concomitant left ventricular hypertrophy,

(c) the presence of a very high degree of left anterior hemiblock.

Diagram 4 of Fig. 56 illustrates the disappearance of the initial q wave in Standard lead I and the initial r waves in Standard leads II and III. The commonest cause of this is the presence of concomitant inferior wall infarction. The final electrocardiographic presentation, as reflected in the Standard leads, is now one of wide, bizarre QRS complexes which are negative in Standard leads II and III, and positive in Standard lead I. This mimics or masquerades as left bundle branch block.

THE SIGNIFICANCE OF MASQUERADING BUNDLE BRANCH BLOCK

The commonest causes of right bundle branch block associated with left anterior hemiblock are coronary artery disease (fibrosis and/or infarction) and long-standing systemic hypertension (Rosenbaum and associates, 1970)[R48]. When myocardial infarction is associated with right bundle branch block and left anterior hemiblock, the usual site of the infarction is anteroseptal. The association has been frequently reported[G6, L18, M6, M7, M88, R49, S136, S147]. At times, the right bundle branch block may be due to a septal infarction, and the left anterior hemiblock may result from an anterolateral infarction[R48].

Other common causes of right bundle branch block with left anterior hemiblock are Lenegre's disease[L19] (idiopathic degeneration of the conducting system) and Lev's disease[L33] (calcarious encroachment on the conducting system from

neighbouring structures, e.g. calcific aortic disease).

Less common causes are cardiomyopathy, and Chaga's myocarditis[R42, R46]. All these aforementioned pathologies may be applicable to masquerading bundle branch block. The commonest cause, however, would seem to be myocardial infarction. Thus, in 12 cases reported by Lenegre[L19] all had massive myocardial infarction. The anterior wall was affected in 10 of these cases. Both bundle branches were severely affected in all 12 of these cases, the right more so than the left. Lenegre also indicated that masquerading bundle branch block may be due to severe fibrosis, in the absence of infarction, which injures both the bundle branch systems.

The presence of masquerading bundle branch block indicates a poor prognosis[C17].

Divisional Peri-infarction Block

Divisional peri-infarction block is characterized electrocardiographically by two basic abnormalities:

1. An abnormality of the initial QRS forces due to the necrosis itself and which is directed *away* from the infarcted area. This is responsible for the inscription of the pathological Q wave in leads orientated to the infarcted area, the genesis of which is considered in Chapters 1 and 3.

2. An abnormality of the terminal forces, the expression of the late activation of the tissues surrounding the necrosis, and which is directed *towards* the infarcted area. These forces are responsible for the inscription of the late R wave in leads orientated to the infarcted zone.

Note: In order to establish the diagnosis of divisional peri-infarction block, it must be evident that the terminal QRS vector abnormalities are related to, dependent upon, or caused by the factors causing the initial QRS vector abnormalities.

Divisional peri-infarction block thus reflects the association of the initial QRS abnormalities of myocardial necrosis with the conduction abnormalities of a left hemiblock. There are two principal forms:

1. Inferior or diaphragmatic peri-infarction block.
2. Anterolateral peri-infarction block.

INFERIOR-DIAPHRAGMATIC-PERI-INFARCTION BLOCK

Inferior diaphragmatic peri-infarction block occurs as a complication of inferior wall myocardial infarction. It is reflected electrocardiographically by a wide angle between the initial 0·04 sec QRS vector and the terminal 0·04 sec

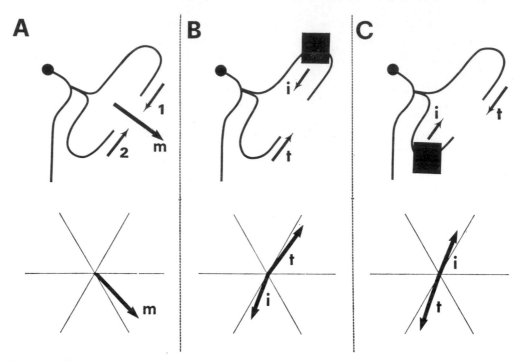

FIG. 57. Diagrams illustrating the genesis of: A, the mean QRS axis (m) with normal intraventricular conduction; B, the initial (i) and terminal (t) QRS vectors with anterolateral peri-infarction block; and C, the initial (i) and terminal (t) QRS vectors with diaphragmatic peri-infarction block.

QRS vector. The necrosis of the inferior wall results in the inscription of an initial 0·04 sec QRS vector which is directed away from the inferior wall, i.e. *superiorly and slightly to the left* in the region of −60° to −80° on the frontal plane hexaxial reference system. This results in wide and deep pathological Q waves (0·04 sec or longer) in Standard leads II and III and lead AVF (initial Vector labelled i in Diagram C of Fig. 57). If the infarction interrupts the posteroinferior division (as illustrated in Diagram C of Fig. 57), terminal activation will be effected through the anterosuperior division of the left bundle branch, thereby resulting in the inscription of a terminal 0·04 sec QRS vector which is directed *downwards and to the right* in the region of +90° to +100° on the frontal plane hexaxial reference system, a left posterior hemiblock. This is reflected by the late *terminal R* waves in Standard leads II and III and lead AVF, which will consequently reflect QR complexes (Diagram C of Fig. 57; Diagram B of Fig. 25; Electrocardiographic Studies 49 and 50). The angle between the initial and terminal QRS vectors is wide and exceeds 110°, being virtually opposite in direction (Grant, 1959)[G33]. The terminal right axis deviation, the left posterior hemiblock, in this case is associated with, and due to, the inferior wall necrosis, as reflected by the initial QRS deformity, thereby establishing the diagnosis of inferior, diaphragmatic, peri-infarction block.

When inferior infarction is associated with left posterior hemiblock, the ratio of the pathological Q waves to the potential ensuing R wave is changed. The R waves become taller and the preceding Q wave constitutes but a relatively small percentage of the QRS deflection (Diagram B of Fig. 25).

ANTEROLATERAL PERI-INFARCTION BLOCK

Anterolateral peri-infarction block may be a complication of anteroseptal and particularly high-lateral myocardial infarction. The necrosis of high anterolateral wall myocardial infarction results in the inscription of:

(a) an initial 0·04 sec QRS vector which is directed inferiorly, i.e. *away* from the anterolateral surface and which is the expression of the anterolateral necrosis;

(b) an interruption of the anterosuperior division of the left bundle branch which results in a terminal vector directed *towards* the anterolateral surface, and is the expression of left anterior hemiblock (Diagram B of Fig. 57; Electrocardiographic Study 41).

The angle between the initial and terminal QRS vectors is wide and exceeds +110°, being virtually opposite in direction.

SUMMARY

TABLE 4 Disturbances of intraventricular conduction

DISTURBANCE	INITIAL 0·04 SEC VECTOR	TERMINAL 0·04 SEC VECTOR
Arterolateral peri-infarction block	Inferior and to the right	Superior and to the left
Diaphragmatic peri-infarction block	Superior and to the left	Inferior and to the right
Uncomplicated left-axis deviation—left anterior divisional hemiblock	Normal	Superior and to the left
Uncomplicated right-axis deviation—left posterior divisional hemiblock	Normal	Inferior and to the right

Further Observations

THE ONSET OF PERI-INFARCTION BLOCK

The complication of peri-infarction block is not invariable in the course of myocardial infarction. When it occurs, it is usually sudden in onset commonly manifesting within a few days after the onset of the infarction. Since serial electrocardiographic tracings are frequently recorded during the first few days of the infarction, pre- and post-block tracings are frequently obtained.

THE MAGNITUDE OF THE TERMINAL 0·04 SEC QRS VECTOR

The magnitude of the terminal R wave in divisional peri-infarction block is usually greater than in focal peri-infarction block (see below). The magnitude is usually greater in anterolateral peri-infarction block (where it may be as much as 15 mm) than in diaphragmatic peri-infarction block (where it usually only reaches a maximum of 10 mm).

PERI-INFARCTION BLOCK WITH QRS PROLONGATION

Diaphragmatic or anterolateral peri-infarction block may be associated with QRS prolongation in about 10 per cent of cases (Grant, 1959)[G33]. This usually occurs late and uneventfully during the course of recovery from the myocardial infarction. The prolongation affects the terminal QRS forces only. The QRS complex may be prolonged and may be 0·14–0·16 sec in duration. The common manifestation is a qR complex with wide and notched terminal R wave. In the case of anterolateral peri-infarction block, this is usually best seen in leads orientated to the left ventricle, Standard lead I, lead AVL and leads V5 and V6 (Electrocardiographic Study 41). The manifestation may mimic left bundle branch block, and the differentiation may be difficult.

In anterolateral peri-infarction block there is always a wide angle between initial and terminal 0·04 sec QRS vectors, whereas this is not necessarily so in left bundle branch block. In anterolateral peri-infarction block the terminal QRS vector is always deviated superiorly and to the left, whereas this is not necessarily so in left bundle branch block. The small initial q wave (in association with the broad and tall notched R wave) in the left precordial leads may mimic infarction of the lower right third of the interventricular septum complicated by left bundle branch block (see p. 89). Such isolated infarction of the lower (right) third of the interventricular septum is rare, since the infarction usually involves the left side of the interventricular septum as well. When this occurs, the first part of the notched R wave will be diminished in amplitude (see Chapter 10). Thus, when a qRR′ complex appears in leads V5 and V6, and the initial R is tall and not attenuated, the diagnosis of anterolateral peri-infarction block is favoured. If the R wave is somewhat attenuated, presenting as a qrR′ complex, then the diagnosis of complete left bundle branch block with septal infarction is suggested (see Chapter 10).

SUMMARY

The Salient Features of Divisional Peri-infarction Block

1. Divisional peri-infarction block is characterized by *both* initial and terminal 0·04 sec QRS vector abnormalities.

2. The initial 0·04 sec QRS vector is directed *away* from the infarction.

3. The terminal 0·04 sec QRS vector is directed *towards* the infarction.

4. Divisional peri-infarction block is commonly associated with specific infarction sites, high-lateral, anteroseptal, and diaphragmatic.

5. Divisional peri-infarction block is associated with specific terminal QRS axes:

(a) Left axis of approximately −60° in anterolateral peri-infarction block.

(b) Right axis of approximately +90° to +100° in diaphragmatic peri-infarction block.

6. The terminal QRS magnitudes, the terminal R waves in leads orientated to the infarction, are relatively large.

7. The complication is not invariable.

8. The onset is sudden, usually occurring within a few days after the beginning of the infarction.

9. The manifestation may be intermittent.

10. Peri-infarction block is associated with prolongation of the terminal QRS vector in 10 per cent of cases.

11. Anterolateral peri-infarction block with terminal QRS prolongation may simulate low septal infarction complicated by left bundle branch block.

12. Diaphragmatic peri-infarction block with prolongation of the terminal QRS vector may simulate inferior infarction complicated by right bundle branch block.

Focal Peri-infarction Block

Focal peri-infarction block is the expression of a *local* conduction disturbance around the area of the infarction. It is also characterized by a terminal QRS force which is directed *towards* the epicardial surface of the infarction and is consequently reflected by a terminal r or R wave in a lead orientated to the infarcted area. Such a lead thus reflects a Qr or QR complex. The activation process reaches the endocardial regions in the neighbourhood of the infarction and circumnavigates the infarction by a circuitous route, to activate the healthy subepicardial area overlying the infarction in a tangential, longitudinal or oblique manner (Fig. 22, and Diagram A11 of Fig. 26). The muscle overlying the zone is, as a result, not activated in the normal endocardial-epicardial direction.

The initial 0·04 sec QRS vector, the basic infarction vector of myocardial necrosis, is directed *away* from the infarction which is dominantly subendocardial.

The terminal 0·04 sec QRS vector of the focal peri-infarction block is directed towards the epicardium overlying the infarction.

The activation of the tissues overlying the infarction may be further complicated by *injury block* (see p. 000). This is because the necrotic material is not completely surrounded by healthy tissue, but by injured tissue which will further delay the activation process. Inscription of the terminal R wave consequently reflects a delay.

The concept governing focal peri-infarction block has been substantiated by the studies of Durrer and associates (1964)[D51] who observed that the activation of muscle overlying the infarction occurred tangentially and that the conduction velocity of such activation could be diminished.

Focal peri-infarction block is usually seen in the neighbourhood of a transmural infarction. The transmural infarct usually extends laterally in the subendocardial regions of the adjacent tissues, having a broad base, i.e. the centre tends to be transmural whereas the edges tend to be subendocardial (Fig. 24). The healthy or relatively healthy tissues overlying the lateral extension of the necrosis are

then in a circuitous fashion, resulting in the focal peri-infarction block. Leads orientated to the centre of the infarction will reflect the QS complex of transmural infarction where adjacent leads will reflect a qR or QR complex (for example leads V5 and V6, Standard lead I and lead AVL of Electrocardiographic Study 18; leads V5 and V6 of Electrocardiographic Study 28).

Thus, focal peri-infarction block may be diagnosed when sequentially adjacent leads show a progression from QS complexes through Qr complex, QR complex, and then to the normal qR complex (Electrocardiographic Study 22).

DIFFERENTIAL DIAGNOSIS BETWEEN FOCAL AND DIVISIONAL PERI-INFARCTION BLOCK

Both focal and divisional peri-infarction block are associated with initial and terminal QRS abnormalities. Their distinction may, at times, be difficult, and is based on the following features:

1. Divisional peri-infarction block is always associated with specific left superior or right inferior frontal plane QRS axes, whereas the terminal frontal plane QRS axes in focal peri-infarction block are non-specific.

2. Divisional peri-infarction block occurs particularly and predominantly with anterolateral and diaphragmatic myocardial infarction, whereas focal peri-infarction block can be associated with infarction at any site.

3. Focal peri-infarction block is reflected by electrodes orientated to the periphery of the infarction, i.e. to the areas of subendocardial infarction with overlying healthy or relatively healthy tissues. Divisional peri-infarction block is reflected by electrodes orientated to the centre, the main region, of the infarction.

BUNDLE BRANCH BLOCK

The significance of bundle branch block, right or left, in relation to coronary insufficiency or myocardial infarction are considered in detail in Chapters 9 and 10.

THE S1 S2 S3 SYNDROME

Anterior myocardial infarction, especially apical myocardial infarction, is sometimes complicated by a terminal QRS vector which is directed *superiorly* and to the *right* in the region of −90° to −150° on the frontal plane hexaxial reference system (Vector 3 of Fig. 49). This will result in terminal negative deflections, S waves, in *all* of the three Standard leads (Electrocardiographic Studies 32, 33, 36, 38 and 102), and has consequently been termed the

'S1 S2 S3' syndrome[G32]. The manifestation, once present, tends to be permanent. The electrocardiographic syndrome may also occur under the following conditions:

AS A NORMAL VARIANT

This occurs in young adults who have no evidence of heart disease. It probably represents the persistence of the physiological dominance of the right ventricular outflow tract which is present during infancy. There are no clinical or other electrocardiographic abnormalities.

AS AN EXPRESSION OF RIGHT VENTRICULAR DOMINANCE

The S1 S2 S3 syndrome is especially prone to occur in cases of right ventricular dominance, particularly those associated with congenital heart disease which have marked right ventricular hypertrophy, and particularly hypertrophy of the infundibulum, the right ventricular outflow tract. It may also occur with cor pulmonale. When the S1 S2 S3 syndrome occurs under these circumstances there will be both clinical and electrocardiographic evidence of right ventricular dominance and possible right atrial enlargement.

CORRELATIVE ESSAY

THE DIFFERENTIAL DIAGNOSIS OF THE TERMINAL AND INITIAL QRS VECTORS IN INFERIOR WALL MYOCARDIAL INFARCTION

Inferior wall myocardial infarction is commonly associated with a terminal *R* wave in one or more of the leads which are orientated to the inferior wall of the heart, Standard leads II and III and lead AVF. The terminal *R* wave(s) may occur in uncomplicated inferior wall myocardial infarction or in inferior wall myocardial infarction complicated by focal peri-infarction block, diaphragmatic (divisional) peri-infarction block, and right bundle branch block. The differential diagnosis is considered below.

The Orientation of the Terminal QRS Vectors

THE TERMINAL VECTORS OF UNCOMPLICATED INFERIOR WALL MYOCARDIAL INFARCTION, AND INFERIOR WALL-MYOCARDIAL INFARCTION ASSOCIATED WITH FOCAL PERI-INFARCTION BLOCK

Uncomplicated inferior wall myocardial infarction may be associated with QS complexes in all three of the inferior leads, Standard leads II and III and lead AVF. This presenta-

tion occurs with extensive inferior wall myocardial infarction, but is uncommon (see below). The usual presentation is a QR complex in Standard lead II, and a Qr complex (or QS complex) in lead AVF, and a QS complex in Standard lead III (Electrocardiographic Studies 4C, 27, 28 and 31). In other words, the terminal QRS vector tends to be orientated *inferiorly and to the left*, and when this occurs the *terminal R wave is tallest in Standard lead II* (Diagram A of Fig. 25). These terminal *R* or *r* waves in Standard lead II, and possibly lead AVF, are most likely the expression of focal peri-infarction block.

THE TERMINAL VECTOR OF DIAPHRAGMATIC PERI-INFARCTION BLOCK

In diaphragmatic peri-infarction block the dominant direction of the terminal vector is inferior towards the region of +90° on the frontal plane hexaxial reference system. There may be a slight rightward deviation to within the region of +90° to +100° (Vector 1 of Fig. 49). The inscription of the terminal vectorcardiographic loop is also slowed. The terminal loop also tends to be relatively wide. These changes are reflected electrocardiographically by the inscription of terminal *R* waves in Standard leads II, III and AVF which, because of the inferior direction and relatively wide terminal loop, tend to be *approximately equal in amplitude in all three leads* (Electrocardiographic Studies 49 and 50; Diagram B of Fig. 25). The deflection in Standard lead III may also be a little taller if the vector is directed more rightward, for example at +120° on the frontal plane hexaxial reference system.

This contrasts with the normal pattern of uncomplicated diaphragmatic infarction complicated by *focal* peri-infarction block. In both these instances the terminal *R* wave is tallest in Standard lead II, Standard lead III usually reflecting no terminal *R* wave at all (Diagram A of Fig. 25).

Differentiation from Right Bundle Branch Block
Diaphragmatic peri-infarction block is, in about 10 per cent of cases, characterized by a marked slowing of the terminal QRS vector[G33].

This is reflected by an increased duration and a widening of the terminal *R* wave and may simulate right bundle branch block. The differentiation is considered below.

THE TERMINAL VECTOR OF RIGHT BUNDLE BRANCH BLOCK

Right bundle branch block is associated with a terminal QRS vector that is usually *more rightwardly directed* than that found in diaphragmatic peri-infarction block, frequently in the region of +150° on the frontal plane hexaxial reference system (Vector 2 of Fig. 49). This means that the terminal R wave *will be considerably taller in Standard lead III than in lead AVF and taller in lead AVF than in Standard lead II* (Diagram C of Fig. 25; Electrocardiographic Study 53), for the Standard lead III axis is more rightwardly orientated than the lead AVF and Standard lead II axes.

The terminal vector of right bundle branch is also anteriorly directed, resulting in an R′ deflection in V1, whereas the terminal vector in diaphragmatic peri-infarction block is posteriorly directed. There is consequently no terminal R′ wave in lead V1 in diaphragmatic peri-infarction block.

THE TERMINAL VECTORS IN INFERIOR WALL MYOCARDIAL INFARCTION ASSOCIATED WITH LEFT ANTERIOR HEMIBLOCK

Inferior wall myocardial infarction may be associated with a terminal QRS vector that is directed in the region of −60° to −90° on the frontal plane hexaxial reference system (Vector 4 of Fig. 49). This may be due to:

(a) Uncomplicated but extensive inferior wall infarction.

(b) Inferior wall infarction complicated by left anterior hemiblock.

The differential diagnosis is considered below.

(a) **Uncomplicated but extensive inferior wall infarction.** The inferior infarction affects both the anterior and posterior regions of the inferior wall (see pp. 110, and Diagrams B of Fig. 26 and Fig. 51). This presentation is uncommon. It will manifest with pure QS complexes in all three of the inferiorly orientated leads (Diagram D of Fig. 25; Electrocardiographic Study 30). There is no modification of the initial QRS deflection, as may occur with a complicating left anterior hemiblock (see below).

(b) **Inferior wall infarction complicated by left anterior hemiblock.** When inferior wall infarction is complicated by left anterior hemiblock, the terminal QRS vector is also directed in the region of −60° to −90° on the frontal plane hexaxial reference system. The electrocardiographic presentation may take one of the following forms:

(1) There are QS complexes in all three of the inferiorly orientated leads (Diagram E of Fig. 25). This stimulates pure uncomplicated, but extensive, inferior wall myocardial infarction as described above. The presence of the associated left anterior hemiblock may, under this circumstance, be inferred when the frontal plane QRS deflections are of relatively large magnitude, the QS complexes are very deep in Standard leads II and III and lead AVF, and the R waves are very tall in

Standard lead I and lead AVL (Electrocardiographic Study 29). QS complexes may also appear in all three inferior leads when inferior infarction is complicated by left anterior hemiblock and incomplete left bundle branch block.

(2) The initial part of the QS complexes in Standard leads II and III and lead AVF may be modified by initial positivities, initial r waves, or initial deformities, and may take one of the following empirical possibilities:

(i) rS complexes in all three inferiorly orientated leads,

(ii) slurring of, or the formation of ledges within, the initial downward deflection of the QS complex.

These manifestations are discussed in greater detail on p. 110 of this chapter.

VECTORIAL CONSIDERATIONS

An understanding of the genesis of the aforementioned phenomena is based on an appreciation of the frontal plane vectorcardiographic loop, and particularly its relationship to the Standard lead II axis. This is considered below.

THE FRONTAL PLANE VECTORCARDIOGRAPHIC LOOP IN UNCOMPLICATED INFERIOR WALL MYOCARDIAL INFARCTION

The frontal plane vectorcardiographic loop in uncomplicated inferior wall myocardial infarction is inscribed in a clockwise direction[B31, B33, H31, H40, Y4] (Diagrams A of Figs. 47, 48 and 26). This means that the initial part of the loop will be dominantly in the negative zone of the Standard lead II axis (Diagram A of Fig. 47), and hence be reflected by a deep, wide pathological Q wave. The terminal part of the loop will enter the positive zone of the Standard lead II axis and be reflected by a terminal R wave (Diagrams A of Figs. 47 and 26). Thus, the common manifestation of uncomplicated inferior wall myocardial infarction in Standard lead II is a QR complex.

The terminal part of the loop may also enter the positive zone of lead AVF (Diagram A of Fig. 47), but the impression will not be as marked as on the positive zone of Standard lead II. Lead AVF will consequently reflect a smaller terminal r wave than Standard lead II and, at times, no terminal r wave at all (Electrocardiographic Study 28). The entire loop is usually situated in the negative zone of Standard lead III (Diagram A of Fig. 47) which consequently reflects a QS complex. The entire or almost the entire loop is situated in the positive zone of Standard lead I and lead AVL (Diagram A of Fig. 48). These leads consequently reflect tall dominant R waves which, in the case of Standard lead I, may be preceded by a small q wave (Electrocardiographic Study 28).

THE FRONTAL PLANE VECTOR LOOP IN LEFT ANTERIOR HEMIBLOCK

The frontal plane vector loop in uncomplicated left anterior hemiblock is inscribed in a counter-clockwise direction (Diagrams C of Figs. 47 and 48)[B32, B33]. The initial part of the loop will thus be in the positive zone of the Standard lead II axis resulting in a small initial *r* wave, whereas the terminal part will be in the negative zone of the Standard lead II axis, resulting in a deep terminal *S* wave (Diagram C of Fig. 47). It is therefore evident that a terminal *R* wave cannot appear in Standard lead II (not in lead AVF or even Standard lead III) in cases of uncomplicated left anterior hemiblock[B33].

In uncomplicated left anterior hemiblock the initial part of the frontal plane vector loop is usually wide and open. This results in initial *r* waves of more or less equal magnitude in Standard leads II and III and lead AVF. This initial *r* wave is frequently most marked in Standard lead II, less prominent in lead AVF, and least conspicuous in Standard lead III (Diagram E of Fig. 25). This contrasts with the situation where inferior wall myocardial infarction is associated with left anterior hemiblock. When this occurs, the initial *r* wave is usually tallest in Standard lead III, and minimal or absent in Standard lead II (Diagram F of Fig. 25, and see below).

If, in addition, the left anterior hemiblock is complicated by incomplete or complete left bundle branch block, the initial *r* waves will disappear completely in Standard leads II and III, and lead AVF, resulting in QS complexes in all these leads, which thus mimics extensive inferior wall myocardial infarction.

THE FRONTAL PLANE VECTORCARDIOGRAPHIC LOOP IN INFERIOR WALL MYOCARDIAL INFARCTION ASSOCIATED WITH LEFT ANTERIOR HEMIBLOCK

When inferior wall myocardial infarction is associated with left anterior hemiblock, the frontal plane vectorcardiographic loop takes the form of a figure-eight (Diagrams B of Figs. 47 and 48)[B33]. A small initial part of the loop is inscribed in a clockwise direction and is directed superiorly and somewhat to the right, whereas the ensuing main body of the loop is inscribed in the usual superior and counter-clockwise direction of left anterior hemiblock. The initial clockwise part of the loop lies in the positive zones of Standard lead III and lead AVF, and will result in the small initial *r* waves in these leads. It is evident from inspection of Diagram B in Fig. 47 that the initial clockwise part of the loop is (a) situated dominantly in the positive zone of Standard lead III, (b) situated minimally in the positive zone of lead AVF, and (c) situated in the negative zone of

Standard lead II. Standard lead III will thus reflect an initial *r* wave (of an rS complex) which is taller than the initial *r* wave in lead AVF. Standard lead II reflects no initial *r* wave at all, or an *r* wave that is barely conspicuous and smaller than that in lead AVF (Diagram F of Fig. 25 and Electrocardiographic Study 44). It is thus evident that the relative magnitudes of the initial *r* waves contrast with those in uncomplicated left anterior hemiblock (as described above).

CORRELATIVE ESSAY

THE MECHANISMS AND SIGNIFICANCE OF LEFT AXIS DEVIATION

Left axis deviation refers to a mean manifest frontal plane QRS axis that is directed superiorly and to the left, in the region of $-30°$ to $-90°$ on the frontal plane hexaxial reference system. There are five basic mechanisms:

1. **Left anterior hemiblock.**
2. **Left anterior parietal block.**
3. **Inferior wall myocardial infarction.**
4. **Some presentations of the Wolff-Parkinson-White syndrome.**
5. **Pacing from the apex of the left or right ventricle.**

Left Anterior Hemiblock

This is due to an interruption or delay in conduction through the anterosuperior division of the left bundle branch. The principles governing this disturbance are discussed in detail on p. 104. The left anterior hemiblock may be due to the following pathological causes.

(a) Interruption of the anterosuperior division of the left bundle branch block by myocardial infarction. This results in anterolateral peri-infarction block; the initial QRS vector being directed away from the left ventricle, i.e. inferior and to the right, and the terminal QRS vector being directed superiorly and to the left.

(b) Interruption of the anterosuperior division of the left bundle branch by fibrosis or calcareous encroachment. This may be due to:

(i) the fibrosis resulting from chronic coronary insufficiency.

(ii) the fibrosis resulting from chronic cardiac failure.

(iii) the fibrosis resulting from chronic left ventricular decompensation in cases of systemic hypertension and other diseases associated with left ventricular failure.

(iv) fibrosis associated with a chronic cardiomyopathy.

(v) calcareous encroachment on the left bundle branch conducting system from neighbouring structures such as aortic valve and interventricular septum, also known as Lev's disease[L33].

Corne and associates (1965)[C47] noted a high incidence of myocardial fibrosis associated with frontal plane axes of −30° or further leftward deviation.

Cerqueira Gomes and associates (1970)[C17], in a study of 13,061 electrocardiograms of a general hospital, noted the following:

(a) Left anterior hemiblock occurred in 2·6 per cent of cases, and was the most common intraventricular conduction defect. The left anterior hemiblock was here used in a broad sense to include the territory of the anterior division of the left bundle branch, and probably included cases of left anterior parietal block.

The conduction disturbance was followed in frequency by complete right bundle branch block, which occurred in 2·1 per cent of cases.

(b) 94 per cent of cases of left anterior hemiblock occurred after the fourth decade.

(c) The condition most often associated with left anterior hemiblock was arteriosclerotic heart disease (55 per cent). Other common associations were hypertensive heart disease, aortic valvular disease, and the cardiomyopathies.

(d) Left anterior hemiblock was frequently associated with anteroseptal and anterolateral myocardial infarction. Some reports have indicated that when isolated left anterior hemiblock or extreme left axis deviation occurs during the course of acute myocardial infarction, it does not increase the mortality or complicate the clinical course of the infarction[K27, M20]. Col and Weinberg (1972)[C37], however, reported a mortality of 29 per cent in patients with left anterior hemiblock as compared with a mortality of 13·6 per cent in patients without intraventricular conduction disturbance. Further study is necessary.

Left Anterior Parietal Block

Left anterior parietal block is due to a delay in conduction in the terminal ramifications of the anterosuperior division of the left bundle branch. This will also result in left axis deviation. There are at present no satisfactory criteria to distinguish this condition from interruption of conduction through the trunk of the left anterosuperior division, as occurs in hemiblock. The vectorcardiogram may, however, be helpful. In both left anterior hemiblock and in left anterior parietal block, the frontal plane vector loop is inscribed in a counter-clockwise direction with the dominant orientation being superiorly and to the left. In left anterior parietal block, however, there is no abnormality of the initial 0·02 sec vector loop, but there is a considerable slowing of the terminal vector loop, whereas in left anterior hemiblock there is an abnormality of the initial 0·02 sec vector which tends to be directed inferiorly and to the right (see p. 106), and there is no associated terminal slurring or slowing. Left anterior parietal block is usually an expression of disease of the myocardium, for example extensive myocardial fibrosis, as would occur with fibrosis of the wall itself. Left anterior hemiblock may be due to a similar pathology, but could also result from a relatively small lesion, for example a minor infarction or calcareous encroachment from a neighbouring structure which interrupts the anterosuperior division at a proximal and critically narrow point.

Inferior Wall Myocardial Infarction

Inferior wall myocardial infarction will result in deep or relatively deep Q waves or QS complexes in Standard leads II and III and lead AVF. There is thus a tendency to left axis deviation. The differential diagnosis from other causes of left axis deviation is based predominantly on the QRS manifestation in Standard lead II. In uncomplicated inferior wall myocardial infarction there is usually a QR complex in Standard lead II, whereas in left anterior hemiblock there is no terminal R wave in Standard lead II. The differential diagnosis is considered further on p. 110.

Some Presentations of the Wolff-Parkinson-White Syndrome

The QRS complex in the WPW syndrome tends to follow, or be orientated in the same direction as, the delta wave axis (Schamroth, 1974)[S18]. Thus, if the delta wave is orientated superiorly and to the left, for example at −70° on the frontal plane hexaxial reference system, then the mean manifest QRS complex will also tend to be similarly directed, but this is not invariably so. This is particularly prone to occur with the Type A WPW syndrome. The resulting negative delta waves and negative QRS complexes in Standard leads II and III and lead AVF may simulate inferior wall myocardial infarction (see Chapter 11).

Pacing from the Apex of the Left or Right Ventricle

When the ventricles are paced from the apex of either the right or the left side, activation of the ventricles must proceed from the distal and proximally, i.e. it must proceed in a superior direction, usually in a superior and leftward direction, thereby resulting in a left axis deviation.

OBSERVATIONS ON LEFT AXIS DEVIATION COMPLICATED BY INCOMPLETE OR COMPLETE LEFT BUNDLE BRANCH BLOCK

Left axis deviation, due to whatever mechanism, is usually associated with an initial *r* wave of an rS complex in Standard leads II and III and lead AVF, the left axis affecting principally the terminal deflection of the QRS complex (Diagram A of Fig. 53). When the left axis deviation is associated with complete or incomplete left bundle branch block, the initial *r* waves disappear, and this results in QS complexes in Standard leads II and III and lead AVF (Diagram B of Fig. 53). This may simulate extensive inferior wall myocardial infarction (see Chapter 5).

When left axis deviation occurs in association with left bundle branch block, it is usually due to left anterior parietal block (Cerqueira Gomes and associates, 1970)[C17].

Chapter 13

The Diagnosis of Myocardial Infarction from Ectopic Ventricular Beats

When ectopic ventricular rhythms such as ventricular extrasystoles, ventricular tachycardia, or a subsidiary idioventricular rhythm in cases of complete A-V block complicate myocardial infarction, the diagnosis of the infarction may be evident from the morphology of the ectopic beats. The manifestations may affect all the parameters of the electrocardiographic deflection, the QRS complex, the S-T segment and the T wave, and may indeed be more obvious, and even more definitive, in the ectopic beats than in the conducted sinus beats[B47, S113].

Relatively few cases have been reported (Anttonen and associates 1962[A12], Cohen 1961[C34], Dressler 1943[D27], Katz and associates 1958[K12], Schamroth 1972[S30], Levenstein and Schamroth 1973[L37], Scherf and Schott Fig. 11, 1953[S53], Silverman and Salomon 1959[S76], Simonson and associates 1945[S82], Sommerville and Wood 1949[S120], Spang 1957, his case 49, [S122], Szilagy and Ginsburg, 1962[S147].

The morphology of the uncomplicated ectopic ventricular beat will be considered first. The principles governing the diagnosis of myocardial infarction from ectopic ventricular beats will be considered thereafter.

THE MORPHOLOGY OF THE UNCOMPLICATED ECTOPIC VENTRICULAR BEAT

The morphology of the uncomplicated ectopic ventricular beat, i.e. an ectopic ventricular beat that is not associated with myocardial infarction, is considered below with reference to a ventricular extrasystole. The principles apply to all the forms of ectopic ventricular rhythm.

The QRS Complex

The QRS complex of a ventricular extrasystole that is dominantly upright is wide, bizarre and notched or slurred (Diagram A of Fig. 58). It frequently has the form of a single, broad, bizarre and notched deflection, an RR' com-

plex with a notched apex, or a wide R wave with a blunted or slurred apex. It may be diphasic in the form of an RS complex. The ventricular extrasystole is rarely triphasic in configuration, as is commonly the case with supraventricular impulses conducted with phasic aberrant ventricular conduction. The conduction in such cases usually reflects a right bundle branch block pattern which is triphasic in form (see Chapter 17, section on Phasic Aberrant Ventricular Conduction). An ectopic ventricular beat with a dominantly upright QRS complex has *no initial q wave*, no matter how small. Further, the initial QRS vector of the ventricular extrasystole is commonly quite different in direction

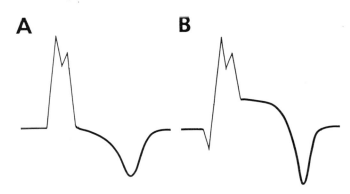

FIG. 58. Diagrams illustrating the QRST complex of: A, an uncomplicated ectopic ventricular beat; and B, an ectopic ventricular beat associated with myocardial infarction.

from that of the conducted supraventricular beat. This contrasts with the QRS complex of phasic aberrant ventricular conduction which usually has an initial vector similar or identical to that of the normally conducted beat. This is considered in greater detail in Chapter 17, section on Phasic Aberrant Ventricular Conduction.

The Secondary S-T Segment and T Wave Changes

The associated S-T segment and T wave of the ectopic ventricular beat reflect changes which are merely secondary to the abnormal intraventricular conduction, i.e. there is no primary abnormality of these parameters. The principles governing these secondary changes are similar to those associated with any form of abnormal intraventricular conduction as, for example, with uncomplicated right or left bundle branch block. They affect:

(a) the direction of the S-T segment and *T* wave vectors,
(b) the shape of the S-T segment, and
(c) the slope of the *T* wave.

THE DIRECTION OF THE S-T SEGMENT AND T WAVE VECTORS

The S-T segment and *T* wave of an ectopic ventricular beat are normally *opposite in direction* to the major QRS deflection or, more accurately, *opposite in direction to the terminal QRS deflection* (Diagram A of Fig. 58). Thus, when the terminal QRS deflection is positive or upright, the S-T segment and *T* wave will be negative or depressed, and vice versa. This may be expressed vectorially in the following manner. The normal angle between the terminal QRS vector and the S-T segment vector is greater than 110° on the frontal plane hexaxial reference system, and may be as wide as 180°. The *T* wave vector, too, is separated from the terminal QRS vector by an angle greater than 110°. Note that the S-T segment and *T* wave vectors are roughly parallel on the frontal plane hexaxial reference system, i.e. they have nearly the same direction.

THE SHAPE OF THE S-T SEGMENT

When the ectopic ventricular beat is reflected by a dominantly upright QRS complex, the S-T segment usually has a straight downward slope or a downward slope that is but slightly convex-upward. The S-T segment does not hug the baseline appreciably, i.e. it is not isoelectric to any appreciable extent. In most cases the S-T segment is not isoelectric at all, beginning its downward course from the QRS complex almost immediately (Diagram A of Fig. 58).

THE SHAPE OF THE T WAVE

The *T* wave of the uncomplicated ectopic ventricular beat has asymmetrical limbs; a shallow proximal limb and a steeper distal limb. The apex tends to be somewhat blunt (Diagram A of Fig. 58).

THE MORPHOLOGY OF THE ECTOPIC VENTRICULAR BEAT COMPLICATED BY MYOCARDIAL INFARCTION

The Basic Prerequisites

The following prerequisites must be satisfied before the diagnosis of myocardial infarction from the morphology of an ectopic ventricular beat can be made.

1. The diagnosis must be made from *an ectopic ventricular beat with a dominantly positive QRS deflection*. In other words, no such diagnosis must be entertained if the ectopic ventricular beat presents with a negative or dominantly negative complex, a QS or rS deflection[B47, S113].

2. The diagnosis must be made from leads orientated to the external—epicardial—surface of the heart. The diagnosis must not be made from such leads as lead AVR or lead V1 which are, or tend to be, orientated towards the cavity of the heart[B47, S113].

The Electrocardiographic Manifestations

MANIFESTATIONS AFFECTING THE QRS COMPLEX

The diagnosis of myocardial infarction is *suggested* when an ectopic ventricular beat with a dominantly positive QRS complex is *preceded by an initial q wave*, no matter how small (Diagram B of Fig. 58). The initial *q* wave may, of course, be of considerable magnitude. The ectopic ventricular beat may thus manifest with a qR, qRR', qRs, QRs or even a QR pattern (Electrocardiographic Studies 40, 66, 67, 68, 71F, 90B and 113). This phenomenon has been demonstrated experimentally in the dog heart. Ventricular extrasystoles arising in either the right or the left ventricle are not associated with an initial negativity unless myocardial infarction is present[S113].

MANIFESTATIONS AFFECTING THE S-T SEGMENT AND T WAVE

The diagnosis of myocardial infarction is suggested when the S-T segment and/or *T* wave manifest with primary changes; changes which are not merely secondary to the abnormal intraventricular conduction of the uncomplicated ventricular extrasystole, but reflect a primary abnormality of repolarization. These primary changes are:

(a) Elevation of the S-T segment.
(b) Coving of the S-T segment.
(c) Slope elevation of the S-T segment.
(d) Symmetry and sharpening of the *T* wave.

ELEVATION OF THE S-T SEGMENT

The S-T segment is deviated in the *same* direction as the terminal or dominant QRS deflection. Thus, in the case of an ectopic ventricular beat with a dominantly positive QRS deflection, the S-T segment will be elevated (Diagram B of Fig. 58; Electrocardiographic Studies 66, 67, 68, 71F, 90B and 113). This may be expressed vectorially as an angle of *less than 110°* between the terminal QRS vector and the S-T segment vector. Note that the normal S-T segment vector very nearly has the same direction as the *T* wave vector, i.e. the two vectors are roughly parallel on the frontal plane hexaxial reference system. Thus, when, in the presence of marked QRS prolongation due to either bundle branch block or ventricular ectopy, the S-T segment vector is not more or less in the same direction as the *T* wave vector, a primary S-T segment change is suggested, and this change may represent the injury pattern of acute myocardial infarction.

COVING OF THE S-T SEGMENT

The S-T segment may, in addition to the elevation, reflect the characteristic upward coving of the myocardial infarction injury pattern (Diagram B of Fig. 58; Electrocardiographic Studies 67, 68, 71F and 113). In other words, the normal almost straight downward slope of the S-T segment of the uncomplicated ventricular extrasystole is changed to an upward convexity.

SLOPE ELEVATION OF THE S-T SEGMENT

The ectopic ventricular beat may, at times, reflect marked elevation of the S-T segment. The configuration of this elevated S-T segment may be straight and horizontal, or straight with a slightly upward slope (Electrocardiographic Studies 66 and 90B). This is analogous to the slope elevation of the hyperacute injury phase of myocardial infarction. This manifestation may also occur as a temporary sign of the variant, Prinzmetal's, atypical angina in the absence of infarction (Electrocardiographic Study 90B).

SYMMETRY AND SHARPENING OF THE T WAVE

The *T* wave tends to become sharply pointed, and its limbs more symmetrical (Diagram B of Fig. 58; Electrocardiographic Studies 67 and 68). This may be the earliest or the only suggestive sign of the infarction. When this occurs, the S-T segment need not be elevated, but nevertheless tends to hug the baseline, i.e. it has an appreciable isoelectric period. This contrasts with the negligible or absent isoelectric period of the S-T segment in the uncomplicated ectopic ventricular beat. This manifestation may also occur as a sign of acute myocardial ischaemia in the absence of infarction.

Further Observations

1. When ectopic ventricular beats complicate the chronic stabilized phase of myocardial infarction, they may only reflect the abnormal initial *q* or *Q* wave without the primary S-T segment and *T* wave changes[S76] (Standard lead III of Electrocardiographic Study 40). The presence of primary S-T segment and *T* wave changes, therefore, reflect the acute or subacute phases of myocardial infarction.

2. The manifestations of infarction as described above may be associated with any form of ectopic ventricular rhythm, ventricular extrasystole (Electrocardiographic Studies 40, 66, 67, 71F and 90B), ventricular parasystole, a subsidiary idioventricular rhythm of complete A-V block, and ventricular tachycardia (Electrocardiographic Study 68).

3. The electrocardiographic signs of myocardial infarction may be present in the conducted supraventricular beat as well as the ectopic ventricular beat, but are frequently more marked in the ectopic ventricular beat[S113] (Electrocardiographic Studies 66 and 67). This infarction pattern may only be evident in the ectopic ventricular beat, the conducted sinus beats being normal or equivocal. The ectopic ventricular beat may reflect the only obvious signs of infarction if the conducted sinus beats are associated with left bundle branch block[D27, S82, S120], or the Wolff-Parkinson-White syndrome[S36] (Electrocardiographic Study 71F), since these complications tend to mask the effects of the infarction. This latter statement must, however, be treated with reserve with respect to left bundle branch block, for the diagnosis of myocardial infarction may still be clearly evident in the presence of left bundle branch block (see Chapter 10).

4. It is further evident from the above account that the principles governing the diagnosis of myocardial infarction from ventricular beats are similar to those governing the diagnosis of myocardial infarction in the presence of left bundle branch block (see Chapter 10).

5. The presence of acute myocardial infarction may even be *suspected* from the shape of the S-T segment when the QRS complex of the ectopic ventricular beat is dominantly negative. When the QRS complex of an ectopic ventricular beat is dominantly negative, the associated S-T segment and *T* wave will be positive, analogous to the pattern recorded by a right precordial lead in left bundle branch block (see Diagram A of Fig. 37). The S-T segment of this uncomplicated ectopic ventricular beat has an upward slope that is straight or minimally concave upward. When such an ectopic ventricular beat occurs during acute myocardial infarction, the S-T segment may become coved or *convex-upwards*. In other words, it becomes coved in the classic form, analogous to that depicted in Diagram E of Fig. 37. (lead V6 of Electrocardiographic Study 34A).

Chapter 14

Atrial Infarction

Infarction of the atria is rarely reported, and relatively few cases reflecting the electrocardiographic features have been documented[B21, B42, C33, C56, D16, F4, F24, H18, H20, L4, L59, P13, S72, S129, W57, Y3]. This is chiefly because there is no distinctive clinical presentation and the electrocardiographic features are small, inconspicuous and difficult to evaluate. The diagnostic criteria have not been defined with precision, and accurate criteria for the localization to a specific wall or surface of the atria have not been established. Furthermore, the atrial infarction is usually associated with ventricular infarction which dominates the clinical and electrocardiographic presentation. There is thus lack of awareness, a low diagnostic suspicion, of the condition.

Nevertheless, pathological studies indicate that atrial infarction may not be as rare as the paucity of clinical and electrocardiographic reports would indicate. Cushing and associates (1942)[C56] found 31 examples of concomitant atrial infarction in 182 cases of myocardial infarction, an incidence of 17 per cent. Wartman and Hellerstein (1948)[W5] encountered 17 atrial infarctions in a total of 235 cases of myocardial infarction, an incidence of 7.3 per cent. In 4 of these, the atrial infarction occurred as an isolated phenomenon, i.e. not associated with ventricular infarction. Earlier reports reflected a much lower incidence[B21, F4, K46, S101]. This is possibly because the atria were not always routinely and specifically examined for evidence of infarction.

In 1939, Langendorf[L4] reported a case of atrial infarction which was diagnosed at autopsy, but which could, in retrospect, have been diagnosed antemortem. Young and Koenig (1944)[Y3] described deviation of the P-R segment in three of their four cases of atrial infarction. They suggested the tentative diagnosis of atrial infarction, which was subsequently confirmed at autopsy. In 1948, Hellerstein[H20] reported another case of atrial infarction which was correctly diagnosed electrocardiographically antemortem, and subsequently confirmed at autopsy. Sporadic reports have since appeared. The diagnosis has, at times, been made with considerable confidence. Thus, Liu (1961)[L59] reported six cases of atrial infarction associated with ventricular in-

farction, the correct diagnosis being made antemortem in all six cases. It was also suggested antemortem in one of the two cases reported by Freundlich and Sereno (1948)[F24]. Atrial injury has also been reported in patients who underwent cardiac catheterization and/or open heart surgery[D15].

THE COMPLICATIONS OF ATRIAL INFARCTION

The accurate diagnosis of atrial infarction may be of considerable clinical import since it is associated with potentially significant complications. These include:

(a) **Mural thrombosis**. This has been reported with an incidence of 80–84 per cent of cases[B21, W5].

(b) **Pulmonary embolism**. This has been reported as occurring in 24 per cent of cases[H20].

(c) **Systemic embolism**.

(d) **Atrial rupture**. This has been reported with a very high incidence, 70 per cent, (Clowe and associates 1934)[C33], and a very low incidence, 5 per cent of the right atrium and 2 per cent of the left atrium (Krimbhaar and Cromwell 1925)[K46]. There were no cases of rupture in the well-studied series of Cushing and associates (1942)[C56]. The latter two studies would make the high incidence reported by Clowe and associates questionable.

(e) **Disturbances of impulse formation**. Atrial infarction may be complicated by atrial extrasystoles, atrial flutter, atrial fibrillation and paroxysmal, extrasystolic, atrial tachycardia.

(f) **Disturbances of intra-atrial conduction**. Atrial infarction may be complicated by sinoatrial block, intra-atrial block, and possibly A-V nodal block.

ELECTROCARDIOGRAPHIC MANIFESTATIONS

The Normal Atrial Complex

THE MODE OF ATRIAL ACTIVATION

The atrial wall, in contrast to the ventricular wall, has no appreciable thickness. This is also evident electrophysiologically, for activation of the atria occurs *longitudinally*, i.e. by contiguity. This is in contrast to the *transverse* form of ventricular activation, the impulse being conveyed relatively quickly by the specialized conducting system to the subendocardial region of the ventricle, and then spreading transversely from endocardium through the thickness of the muscle wall. The shape and duration of the *P* wave therefore have no bearing on the degree of atrial muscle thickness, and atrial hypertrophy cannot be diagnosed electrocardiographically. One can only refer, in an electrocardiographic sense, to *atrial enlargement*.

Atrial Depolarization—the P Wave

Activation of the atria tends to occur from above downwards, and from right to left. This results in a mean activation front that is directed downward and to the left, and is reflected by a mean *P* wave axis in the region of $0°$ to $+60°$, more commonly in the region of $+30°$ to $+60°$ on the frontal plane hexaxial reference system. The *P* wave therefore tends to be tallest in Standard lead II. It is normally pyramidal in shape with a smooth apex in Standard lead II, and is normally diphasic in lead V_1.

Atrial Repolarization—the Ta Wave

Atrial repolarization is reflected by the P-Ta segment (see below) and the *Ta* wave. The *Ta* (*Tp*) wave, the *T* wave of atrial repolarization, is normally opposite in direction to the *P* wave, i.e. it is *normally* negative in Standard lead II (Diagrams A and B of Fig. 59). This is in contrast to ventri-

cular repolarization, which is reflected by a *T* wave in the same direction as the QRS complex. The Ta wave is, however, usually obscured by the QRS complex, and may even encroach on the junctional part of the S-T segment, thereby causing some degree of junctional S-T segment depression (see Chapter 16, p. 160).

The P-Ta Segment

The P-Ta segment was named as such by Abramsen and associates (1938)[A3]. It reflects part of atrial repolarization, and is analogous to the S-T segment of ventricular depolarization (Diagram A of Fig. 59). When associated with an upright *P* wave, it slopes gently downward from the distal limb of the *P* wave and tends to merge smoothly with the proximal limb of the *Ta* wave. As with the *Ta* wave, the P-Ta segment too is masked, distorted or obscured to a considerable degree by the superimposition of the QRS complex, the only part which is normally visible being reflected by the *P-R (P-Q) segment*, the interval between the *end* of the *P* wave and the beginning of the QRS complex. The P-Ta segment and *Ta* wave are best seen, in its entirety, when the QRS complex is absent, as in second degree and third degree A-V block.

The Effect of Tachycardia

Tachycardia as it occurs, for example, in response to normal exercise, results in an increase in *P* wave amplitude (Diagram B of Fig. 59). This is particularly so in Standard lead II and is, in part, due to a slight right axis deviation of the *P* wave axis, so that it tends to become more aligned with, and hence taller in, Standard lead II. The associated *Ta* wave becomes deeper, i.e. more accentuated. The P-Ta segment acquires a steeper downward slope and is consequently a little depressed, particularly at its distal end (Diagram B of Fig. 59). It is thus important, in the evaluation of pathological P-Ta segment deviation, to appreciate that, in the presence of tachycardia and a dominantly upright *P* wave, the P-Ta segment depression may be minimally accentuated, and that this may be a normal physiological phenomenon.

The Abnormal Atrial Complex: The Complex of Atrial Infarction

Atrial infarction may manifest with abnormalities affecting the three basic electrocardiographic parameters of atrial activity:

1. There may be a **disturbance of atrial depolarization** manifesting as a change in the shape of the *P* wave.

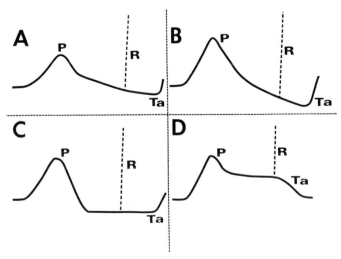

FIG. 59. Diagrams illustrating the *P* wave and the *Ta* wave in: A, a normal tracing; B, a normal tracing with normal accentuation of the height of the *P* wave, C and D, atrial infarction. The position of the QRS complex is indicated by the dotted line.

2. There may be a **disturbance of atrial repolarization** manifesting as a change in the P-Ta segment.

3. There may be a **disturbance of atrial rhythm**.

The changes affecting repolarization are the more characteristic, and will be considered first.

ABNORMALITIES OF THE P-Ta SEGMENT

Atrial infarction may be associated with **elevation or depression of the P-Ta segment.**

THE DIRECTION OF THE P-Ta DEVIATION

It would appear from most published cases of atrial infarction, that the deviation of the P-Ta segment vector tends to occur superiorly or inferiorly in the frontal plane. It is therefore best reflected in Standard leads II and III and lead AVF, where it appears either as a slight elevation of the P-R segment (Electrocardiographic Studies 7 and 8) or as a slight depression of the P-R segment (Electrocardiographic Studies 9, 17, 41 and 51).

Various authors[F24, H20, L59] have attempted to localize the infarction by the direction of the P-Ta segment vector. It has, for example, been postulated that the P-Ta segment is deviated to the surface of injury, analogous to the deviation of the S-T segment to the surface of injury in ventricular infarction. Hypothetically, this would result in elevated P-Ta (P-R) segments in Standard leads II and III and lead AVF in cases of inferior atrial infarction, and depressed P-Ta (P-R) segments in Standard lead II and III and lead AVF in cases of superior atrial infarction. Analysis of all published examples, however, fails to reveal a consistent or clear-cut pattern. The problem is further complicated by the rather complex and irregular external architecture of the biatrial chamber, which contrasts with the relatively smooth external architecture of the biventricular chamber. As a result, there has hitherto not been any accurate designation of atrial surfaces with relevance to electrode placement. Furthermore, an analogy of P-Ta segment displacement as a result of atrial injury to the S-T segment displacement as a result of ventricular injury may be fallacious. This is because the atria are activated longitudinally, whereas the ventricles are activated transversely. Moreover, the atria are low pressure chambers. It is thus unlikely that a significant differential state of polarization will exist between cells of the inner endocardial and outer epicardial layers of the relatively thin wall, as occurs in the case of ventricular injury (see Chapter 2). The differential polarization resulting from atrial injury probably results in a longitudinal or surface abnormality. Should this hypothetical state in fact occur, the differential depolarization would exist between the injured tissue of the infarction, and the adjacent healthy area. Such an adjacent healthy area could be sited inferiorly, superiorly, or laterally. The P-Ta segment depolarization could thus, theoretically, be displaced in any direction. The problem obviously requires much further study.

THE DEGREE AND FORM OF P-Ta (P-R) SEGMENT DEVIATION

The displacement of the P-Ta segment, as reflected by the deviation of the P-R segment, is usually slight. It is commonly about 0·5 mm and rarely exceeds 1 mm in amplitude (Electrocardiographic Study 9). It is less than half the amplitude of the preceding P wave[J10]. Displacement of the P-Ta vector segment in the *same direction as the* P *wave* vector is usually very much more significant than duration of the P-Ta segment in an opposite direction to the P wave. In other words, *elevation* of the P-Ta (P-R) segment, no matter how slight, is usually significant when associated with an upright P wave (Diagram D of Fig. 59; Electrocardiographic Study 8). This is because the P-Ta segment tends to be slightly opposite in direction to the P wave, and this is exaggerated by exercise and tachycardia.

Contrariwise, a slight depression of the P-R segment in association with an upright P wave may be physiological, especially in the presence of tachycardia. Under these circumstances, it is necessary to have an appreciable depression, for example, of 1 mm or more, and/or a concomitant change in the shape of the P-Ta segment (see below) before the diagnosis of atrial infarction can be entertained with confidence. The angle between the P wave and the P-R segment may be helpful in these equivocal cases of P-Ta depression. The angle is virtually non-existent in the P-Ta physiological depression which occurs as a response to tachycardia; the distal limb of the P wave tending to merge smoothly and imperceptibly with the P-R segment. With atrial injury, however, the P-R segment tends to be *horizontally depressed*, thereby resulting in a sharp-angled P:P-R junction (Diagram C of Fig. 59; Electrocardiographic Study 51). Compare this manifestation with the plane depression of the S-T segment in cases of subendocardial ventricular injury (Chapter 2).

ABNORMALITIES OF THE P WAVE

As can be readily appreciated, atrial infarction will distort the pathway of normal atrial activation, manifesting with abnormalities of the P wave. The P wave may be *widened, notched, slurred, 'W' or 'M'* shaped. The P wave may even become transiently taller and/or peaked[B57, G43, M29].

Several authors have described an atrial Q wave, an initial prominent negative deflection associated with a dominantly upright *P* wave, a mechanism which has been postulated to be analogous to the genesis of the pathological wave of ventricular infarction[F24, L59, S10]. It is doubtful, however, whether such a postulate is valid, for the pathological *Q* wave of ventricular infarction reflects a disturbance of transverse, endocardial to epicardial, activation, and activation of the atria occurs longitudinally. See also comment above on the questionable analogy of S-T segment and P-Ta segment deviation.

Thus, while the atrial infarction may certainly distort the *P* wave, an initial negative deflection usually reflects a disturbed course of activation and not a true pathological *Q* wave which connotes a loss of full thickness myocardial tissue.

Disturbances of Atrial Rhythm

Atrial infarction may precipitate disturbances of atrial rhythm. These include disturbance of impulse formation and impulse conduction.

The disturbance of impulse formation may manifest as atrial fibrillation, the commonest manifestation[C56], atrial extrasystoles, extrasystolic atrial tachycardia, atrial flutter, sinus bradycardia, sinus arrest, and possibly idionodal tachycardia[S78].

The disturbance of impulse conduction may manifest as *sinoatrial or atrioventricular* block (Electrocardiographic Studies 8 and 9). Furthermore, the associated abnormal *P* wave must, in part, be due to *abnormal intra-atrial conduction*, an intra-atrial conduction disturbance.

Overall Evaluation

The diagnosis of atrial infarction is based on the presence of one or more of the electrocardiographic parameters outlined above, which occur in association with a clinical presentation and with biochemical changes (the enzyme changes of tissue necrosis) suggestive of infarction. The diagnosis is very suggestive when the clinical and biochemical presentation are associated with abnormalities of the *P* wave and the P-Ta segment, especially a deviation of the P-Ta segment in the *same* direction as the *P* wave. The diagnosis is further considerably strengthened if all three parameters of electrocardiographic abnormality are present. Indeed, the presence of complicating atrial infarction should be suspected whenever ventricular infarction is complicated by a disturbance in atrial rhythm.

It must again be emphasized that the electrocardiographic criteria of atrial infarction have not been definitively established, and that much further study is required.

Section 3 Coronary Insufficiency

Chapter 15

The Electrocardiographic Manifestations of Coronary Insufficiency

Coronary insufficiency is here defined, from the electrocardiographic viewpoint, as an impairment of blood flow through the coronary arteries short of complete obstruction, and which may manifest with the electrocardiographic effects of injury and/or ischaemia but not those of necrosis.

Coronary insufficiency may manifest both clinically and electrocardiographically in acute and chronic forms. Acute coronary insufficiency usually occurs in the symptomatic patient, being associated with pain, angina pectoris, which may be preinfarctional, and which may be precipitated by effort. The acute electrocardiographic manifestation may also be precipitated by the exercise test in the absence of symptoms. The electrocardiographic manifestations of acute coronary insufficiency tend to be transient but conspicuous. Chronic coronary insufficiency may be present electrocardiographically and be clinically latent. The manifestations tend to be more stable, and they may be exaggerated by effort or by an attack of angina pectoris. While the various electrocardiographic manifestations are common to both forms, there is a tendency to a different emphasis in each type.

The general electrocardiographic manifestations of coronary insufficiency will be presented first. Their special emphasis in acute coronary insufficiency will be considered later.

The Electrocardiographic Manifestations

Coronary insufficiency may manifest electrocardiographically as follows:

1. Manifestations which affect repolarization: abnormalities of the S-T segment, the T wave, the U wave, and the Q-T interval.

2. Manifestations which affect depolarization: abnormalities of the QRS complex.

3. Manifestations which affect the vectorial relationship of depolarization to repolarization: abnormalities of the QRS-T angle.

4. Disorders of cardiac rhythm.

THE MANIFESTATIONS OF CORONARY INSUFFICIENCY AFFECTING REPOLARIZATION

The first signs of coronary insufficiency are usually evident in the repolarization process as abnormalities of the S-T segment, the T wave, the U wave, or the Q-T interval. These abnormalities may be stable or transient. The early manifestations are usually transient. They may be aggravated by an attack of angina pectoris, and precipitated or aggravated by the exercise test.

ABNORMALITIES OF THE S-T SEGMENT

The normal S-T segment usually merges smoothly and imperceptibly with the proximal limb of the T wave so that it is impossible to separate them and to tell where the S-T segment ends and the proximal limb of the T wave begins (Diagram A of Fig. 60; Standard lead I of Electrocardiographic Study 77, and Electrocardiographic Study 93a). Furthermore, the normal S-T segment does not remain isoelectric for any appreciable duration. It does not hug the baseline for more than 3 mm (0·12 sec). Indeed, it usually begins to rise almost immediately after leaving the QRS complex to merge with the T wave.

The advent of coronary insufficiency is frequently characterized by the development of a **sharp-angled ST-T junction**. This is due mainly to a **straightening or horizonatality of the S-T segment** which results in a distinct angle between the S-T segment and the T wave (Diagram E of Fig. 60). The S-T segment tends to be isoelectric for 0·12 sec or longer, hugging the baseline (Standard lead II and lead V6 of Electrocardiographic Study 83; see also Electrocardiographic Study 92). The manifestation is due to anterior or apical wall subendocardial electrical injury, this being the characteristic site for development of the injury pattern, since it constitutes the greatest muscular mass of the heart (Fig. 61). This causes

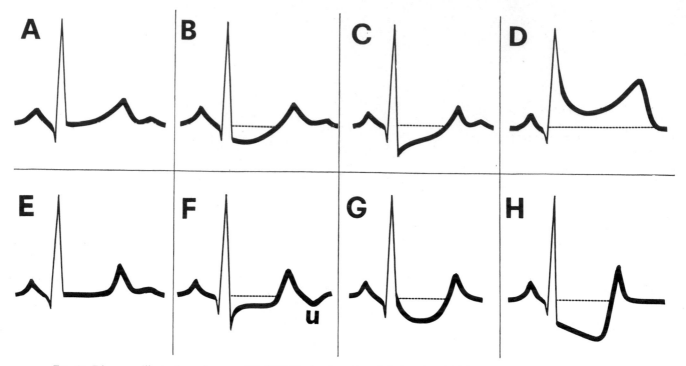

FIG. 60. Diagrams illustrating: A, normal P-QRS-T complex; B and C, junctional S-T segment depression; D, S-T segment elevation and increase in T wave amplitude of the variant form of angina pectoris; E, horizontality of the S-T segment with a sharp angled ST-T junction; F, plane S-T segment depression with U wave inversion; G, sagging S-T segment depression with U wave inversion; G, sagging S-T segment depression; and H, downward-sloping S-T segment depression.

the S-T segment vector to deviate to the endocardial surface of the apex and thus away from the precordial leads which are orientated to the epicardial surface of the apex (see Chapter 2). The earliest sign of this deviation is the sharp angled ST-T junction, and this will be most evident in leads orientated to this greatest muscle mass and which reflect the electrical centre of gravity of the heart. In other words, the manifestation will be most evident in leads with the tallest R wave. These are usually lead V5 in the horizontal plane and Standard lead II in the frontal plane (Fig. 61).

While the hazard of false positive diagnosis of coronary insufficiency on the basis of minor electrocardiographic changes and its attendant iatrogenic sequelae must always be guarded against, the presence of such a sharp angled ST-T junction, even in the absence of S-T segment depression, constitutes a significant pointer to the potential or actual presence of coronary insufficiency. If it is the only abnormal sign present, and the diagnosis is in doubt, confirmation may be obtained by the exercise test. This may accentuate the S-T segment abnormality, causing S-T segment depression (see below), and may also elicit other electrocardiographic abnormalities.

Note: 1. A normal transition S-T segment and T wave may

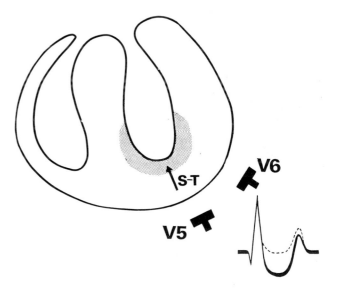

FIG. 61. Diagram illustrating the typical subendocardial location of the injured zone in the classic form of angina pectoris.

produce the effect of a sharp angled ST-T junction. For example, if the T wave is upright in Standard lead I but inverted in Standard lead III, then Standard lead II may reflect a transitional T wave which may manifest as a sharp angled ST-T junction. This does not necessarily signify abnormality (Electrocardiographic Study 77).

A similar phenomenon may occur in the horizontal plane. If the *T* wave in the right precordial leads is opposite in direction to the *T* wave in the left precordial leads, the transition lead (usually lead V4) may reflect a horizontal S-T segment with a sharp angled ST-T junction. This is not significant of coronary artery disease unless the S-T segment horizontality with sharp angled ST-T junction also appears in leads V5 and V6.

2. Horizontality of the S-T segment with a sharp angled ST-T junction may also occur with hypocalcaemia (Electrocardiographic Study 104). The Q-T interval is prolonged, and the *T* wave is normal or diminished in duration. The prolonged Q-T interval is thus due to prolongation of the S-T segment which consequently also hugs the baseline for longer than 0·12 sec. The manifestation is usually seen in all leads (Electrocardiographic Study 104).

Progression, deterioration, of the electrical injury is characterized by the following.

An Increase in the Sharpness or Angulation of the ST-T Junction
This is due to an even greater horizontality of the S-T segment, the S-T segment remaining isoelectric for an even longer period.

Depression of the S-T Segment Below the Baseline
This may take one of the following forms:

Plane depression. The S-T segment is depressed but the horizontality is maintained (Diagram F of Fig. 60; Electrocardiographic Studies 79, 80, 81, 82, 92 and 93).

Downward-sloping S-T segment depression: exaggeration of the distal angle. At times, the depression of the distal part of the S-T segment is more marked than the proximal part. In other words, the distal angle, the angle between the S-T segment and the *T* wave, is even more pronounced (more acute) than the proximal angle, the angle with the QRS complex (Diagram H of Fig. 60; Electrocardiographic Studies 82 and 94). The S-T segment will then have a downward slope.

Sagging — concave-upward — S-T segment depression. The depression may affect the centre of the S-T segment predominantly, giving it a sagging, concave-upward appearance (Diagram G of Fig. 60; Electrocardiographic Studies 34C and 81). An attack of angina pectoris may occur during the course of a myocardial infarction. This will be reflected by the advent of the classic S-T segment depression (Electrocardiographic Study 34C), this being

superimposed upon, or modifying, the parameters of infarction.

Comments and Further Observations
1. The S-T segment depression of chronic coronary insufficiency may increase with the exercise test or with an associated attack of angina pectoris (Electrocardiographic Studies 92 and 94).

2. The degree of S-T segment depression correlates roughly with the severity of the coronary insufficiency (Robb and Marks, 1964)[R20], see also p. 166.

3. S-T segment depression of moderate or marked degree is usually an expression of *acute* coronary insufficiency, as occurs during angina pectoris or when precipitated by the exercise test. Marked S-T segment depression is seldom seen when the patient is asymptomatic at the time of the electrocardiographic recording. However, horizontality of the S-T segment and sharp angled ST-T junction without depression or with minimal depression are common manifestations of chronic coronary insufficiency, and may occur in the absence of symptoms or physical stress (Electrocardiographic Studies 37, 79, 81, 82 and 83).

4. The diagnosis of coronary insufficiency from abnormal S-T segment and *T* wave changes in the presence of left bundle branch block is considered on p. 164.

Junctional S-T segment depression. Junctional S-T segment depression refers to depression of the *proximal* part of the S-T segment, viz. its junction with the QRS complex. While the proximal part of the S-T segment is depressed, the distal part still rises to merge smoothly and imperceptibly with the *T* wave (Diagrams B and C of Fig. 60).

Junctional S-T segment depression is frequently a physiological phenomenon, and may indeed be an expression of a normal and healthy heart. It may also, at times (though rarely), be an expression of coronary insufficiency. The significance of junctional S-T segment depression may thus be difficult to evaluate, and is considered further below. It must, however, be emphasized at the outset that the diagnosis of coronary insufficiency should rarely, if ever, be based solely on the presence of junctional S-T segment depression.

Junctional S-T Segment Depression of Physiological Origin
Physiological depression of the S-T segment junction is usually due to the depressing effect of the deflection representing atrial repolarization; the P-Ta segment, and the *Ta* or *Tp* wave, the atrial *T* wave (see Chapter 14). Atrial depolarization, as represented by the *P* wave, is followed by atrial repolarization, which is represented by a *T* wave

analogous to that of the T wave of ventricular repolarization. However, unlike the T wave of ventricular repolarization wave, which is in the *same* direction as the depolarization process (the T wave and QRS complex being similarly directed), the atrial T wave (the Ta wave) is *opposite in direction to the* P *wave*. The Ta wave occurs coincidentally with, and is thus superimposed upon, the QRS complex. It is therefore masked or obscured by the QRS complex. It is best seen when the P wave occurs in isolation, as in second degree or complete A-V block, when it appears as a shallow depression following the P wave. The distal limb of the P wave usually continues in an almost unbroken downward slope with the proximal limb of the Ta wave (Diagrams A and B of Fig. 59). Furthermore, the taller the P wave, the deeper the associated Ta wave. The Ta wave may, at times, extend onto, and thus be superimposed upon, the proximal or junctional part of the S-T segment. This is particularly likely when the associated P-R interval is relatively short, so that the atrial events are brought closer to the ventricular events. When this occurs, the Ta wave will tend to encroach upon and depress the proximal or junctional part of the S-T segment. The longer the P-R interval, the less likely the extension of the Ta wave onto the S-T junction. Such depression is physiological and not the expression of coronary insufficiency.

This physiological form of junctional S-T segment depression is commonly associated with sinus tachycardia, either inherent or when precipitated by exercise. This is because:

(a) sinus tachycardia will tend to shorten the P-R interval and hence favour a shift of the Ta wave onto the S-T segment, and

(b) sinus tachycardia is frequently associated with a slight right axis deviation of the P wave. This will cause the P wave axis to shift maximally to its normal rightward limit which is $+60°$. The P wave thus becomes taller in Standard lead II, and the depressing effect on the S-T segment will tend to be greater in Standard lead II, a lead commonly used for interpretation of S-T segment abnormalities, particularly those precipitated by exercise.

A method for distinguishing between the junctional depression of physiological origin and pathological origin is discussed in Chapter 16, p. 160 and 161.

ABNORMALITIES OF THE T WAVE

With the advent of coronary insufficiency, the T wave may become more symmetrical, pointed and arrow-head in appearance. Since it is directed away from the surface of ischaemia, it will become inverted in the left lateral leads, leads V4–V6, Standard lead I, lead AVL, and possibly

Standard lead II, in cases of left ventricular subepicardial ischaemia (Electrocardiographic Studies 40 and 88). In such cases it is frequently associated with a prolonged Q-T interval and possibly some slight elevation of the S-T segment. The manifestation tends to occur more commonly in chronic coronary insufficiency. In cases of subendocardial ischaemia the T wave may become taller and more symmetrical in the left lateral leads, since the T wave vector is now directed away from the subendocardium towards the left lateral leads (Electrocardiographic Studies 55, 78, 81, 83, 85 and 86). In such cases it is frequently associated with a depressed S-T segment and a *shortened* Q-T interval (see section on Acute Coronary Insufficiency, p. 142).

The localization of the T wave changes of myocardial ischaemia are discussed in greater detail in Chapter 3.

Post-extrasystolic T *Wave Change*

Post-extrasystolic T wave change refers to a change in the form or direction of the T wave which occurs in the first conducted beat *after* an extrasystole (ventricular or supraventricular). The manifestation usually occurs without any change in the associated antecedent QRS complex. The change commonly occurs for one beat only, and the pattern then reverts to that of the basic uncomplicated sinus rhythm.

The post-extrasystolic change is not due to the extrasystole as such, but rather to the pause which it evokes. Thus, a similar change may occur with the pause resulting from a blocked atrial extrasystole, or a relatively long ventricular cycle during atrial fibrillation.

The change is frequently best seen in leads of the transition zone, for example lead V3 and V4, and may take the form of:

(a) a frank inversion of the T wave (Electrocardiographic Study 96),

(b) a diminution in the amplitude of the T wave,

(c) an increase in the amplitude of the T wave.

Moreover, when the change is due to coronary insufficiency, the T wave is not only changed in amplitude and direction but also in form. Thus, when the T wave becomes inverted, it frequently tends to adopt the features of coronary insufficiency, being symmetrical, sharply pointed and arrow–head in appearance (Electrocardiographic Study 96). When inverted, it is also frequently associated with a *prolongation of the Q-T interval*. All these features contribute to the so-called characteristic 'coronary contour'.

At times, the T wave may be increased in amplitude, also tending to become symmetrical. It is then usually associated with some S-T segment depression, and possibly a shortened Q-T interval.

The post-extrasystolic T wave change may be accentuated if it occurs immediately after exercise[M90].

Significance

The phenomenon is generally associated with myocardial disease, and may be associated with such conditions as hypertensive heart disease and coronary insufficiency[L42, M12, M81]. It correlates well with the abnormal manifestations elicited by the exercise test in cases of myocardial ischaemia[L42], and has indeed been termed the 'poor man's exercise test' by Harold Levine (1958)[L39], since it gives immediate evidence of abnormality and obviates the necessity for a more expensive exercise test.

The dominant manifestation in leads V3 and V4 suggests myocardial ischaemia of the anterior wall of the left ventricle and an impairment of blood flow through the anterior descending branch of the left coronary artery.

Mechanism

The exact mechanism is still speculative. It has been postulated that it may be due to changes in diastolic filling[L42, S46], an increase in ventricular gradient secondary to the increased cycle length[L42], the mechanical impact of the heart against the chest wall after a long pause[L42], and an asynchrony of repolarization[M12]. Recent work has indicated that the phenomenon may be due to an asynchronous adjustment of the action potential to the new cycle length[J11], there being, in effect, a hysteresis of the action potentials to the abrupt change in rate. See also section on Post-extrasystolic U Wave Change on p. 140).

ABNORMALITIES OF THE U WAVE

The U wave is the smallest, the most ill-defined, and the most inconspicuous of the electrocardiographic deflections. It is therefore frequently unobserved or overlooked. Yet, the U wave is probably one of the most important of the electrocardiographic deflections, since changes in its configuration and/or vectorial direction are usually associated with heart disease that is frequently advanced.

The Normal U Wave

The normal U wave is a small, rounded deflection which appears just after the T wave, and is similarly directed to the T wave (Diagrams A, B, C and E of Fig. 60, and Fig. 65). In other words, the U wave is upright in leads where the T wave is upright.

The U wave axis is commonly directed at $+60°$ on the frontal plane hexaxial reference system. It is directed anteriorly and slightly to the left in the horizontal plane (Fig. 62). It is therefore of greatest magnitude, and is consequently most conspicuous, in Standard lead II, and in the precordial leads of the transition zone, particularly leads V3 and V4. Since it is directed at $+60°$ it is least conspicuous (equiphasic or isoelectric) in lead AVL (Fig. 62). This is the reason why measurement of the Q-T interval is best done in lead AVL; for the isoelectric U wave means that the end of the T wave is not distorted by the effects of the U wave, and accurate measurement of the Q-T interval is thereby facilitated. The T-U segment is the isoelectric period between the end of the T wave and the beginning of the U wave.

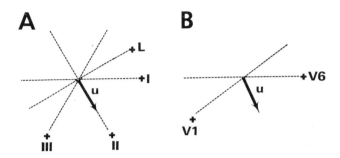

FIG. 62. Diagrams illustrating the typical direction of the U wave vector in: A, the frontal plane; and B, the horizontal plane.

The Genesis of the U Wave

Many theories have been advanced as to the genesis of the U wave. These include the following:

(a) The U wave may represent an after-potential.

(b) The U wave may represent the longer duration of the action potential of Purkinje tissues, and possibly the conducting system.

(c) The U wave may represent repolarization of the papillary muscles. This appears to be the most likely explanation at present, since the papillary muscles, because of their structure and function, are repolarized late, i.e. after the main muscle mass.

The Abnormal U Wave

An inverted U wave, i.e. a U wave that is opposite in direction to an upright T wave, is abnormal and is always associated with heart disease (Diagram F of Fig. 60). It is usually a manifestation of myocardial ischaemia but may also occur in association with left ventricular hypertrophy.

The inverted U wave may occur as an isolated phenomenon (Electrocardiographic Study 84), or it may be associated with other manifestations of heart, and particularly coronary artery, disease such as tall symmetrical T waves and abnormalities of the S-T segment (Electrocardiographic Studies 83, 91 and 92). Thus, the presence of an inverted U wave in Standard lead I, II, lead AVL, and leads V4–V6 is *always* abnormal.

The inverted, abnormal, *U* wave may be present as a stable manifestation of chronic coronary insufficiency (Electrocardiographic Studies 83 and 84), or it may be precipitated by the exercise test as a transient manifestation of acute coronary insufficiency (Electrocardiographic Studies 91 and 92). It may also manifest as a post-extrasystolic phenomenon (see below, and Electrocardiographic Study 97).

The Significance of Abnormal U Waves

An abnormal, inverted, *U* wave is always a sign of heart disease. In a review of 11,000 cases, Furbetta and associates (1956)[F36] found that every case was associated with cardiovascular pathology and with definite involvement of the papillary muscles.

Post-extrasystolic U Wave Change

The first beat after a long pause as associated, for example, by an extrasystole, may also result in changes of the *U* wave. The usual manifestation is an increase in the amplitude of the *U* wave[L42]. The change is best seen in the same leads which reflect the post-extrasystolic *T* wave change, viz. leads V3 and V4. There may also be an associated post-extrasystolic *T* wave change (see p. 138).

The *U* wave may also become *inverted* in the first, and occasionally the second, sinus beats following an extrasystole[S19] (Electrocardiographic Study 97). This is always indicative of myocardial disease and is most commonly due to coronary insufficiency.

ABNORMALITIES OF THE Q-T INTERVAL

The Q-T interval represents the duration of electrical systole and diastole. Its duration may change with both subacute and acute coronary insufficiency.

The Q-T interval may be prolonged with the advent of subacute coronary insufficiency. Prolongation may also occur during the evolution of acute myocardial infarction, appearing after the regression of the early hyperacute injury phase. It is usually observed on about the third or fourth day of acute myocardial infarction (Electrocardiographic Studies 14, 15, 16 and 20). The duration of the Q-T interval may, at times, be very prolonged, and such prolongation may remain for hours or even days.

Acute coronary insufficiency most commonly results in a *shortening of the Q-T interval*. This is usually associated with depressed S-T segments and tall *T* waves in the left lateral leads. The shortening is usually transient, lasting but a few minutes during the duration of an attack of chest pain, or for a few minutes when the changes of myocardial ischaemia are precipitated by the exercise test.

It is of interest to note that when a patient has a re-crudescence of chest pain during the course of acute myocardial infarction, the prolonged Q-T interval of the subacute phase may show considerable shortening (Electrocardiographic Study 16). Thus, with repeated attacks of chest pain during the course of acute myocardial infarction, the Q-T interval may fluctuate between durations which are long and short.

MANIFESTATIONS OF CORONARY INSUFFICIENCY AFFECTING DEPOLARIZATION

THE QRS COMPLEX IN CORONARY INSUFFICIENCY

The QRS changes of coronary insufficiency are most commonly due to chronic coronary insufficiency and, once present, tend to be permanent. Nevertheless, QRS changes may occasionally also be associated with acute coronary insufficiency, and these tend to be transient.

Manifestations of coronary insufficiency which affect the QRS complex are:

1. **Complete or incomplete right bundle branch block.**
2. **Complete or incomplete left bundle branch block.**
3. **Left hemiblock.**

Right Bundle Branch Block

Right bundle branch block may occur in the absence of heart disease, the incidence of normal individuals being 1·5/1000 under the age of 40 years[J17]. The incidence in individuals over 40 years of age is slightly higher, it being 2·9/1000[J17]. This would suggest the possibility of some degree of latent of hidden coronary insufficiency in the older, though asymptomatic, age group.

It is thus evident that right bundle branch block *per se* does not necessarily connote coronary artery disease unless there is other concomitant clinical or electrocardiographic evidence of coronary insufficiency present, such as primary S-T segment and *T* wave change (see Chapter 9, and Chapter 16, p. 164).

Right bundle branch block may also be precipitated as a transient phenomenon in response to exercise. It is then usually an expression of phasic aberrant ventricular conduction (see Chapter 17), although not invariably so. Bauer (1964)[B14] reported the presence of ischaemic heart disease in 13 of 14 such patients.

Left Bundle Branch Block

The presence of established left bundle branch block should always be regarded as pathological. It may be due to myocardial fibrosis as associated for example with long standing congestive cardiac failure or cardiomyopathy, and is frequently an expression of coronary insufficiency. To establish a causal relationship to coronary artery disease, it is necessary to have other clinical and/or electrocardiographic evidence of coronary insufficiency.

The diagnosis of coronary insufficiency from the abnormal S-T segment and *T* wave changes in the presence of left bundle branch block is considered on p. 146 and in Chapter 16. p. 164.

Hemiblock

Block of one of the divisions of the left bundle branch is commonly due to the effects of coronary artery disease. The disease process nearly always affects the anterosuperior division of the left bundle branch resulting in a left anterior hemiblock, a left axis deviation (see Chapter 12).

Left anterior hemiblock is probably the commonest electrocardiographic manifestation of coronary artery disease, and may indeed be the first manifestation of the disease. It is however necessary to observe other electrocardiographic abnormalities of coronary artery disease in order to establish a causal relationship (see also Correlative Essay, Chapter 12, p. 121).

The posteroinferior division of the left bundle branch is very rarely affected because it is more resistant to disease processes enjoying, *inter alia*, a double blood supply (see Chapter 12).

Both left anterior hemiblock[K50] and eft posterior hemiblock[B64, K50] may occur as transient phenomena during the exercise test.

Transient left hemiblock has also been observed during episodes of chest pain in patients with the variant form of angina pectoris[J19], and after opacification of the coronary arteries with radio-opaque substances[F10, M62].

MANIFESTATIONS OF CORONARY INSUFFICIENCY AFFECTING THE VECTORIAL RELATIONSHIP OF DEPOLARIZATION TO REPOLARIZATION

ABNORMALITIES OF THE QRS:T ANGLE

The effects of coronary insufficiency may be evident from the vectorial relationship of the depolarization to repolarization processes. In other words the relationship of the mean manifest QRS and *T* wave vectors—the QRS-T angle.

The Normal QRS: T Relationship

The QRS and *T* wave vectors tend to be similarly directed on both the frontal and horizontal planes, and the QRS-T angle is consequently narrow. The QRS and *T* wave

vectors are usually directed to the region of $+30°$ to $+40°$ (range $0°$ to $+90°$) on the frontal plane hexaxial reference system, and the QRS-T angle is usually less than $45°$, rarely exceeding $60°$ (Diagram A of Fig. 63). Furthermore, the mean manifest frontal plane *T* wave vector tends to follow any deviation of the mean manifest frontal plane QRS vector, so that the narrowness of the QRS-T angle is maintained. Such deviations of the *T* wave vector are less marked than those of the QRS vector. This close relationship between the mean manifest frontal plane QRS and *T* wave vectors means that the *T* wave is upright where the QRS is dominantly upright, and vice versa.

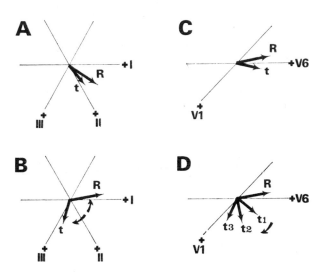

FIG. 63. Diagrams illustrating: A, a normal QRS-T angle on the frontal plane; C, a normal QRS-T angle on the horizontal plane; B, a wide frontal plane QRS-T angle; and D, the development of a wide horizontal plane QRS-T angle.

Occasionally, a wide frontal plane QRS-T angle may manifest in a normal individual. This is particularly likely to occur in the tall and thin individual. It is associated with specific locations of the frontal plane QRS and *T* wave axes—*a half-past-two syndrome*. The QRS axis is usually directed to the vicinity of $+90°$ (the long arm of the clock), and the *T* wave axis (the short arm of the clock) is directed to $-30°$ (Electrocardiographic Study 102A).

The QRS-T angle is also normally narrow on the horizontal plane (Diagram C of Fig. 63). Accurate measurement of these vectors is, however, more difficult because of the proximity of the precordial leads, and the variations in body build. Nevertheless, both mean QRS and *T* wave vectors are usually directed to the left and somewhat posteriorly, towards the positive pole of the lead V6 electrode and away from the V1 electrode (Diagram C of Fig. 63). Thus, both the QRS complex and *T* wave are normally upright in lead V6 and inverted in lead V1.

The Effect of Coronary Insufficiency

As indicated in Chapter 2, the *T* wave vector deviates away from the area of mischief. As coronary insufficiency affects mainly the left ventricle, the *T* wave vector will deviate or tend to deviate away from the left. The result is a widening of the QRS-T angle, which may be evident on both the frontal and horizontal planes. This deviation may, in the presence of chronic coronary insufficiency, be permanent.

The Effect on the Frontal Plane

The *T* wave vector tends to deviate inferiorly and to the right, whereas the QRS vector is stationary or may even be deviated slightly or more markedly to the left, due to the development of a concomitant left anterior hemiblock, a frequent manifestation of coronary insufficiency (Diagram B of Fig. 63). The mean manifest QRS vector thus becomes more aligned with the lead axis of Standard lead I, and hence dominantly positive, and possibly tallest, in this lead. The *T* wave axis deviates towards the positive pole of Standard lead III and away from the Standard lead I electrode. It therefore tends to become relatively tall in Standard lead III, and relatively low or inverted in Standard lead I (Electrocardiographic Studies 37, 83, 88 and 89).

This manifestation is also known empirically as the 'T III greater than T I' syndrome[D28, D31]. It is evident, however, that this empirical observation must be further qualified by the presence of a dominantly positive QRS complex in Standard lead I. For example, the T III greater than T I syndrome has little meaning if the QRS axis is also deviated to the right. It is also evident that the T III greater than T I syndrome, in the presence of a dominantly upright QRS complex in Standard lead I, is merely an expression of a wide QRS-T angle, and is more accurately expressed as such.

The Effect on the Horizontal Plane

With the advent of coronary insufficiency, myocardial ischaemia, the *T* wave deviates away from the left and towards the right (Diagram D of Fig. 63). Thus, with progressive deviation, the *T* wave becomes progressively lower in lead V6 and eventually becomes frankly inverted in lead V6 (Electrocardiographic Study 88). It also becomes progressively taller in lead V1. It is further evident that during this progression a stage will be reached when the *T* wave vector is directed towards both the lead V6 and the lead V1 electrodes but is more aligned with the V1 electrode. The *T* waves, under this circumstance, will be taller in lead V1 than in lead V6, although both will be upright. This is known as the 'T V1 greater than T V6' syndrome[G31, W31] (Electrocardiographic Studies 37, 46 and 89). This is merely an expression of a wide QRS-T angle,

and may be the only, and earliest, manifestation of coronary insufficiency.

DISORDERS OF CARDIAC RHYTHM

Coronary insufficiency may manifest with almost any form of abnormal cardiac rhythm. There may be abnormalities of impulse formation such as ventricular extrasystoles (Electrocardiographic Study 91), or there may be abnormalities of impulse conduction, particularly first and second degree A-V block. The advent of acute A-V block in patients with coronary artery disease is usually due to myocardial ischaemia, whereas chronic A-V block is due to a combination of myocardial ischaemia with a mechanical factor such as fibrosis or calcification of the interventricular septum[L34] (see Chapter 17). To establish a causal relationship with coronary insufficiency, there must by other clinical and/or electrocardiographic abnormalities of coronary insufficiency present.

ACUTE CORONARY INSUFFICIENCY

Acute coronary insufficiency is defined as that which is precipitated suddenly, and which manifests in the symptomatic patient as angina pectoris, or that which occurs when electrocardiographic changes are precipitated acutely by, and related to, exercise (with or without associated angina pectoris) as in the exercise test.

The electrocardiographic manifestation of acute coronary insufficiency may develop or be precipitated in a patient whose tracing during the non-acute phase is completely normal. Or, the manifestation of the acute phase may be superimposed upon the manifestation of chronic coronary insufficiency.

Whereas the changes of chronic coronary insufficiency tend to be more stable and permanent, the changes of acute coronary insufficiency tend to be unstable and transient.

Manifestations Affecting the S-T Segment

Acute coronary insufficiency commonly results in subendocardial injury and less commonly in subepicardial injury, affecting in particular the apical and adjacent anteroseptal regions of the left ventricle (see Chapter 2; Diagram B of Fig. 9 and Fig. 61).

ACUTE SUBENDOCARDIAL INJURY

This is one of the commonest manifestations of angina pectoris, and is reflected by the depression of the S-T segment which may, at times, be marked (see Chapter 16). Subendocardial injury will manifest with depression of the

S-T segment in leads orientated to the apical region, particularly leads V5 and Standard lead II. The manifestations not infrequently appear in Standard leads I, II, lead AVL and leads V4–V6, thereby indicating considerable extension of the injury. The S-T segment depression is more marked in the precordial leads (V4–V6) than in the extremity leads (Standard leads I, II and AVL) (Electrocardiographic Study 94). The depression may, for example, be as much as 4 mm below the baseline in lead V5, but is usually about 1 mm below the baseline in Standard lead II. See also the section dealing with the criteria for a positive exercise test in Chapter 16. The depression may be of the plane (horizontal) type (Electrocardiographic Studies 93 and 94), or of the sagging type (Electrocardiographic Study 34C). There is also some evidence that the degree of depression is roughly proportional to the degree of coronary insufficiency (Robb and Marks, 1964)[R20]. The depression may be associated with angina pectoris, particularly if marked, but may also occur in the absence of angina pectoris.

The S-T segment depression may occur as an isolated phenomenon (Electrocardiographic Studies 93 and 94), or it may be accompanied by other manifestations of acute coronary insufficiency such as U wave inversion (Electrocardiographic Studies 79 and 92).

ACUTE SUBEPICARDIAL INJURY

THE VARIANT FORM OF ANGINA PECTORIS: PRINZMETAL'S—ATYPICAL—ANGINA PECTORIS

Acute angina pectoris may occasionally be due to acute subepicardial injury, and manifest characteristically with *elevated S-T segments* in leads orientated to the injured surface. This is in contrast to the more common and classic form of angina pectoris which is due to subendocardial injury and which manifests with depressed S-T segments in the left lateral leads. Attention was first focused on this unusual form of angina pectoris by Prinzmetal and associates[P30], who termed it the variant form of angina pectoris. Sporadic reports had previously appeared in the literature. For example, Kroop and Master (1949)[K45] drew attention to the fact that elevation of the S-T segment was occasionally seen as a response to exercise, and that this was an unusual manifestation of myocardial ischaemia. The condition, although not uncommon in clinical practice, has nevertheless been poorly reported, there being only 51 cases until 1970[R65]. This is probably because it is difficult to document the attacks, since they usually occur spontaneously. The phenomenon is, however, receiving increasing attention[E3].

ELECTROCARDIOGRAPHIC CHARACTERISTICS

Elevated S-T Segments

Since the S-T segment vector is always directed towards the surface of injury, the epicardial injury of the variant form of angina pectoris manifests characteristically with *elevation* of the S-T segment in leads orientated to the epicardial surface of the left ventricular apex and adjacent regions. The elevated S-T segments are thus usually seen in leads V2–V6, particularly leads V4–V6 (Electrocardiographic Studies 90 and 91), but may occasionally be most marked in the mid-precordial leads, leads V2–V4[C30]. At times, it may also manifest in the inferiorly orientated leads, Standard leads II and III, and lead AVF[B65]. This is especially likely to occur in patients with vertical hearts.

The S-T segment elevation is usually marked, and may be as much as 4 mm in magnitude. The elevation is most commonly associated with an upright T wave, in which case it tends to be concave-upward or to have an upward slope towards the T wave. The manifestation is identical to the slope elevation of the hyperacute early injury phase of acute myocardial infarction. The manifestation may also appear as a primary S-T segment and T wave change in complicating ventricular extrasystoles (Electrocardiographic Study 90[S37]; see Chapter 13).

The S-T segment elevation may, at times, also be associated with inverted T waves, in which case it is convex-upward and simulates the S-T segment and T wave presentation of the fully evolved phase of acute myocardial infarction.

The T Wave Abnormality

The upright T waves are usually increased in amplitude. They also tend to become pointed and widened, as in the early hyperacute phase of myocardial infarction (Electrocardiographic Studies 90 and 91). Less frequently, the T wave may be inverted, pointed and symmetrical as in the fully evolved phase of acute myocardial infarction.

Manifestations Affecting the QRS Complex

Increase in the Amplitude of the R Wave

The R wave may become taller than normal. This is probably a manifestation of acute injury block (Electrocardiographic Study 90; see also Chapter 12, p. 101).

Diminution in the Depth of the S Wave

There may be a diminution in the depth of the S wave of an RS complex. When the left lateral or inferior leads reflect a tall R wave followed by a terminal S wave, the S wave may be diminished in size during an attack of the variant form of angina pectoris (Electrocardiographic Study 91).

Transient Left Anterior Hemiblock: Transient Left Axis Deviation

A transient left axis deviation during the attack is occasionally evident (Case of Ruser[R65], and Case 3 of Bobba and associates, 1972[B65]).

U Wave Inversion

Inversion of the U wave, particularly in the left lateral precordial leads, may also occur during an attack of the variant form of angina pectoris (Electrocardiographic Study 91).

Ventricular Extrasystoles and Extrasystolic Ventricular Tachycardia

Ventricular extrasystoles, either singly (Electrocardiographic Study 90), in pairs, or three or more consecutive ventricular extrasystoles in a row—an extrasystolic ventricular tachycardia (Electrocardiographic Study 91)—may be associated with an attack of the variant form of angina pectoris. The typical S-T segment changes may also be evident in the S-T segments of the complicating ventricular extrasystoles, and may indeed be more marked in the ventricular extrasystoles than in the conducted sinus beats (Electrocardiographic Study 90)[S37].

A-V Block

Various and varying degrees of A-V block have also been reported in association with the variant form of angina pectoris. These include transient complete A-V block.

FURTHER OBSERVATIONS

1　*Apparent Normalization of the Electrocardiographic Manifestations of Subendocardial Injury*

Where the electrocardiogram recorded before an attack of the variant form of angina pectoris shows depressed S-T segments and/or T wave inversion in the lateral precordial leads (manifestations of the classic form of angina pectoris or the expression of chronic subendocardial injury), the advent of the variant form of angina pectoris may erroneously appear to improve the electrocardiographic presentation. This is because there is elevation of the depressed S-T segment and reversion of the inverted T wave, thereby correcting or neutralizing the abnormal features.

2　*Relationship to Physical Effort*

The original description of the variant form of angina pectoris emphasized that it occurred spontaneously, at rest, and was not related to physical effort. Nevertheless, recent reports have indicated that the variant form of angina pectoris and the typical electrocardiographic manifestations may also be precipitated by effort[B90, H21, M26, M55, S34, S37]

(Electrocardiographic Study 91). Moreover, the prognosis (see below) appears to be the same whether it occurs spontaneously or is precipitated by effort.

3　*Relationship to the Electrocardiographic Manifestations of Acute Myocardial Infarction*

It is evident that the classic electrocardiographic presentation of the variant form of angina pectoris, slope elevation of the S-T segment with tall, wide T wave, is identical to that of the early hyperacute injury phase of acute myocardial infarction (see Chapter 2), the only difference being that the electrocardiographic changes of the variant form are transient and reversible, whereas the manifestations in acute myocardial infarction progress to the fully evolved phase of acute myocardial infarction. The mechanism is probably the same. The coronary artery occlusion in the case of myocardial infarction, and the near-total obstruction in the case of the variant angina pectoris, effect a loss of intracellular potassium which brings about the electrocardiographic manifestations of injury and ischaemia. The transient nature of the variant form of angina pectoris indicates that these manifestations are still reversible. Indeed, the classic coved and elevated S-T segment with inverted T wave of the fully evolved phase of acute myocardial infarction may also appear as a transient manifestation of the variant form of angina pectoris. Even the added manifestation of myocardial necrosis may appear as a single transient manifestation in a ventricular extrasystole complicating the variant form of angina pectoris (Electrocardiographic Study 90)[S37].

CLINICAL CHARACTERISTICS OF THE VARIANT FORM OF ANGINA PECTORIS

The character and distribution of the pain of the variant form of angina pectoris are identical to that of the classic form of angina pectoris, being substernal with the typical radiation to the jaw and down the ulnar surfaces of the arms. It is also typically oppressive in character. Unlike the classic form of angina pectoris, the pain frequently occurs *spontaneously* and is not necessarily related to effort or emotion. A prominent feature of the pain is its *unusual severity* and *longer duration* when compared to the classic form of angina pectoris. The condition usually presents with a series of attacks which tend to be cyclical; the pain recurs every few minutes, with peaks of remarkable constancy, and frequently at the same time or times of each day. The waxing and waning periods of chest pain are often of equal duration, unlike the typical form of angina pectoris where the waning period is shorter and more abrupt than the waxing period. The attacks frequently progress to myocardial infarction, after which the severe angina pectoris often disappears dramatically. In about half the cases, the variant form of angina pectoris is preceded by the classic angina pectoris of effort.

The clinical associations closely mirror those of classical angina pectoris and myocardial infarction. Hence, in a recent review Ruser[R65] reported that 90 per cent of the cases occurred in men, the average age being 59 years. Associated factors included diabetes, systemic arterial hypertension, obesity, and a smoking habit.

PROGNOSIS

The very grave prognosis of the variant angina pectoris is well documented. Infarction and death occur in more than one half of the patients in less than 1 year after the onset of symptoms (see p. 166).

PATHOLOGY

In the majority of cases, the disorder is due to a marked narrowing of a major coronary artery or branch. On the basis of autopsy material and animal experimentation, Prinzmetal and associates [P28,P30] showed that the variant angina pectoris is associated with severe narrowing of a single major coronary artery. Most of the available evidence supports the concept that the clinical findings characteristic of the variant angina pectoris constitute presumptive evidence that there is a single severe obstruction of a major coronary artery or branch[F18, M1, M2]. Thus. MacAlpin[M1], in all 12 of a group of patients with the variant angina pectoris, reported focal stenotic lesions of a major coronary artery on angiography precisely in the area predicted from the distribution of the abnormal S-T segments during pain. Fortuin and Friesinger[F18] reported a near-total occlusion of a major coronary artery in 11 of 12 patients with the variant angina pectoris.

The pathological nature of the obstruction is not always clear. Prinzmetal suggested that it may be due to an increase in vascular tone in an already narrowed major coronary artery. The syndrome thus represents a more severe and usually more focal form of coronary atherosclerosis. For example, angiographic studies in six patients revealed a single stenotic lesion in one major artery without significant disease elsewhere[M2]. It has, however, become clear from recent reports that the severe focal stenosis is not necessarily due to an isolated patch of atherosclerosis, but rather a grossly affected region of a major coronary artery, as part of more diffuse coronary atherosclerosis. Superimposed hypertonus or spasm of the coronary artery may aggravate the narrowing, and thus precipitate an attack. This may have been the mechanism in two recent reports[G11, W37]

which showed normal or nearly normal coronary arteries on coronary angiography.

Experimental observations are similar to those in man. Near-total obstruction of a major coronary artery results in S-T segment elevation[B19, B60, E8, W19, W62]. Such changes do not occur until coronary blood flow has been reduced by 70 per cent or more[W19], and are rapidly reversible by the re-establishment of blood flow.

Manifestations Affecting the T Wave

Acute coronary insufficiency frequently results in temporary subendocardial or subepicardial *ischaemia* of the anterior myocardial wall which manifests with *T* wave changes. Such *T* wave changes are, in the acute context, usually marked and transient.

ACUTE ANTERIOR WALL SUBENDOCARDIAL ISCHAEMIA

Acute coronary insufficiency frequently results in acute subendocardial ischaemia which commonly affects the anteroseptal and apical regions of the left ventricle. The electrocardiogram consequently manifests with *tall symmetrical* T *waves* which appear in leads V3–V6 (possibly Standard leads I and II), and which thus reflect a *T* wave vector directed away from the subendocardial surface of the left ventricle (see Chapter 3; Electrocardiographic Studies 85 and 86). The *T* waves may be very tall and may reach 10–15 mm in height. The manifestation may occur as an isolated phenomenon (Electrocardiographic Studies 85 and 86), or it may be associated with other signs of coronary insufficiency such as *U* wave inversion of S-T segment elevation (Electrocardiographic Study 97). The associated Q-T interval is not infrequently shortened.

Note: Tall symmetrical *T* waves may also appear in leads V2–V6 in posterior wall subepicardial ischaemia. The differential diagnosis is discussed in Chapter 3. The differential diagnosis of other causes of tall symmetrical *T* waves in the precordial leads is discussed in a Correlative Essay in Chapter 3 p. 29.

ACUTE ANTERIOR WALL SUBEPICARDIAL ISCHAEMIA

Acute coronary insufficiency may be associated with acute subepicardial ischaemia. This is far less common than acute subendocardial ischaemia. It results in a *T* wave vector which is directed away from the left epicardial surface, and which is reflected by inversion of the *T* waves in the left lateral leads V4–V6, Standard lead I and lead AVL, and not infrequently in Standard lead II. The *T* waves tend to be symmetrical. The associated Q-T interval is often *prolonged.*

THE ELECTROCARDIOGRAPHIC DIAGNOSIS OF CORONARY INSUFFICIENCY IN THE PRESENCE OF LEFT BUNDLE BRANCH BLOCK

Acute or chronic coronary insufficiency may result in anterolateral subendocardial injury and ischaemia, or anterolateral subepicardial ischaemia. The diagnosis of these electropathological phenomena in the presence of left bundle branch block is considered below. The S-T segment and *T* wave manifestations of uncomplicated left bundle branch block will be presented first.

The S-T Segment and T Wave Manifestations in the Left Lateral Leads of Uncomplicated Left Bundle Branch Block

In uncomplicated left bundle branch block, leads orientated to the left ventricle, leads V5 and V6, Standard lead I and lead AVL, will reflect the following secondary changes of repolarization (Diagram B of Fig. 37 and Diagram D of Fig. 67).

(a) The S-T segment is depressed with a slight, though characteristic, minimal *upward convexity.*

(b) The associated *T* wave has a blunt apex with asymmetrical limbs, the proximal limb being shallower than the distal limb.

THE DIAGNOSIS OF ANTEROLATERAL SUBENDOCARDIAL INJURY AND ISCHAEMIA IN THE PRESENCE OF LEFT BUNDLE BRANCH BLOCK

With the advent of anterolateral subendocardial injury and ischaemia, the following primary changes in repolarization occur:

1. The depressed S-T segment in the left lateral leads may become *concave-upward* (Diagrams E and F of Fig. 67; Electrocardiographic Study 57).

2. The S-T segment may become more depressed as, for example, in the acute coronary insufficiency precipitated by the exercise test (Diagrams E and F of Fig. 67; see also Chapter 16, p. 164).

3. The associated *T wave in the left lateral leads may become upright* (Electrocardiographic Study 57).

THE DIAGNOSIS OF ANTEROLATERAL SUBEPICARDIAL ISCHAEMIA IN THE PRESENCE OF LEFT BUNDLE BRANCH BLOCK

When left bundle branch block is complicated by left axis deviation due, for example, to a complicating left anterior hemiblock or left anterior parietal block, the QRS complexes will be dominantly negative in Standard leads II and III, and lead AVF. The associated secondary changes of repolarization will be reflected by upright *T* waves. Under this circumstance, the advent of anterolateral subendocardial ischaemia will result in a primary *T* wave change manifesting with *inverted T* waves in Standard leads II and III, and lead AVF.

The advent of anterolateral subepicardial ischaemia in the presence of left bundle branch block, is characterized by the following primary changes in repolarization:

1. The *T* wave becomes deeper, more symmetrical and sharply pointed (Electrocardiographic Study 56).

2. The S-T segment may become more convex-upward, and perhaps even isoelectric.

CORRELATIVE ESSAY

The Differential Diagnosis of T Wave Changes

The *T* wave is the most fickle of the electrocardiographic deflections, and may reflect changes in form and direction under both physiological and pathological conditions. *T* wave changes may occur as:

A. Normal variants.

B. Expression of extracardiac disease.

C. Secondary phenomena, secondary to abnormal intraventricular conduction.

D. Primary phenomena, the expression of primary myocardial disease.

E. A post-tachycardia phenomenon.

The following account, while not exhaustive, reflects the important characteristics of the major categories outlined above.

A NORMAL VARIANTS OF THE T WAVE

Normal *T* wave variants may present under the following circumstances:

1. As a persistent 'Juvenile' pattern.
2. As a response to anxiety or fear.
3. As an expression of vagotonia.
4. As an orthostatic response.
5. As a postprandial response.

6. As a result of hyperventilation.

7. As a 'half-past-two' syndrome.

The reader is referred to a classic paper on this subject by Marriott (1960)[M14].

THE PERSISTENT JUVENILE PATTERN

Inversion of the T wave in the right precordial leads, leads V1–V4, is common in infancy and childhood. This may persist into adulthood, and is then known as the 'persistent juvenile pattern'. This occurs more commonly in Negroes than in Caucasians[G28], having been observed in about 1·2 per cent of Caucasians and in about 11–12 per cent of Negroes[W6, W11]. These changes have been observed in American negroes[G23, L55] as well as South African negroes[G45].

T wave abnormalities have been noted with an incidence of 0·5–4·2 per cent of normal individuals in various population samples[H25, K23, S90, S134, V10]. For example, they have been noted in 0·2 per cent[L56] and 0·7 per cent[F30] of hospital patients, and in 0·4 per cent of a large group of life insurance applicants[K23]. The largest of such group studies (Hiss and Lamb 1962)[H25] comprised 122,043 individuals. The overall incidence of so-called T wave abnormalities was 1·15 per cent. The incidence of T wave variants confined to the right precordial leads was 0·6 per cent. The precordial T wave inversion may, at times, be very marked, greater than 5 mm, in the absence of demonstrable heart disease[P34]. The pattern may disappear with deep inspiration[B53]. It has been suggested that this pattern is due to the transmission of local potentials from the cardiac surface[B53], since local electrocardiograms recorded from the epicardial surface frequently reflect negative T waves[B4]. It is thus possible that these negative epicardial T waves are transmitted to the chest wall from areas not covered by lung, the 'cardiac notch'[B53]. The cardiac notch usually covers an area equivalent to the electrodes of leads V2–V4. The hypothesis may also explain the inverted T waves which may at times appear in the right precordial leads in cases of pectus excavatum[E9].

T WAVE CHANGES PRECIPITATED BY ANXIETY AND FEAR

Fear or anxiety may precipitate T wave changes in individuals who have no evidence of organic heart disease[B39, G39, H22, K5, L25, L36, L60, L62, M5, M8, M51, M85, S81, T1, W25, W28, W32, W36, W51]. Thus, a sudden fright, as induced by the firing of a nearby pistol, may be followed by T wave inversion[G38]. Hypnotically induced anxiety or fear may result in similar changes[B39, L25]. Patients with neurocirculatory asthenia (synonym: Da Costa's Syndrome, Soldier's Heart) and with other forms of psychoneurosis

may reflect low to inverted T waves, particularly in Standard leads II and III[G39, W51]. An increased incidence of minor electrocardiographic abnormalities of the T waves, particularly in Standard leads I and II, has also been reported in patients with psychoneurotic disorders[H22, L25].

THE T WAVE CHANGES ASSOCIATED WITH VAGOTONIA

Increased vagotonia, as occurs, for example in an athlete, is frequently associated with tall symmetrical T waves and minimally elevated S-T segments, particularly in the left precordial leads, leads V4–V6 (Electrocardiographic Studies 100 and 101). The presentation is discussed in greater detail in Chapter 3, p. 30.

ORTHOSTATIC VARIATIONS OF THE T WAVE

The configuration and direction of the T wave may reflect differences with changes in posture.

The assumption of the upright position may be accompanied by inversion of the T wave in Standard lead II. This is especially prone to occur in asthenic individuals[W35], and may be associated with slight prolongation of the P-R interval[M61]. The T wave may occasionally be normally inverted in Standard lead II in the supine position, and the inversion may be accentuated by the upright posture and by deep inspiration. Conversely, the inverted T wave which occurs as a normal variant may become upright upon full expiration and the assumption of the supine posture. The T wave in Standard lead II may at times also become inverted on passive tilting as well as during active changes in position[H39]. The QRS-T angle may widen in the upright position[S60].

Orthostatic T wave changes were found to occur in 30 per cent of subjects who showed junctional S-T segment depression following the exercise test, and in 23 per cent of patients with a positive, ischaemic, response to exercise (Lepeschkin and Surawicz 1958)[L30].

Orthostatic T wave abnormalities have also been observed in 63 per cent of women and 30 per cent of men with neurocirculatory asthenia[L36].

Elevation of the diaphragm in conditions such as obesity or pregnancy may result in loss of amplitude or even inversion of the T waves in the left precordial leads, leads V5 and V6, leads which are orientated to the apex[J3]. These T waves may become upright following a loss of weight[K1].

These transient orthostatic T wave changes have been attributed to increased sympathetic activity[W28]. This is supported by the observations that beta adrenergic blockade decreases the QRS-T angle in the upright posture[S60] and also suppress the orthostatic T wave changes[F34, N13, P12].

POSTPRANDIAL *T* WAVE VARIANTS

A diminution in *T* wave amplitude, or frank inversion of the *T* wave, may occur in Standard leads I and II and leads V2–V4 after a meal[L57, R28, S63, S83, S85]. They have been observed in 3·9 per cent of 2000 young, healthy airmen[S63]. The changes are apparently related to the carbohydrate content of a meal, and has been observed within 30 minutes after a meal of 1200 calories[S85]. It is likely to occur in the dumping syndrome where absorption of sugar is rapid.

These *T* wave variants frequently disappear when the electrocardiograph is recorded after fasting[S90] and may be forestalled by the addition of 3 g of potassium chloride to the meal[R28].

THE EFFECTS OF HYPERVENTILATION

Hyperventilation may result in a diminution in amplitude or frank inversion of the *T* waves in the precordial leads in individuals without heart disease[B44, S6, W11, W12]. It has been reported with an incidence of 11 per cent in normal subjects[W12]. The changes may be more marked after 20 sec hyperventilation than after 60 sec hyperventilation[B44]. Similar observations were noted by Lewis (1964)[L48], and by Crede and associates (1951)[C52].

Hyperventilation may unmask latent examples of the juvenile pattern[W7].

The phenomenon has been variously attributed to tachycardia[S6], a change in the extracellular potassium concentration[Y9], and respiratory alkalosis[B8, B77, C28, C29, L48, T8, Y9], and to a change in heart position[S55].

It is clear, however, that the changes cannot be due to tachycardia, since in individuals who have *T* wave inversion after hyperventilation, no such changes follow the tachycardia induced by exercise[S6, Y9], propantheline bromide[W50, Y9], or breathing air with a 59 per cent concentration of carbon dioxide[C28, C29].

The phenomenon has been attributed to asynchronous shortening of ventricular repolarization during the early phase of sympathetic stimulation, there being a hysteresis of the Q-T interval, with an associated prolongation of the QTc interval[B44]. The changes are analogous to those produced by the infusion of isoproterenol[B44]. Similar abnormalities have also been observed following the intravenous administration of 20 μg of epinephrine[Y9].

Moreover, these changes can be prevented by the prior administration of a beta receptor blocking agent[F35, P12].

THE HALF-PAST-TWO SYNDROME

Occasionally, a wide frontal plane QRS-T angle may manifest in a normal individual, particularly one who is tall and thin. The manifestation is associated with specific locations of the mean manifest frontal plane QRS and *T* wave axes, a 'half-past-two' syndrome. The QRS axis (the long arm of the clock) is commonly directed at $+90°$, and the *T* wave axis (the short arm of the clock) to $-30°$ (Electrocardiographic Study 102A). The phenomenon is sometimes normalized by the exercise test (Electrocardiographic Study 102B).

THE DIAGNOSIS OF NORMAL T WAVE VARIANTS

METHODS USED TO NORMALIZE *T* WAVE VARIANTS

The diagnosis of an apparently abnormal *T* wave as a normal variant is dependent upon the exclusion of any evidence of cardiac or extracardiac disease. When such *T* wave abnormalities occur in isolation and are suspected to be normal variants, the following methods may be used to correct the abnormal manifestation:

1. The electrocardiogram is recorded with the patient in a fasting state.

2. The electrocardiogram is recorded with the patient in a change of posture, i.e. the electrocardiogram is recorded with the patient in the upright position.

3. The electrocardiogram is recorded following hyperventilation.

4. The electrocardiogram is recorded following the induction of tachycardia by exercise, atropine, propantheline bromide, hyperventilation, epinephrine. The resulting tachycardia may normalize the *T* waves[S90, S42, W11].

5. The electrocardiogram may be recorded following a slowing of the heart rate by beta receptor blockers, *ergot* alkaloids such as ergotamine and dihydroergotamine. The intravenous injection of 0·5–1 mg of ergotamine tartrate or 0·25–1 mg of dihydroergotamine will tend to normalize orthostatic and exercise-induced *T* wave abnormalities[H17, L36, L38, Z3]. It should, however, be borne in mind that ergotamine may have a coronary vasoconstricting effect, and may thus induce an attack of angina pectoris in a patient with coronary insufficiency[S52].

6. The electrocardiogram is recorded following the administration of potassium salts by mouth. This may normalize orthostatic *T* wave variants and those induced by hyperventilation[D18, W9], and may also normalize the *T* wave variants in patients with neurocirculatory asthenia, anxiety and psychiatric disturbance[W27]. The abnormal frontal or horizontal plane QRS-T angle of functional *T* wave variants will tend to be normalized, whereas those of left ventricular hypertrophy and myocardial infarction will be unaffected[D18, S58, W9].

The administration of potassium salts may, however, be potentially hazardous in patients with organic heart disease, and should therefore only be done in cases where there is no organic evidence of heart disease, and where it is desired to prove the T wave change as a functional variant.

7. The electrocardiogram is recorded following the administration of isoproterenol. This procedure should only be entertained when there is definitely no evidence of cardiac or extracardiac disease, and where it is desired to establish the T wave change as a functional variant.

B EXTRACARDIAC CAUSES OF T WAVE ABNORMALITIES

Many extracardiac diseases may result in abnormalities of the T wave. These include the following:

1. Acute and chronic abdominal disorders.
2. Endocrine disorders.
3. Cerebrovascular accidents.

ACUTE AND CHRONIC ABDOMINAL DISORDERS

Acute and chronic abdominal disorders[B16, B75, C41, L25, W41] include acute appendicitis[C41], acute pancreatitis[B16, F33, G27, K23, L50, P24, S128], cholecystitis and experimental gall bladder disease[B75, C32, G14, H1, H28, K14, M64, S13, S86, W18, W23, W41] and acute peritonitis[A15], which may simulate the T wave change of acute coronary insufficiency and even myocardial infarction. An electrocardiographic presentation resembling the cerebrovascular accident (CVA) pattern following truncal vagotomy has also been reported[G1].

ENDOCRINE DISORDERS

T wave abnormalities may occur in association with the following endocrine disorders:

Hypothyroidism. This causes a generalized diminution of the T wave amplitude with a deviation of the T wave vector posteriorly and to the right[U4, Z5].

Hypoadrenalism. Adrenal insufficiency may be associated with low to inverted T waves, and a prolonged Q-Tc[R63, S119, T12, W56].

Hypopituitarism. Hypopituitarism may be associated with low to inverted T waves, and a prolonged Q-Tc[B22, B40, D12, H9, K36, Q1, S69, S133]. Such changes are similar to those associated with hypothyroidism and hypoadrenalism. They may be reversed by the administration of corti-

costeroids[B22, H9, K36], and the intravenous administration of isoproteranol[D2].

Phaeochromocytoma[S14, S142]. This may result in T wave inversion with Q-Tc prolongation, and even S-T segment depression. The changes may simulate the electrocardiographic effects of myocardial ischaemia[S142]. The effects may be blocked by alpha adrenergic blocking agents. They will regress after removal of the tumour.

THE ELECTROCARDIOGRAPHIC MANIFESTATIONS OF CEREBROVASCULAR ACCIDENTS: THE CVA PATTERN

Intracranial disease may cause significant electrocardiographic changes of the T wave, the U wave, the S-T segment, and the Q-T interval. This has been termed the 'CVA pattern', and may present as follows:

(a) An increase in the amplitude of the T wave.
(b) An inversion of the T wave.
(c) Marked widening of the T wave (Electrocardiographic Study 105).
(d) An increase in the amplitude of the U wave.
(e) Minor degrees of S-T segment depression.
(f) Prolongation of the Q-T interval (Electrocardiographic Study 105).

The Q-Tc is frequently prolonged by 20 per cent or more. The widening of the T wave is in part due to the prolongation of the Q-T interval. It has also been suggested that the incorporation of the U wave contributes to the widening of the T wave[J12]. The T wave amplitude always exceeds 5 mm and may be particularly marked. The combination of a widened T wave, increased amplitude and prolonged Q-T interval results in the so-called massive or giant T wave.

The increased amplitude of the U wave, when present, exceeds 1·5 mm and is usually associated with an increase in the height of the upright T wave.

The associated S-T segment may reflect minor degrees of deviation, either depression or, less commonly, elevation. Attention was first focused on this pattern by Burch and associates in 1954[B89]. It occurs in association with intracranial haemorrhage, particularly within the anterior fossa[A2, B89, C31, C39, C45, C53, C54, F8, J13, K35, L44, S74, S139, S142], cerebral thrombosis[F8, H8], neurosurgical procedures[F13], cryohypophysectomy[S141]. Indeed, it has been shown that even minor repolarization abnormalities such as low or notched T waves, S-T segment depression and prolongation of the Q-T interval, occur more frequently in patients with disorders of the central nervous system than in a control population[M82].

The massive T wave inversion may also be associated

with sudden cerebral anoxia, as occurs in syncope. This is particularly associated with the Stokes-Adams syncopal attacks of complete A-V block with ventricular standstill, or complete A-V block complicated by ventricular flutter [I3, J2]. It has also been reported in association with partial A-V block[S148]. The condition may also occur in acute myocardial infarction, when the Q-Tc in particularly prolonged[F15, I3, J2], and occasionally in association with an acute abdomen[D21]. The pattern may, very rarely, be associated with hypertensive encephalopathy, primary cerebral tumours and cerebral metastases[S142].

Experimentally, repolarization abnormalities resembling the so-called CVA pattern have been elicited by cerebral stimulation[M77, P35], including stimulation of the hypothalamus[M77]. Similar manifestations have also been reproduced by stimulation of the stellate ganglion or stellate ganglionectomy[Y1]. The CVA pattern elicited by unilateral ganglionectomy in dogs was abolished after contralateral ganglionectomy[Y1].

It would appear that the phenomenon is due to transient injury or ischaemia of the cerebral centres representing the autonomous nervous system[C54], particularly the hypothalamus[S142].

C   SECONDARY T WAVE ABNORMALITIES

Abnormalities of the T wave may be secondary to abnormal ventricular depolarization, as reflected by abnormalities of the QRS complex. These T wave abnormalities occur secondary to bundle branch block, the Wolff-Parkinson-White syndrome, the abnormal ventricular depolarization resulting from ectopic ventricular beats, and the hemiblocks. As such, they have no primary clinical significance, since they do not connote primary myocardial disease. Secondary T wave abnormalities are always associated with abnormalities of the QRS complex. Their characteristics are discussed in each of the chapters dealing with abnormal intraventricular conduction, Chapter 9 (right bundle branch block), Chapter 10 (left bundle branch block), Chapter 11 (the WPW syndrome), Chapter 12 (the hemiblocks), and Chapter 13 (ectopic ventricular beats).

D   PRIMARY T WAVE ABNORMALITIES

Abnormalities of the T wave may be due to myocardial disease, a disease which causes a primary abnormality of repolarization. Such primary T wave abnormalities are not necessarily associated with abnormality of the QRS complex.

Primary T wave abnormalities may reflect the following changes:

(a) A change in the direction of the T wave vector, and/or

(b) a change in the configuration of the T wave.

These may be associated with an abnormality of the Q-T interval: a prolongation or a shortening.

The electrocardiographic characteristics of primary T wave abnormalities are considered in Chapter 1. Their clinical import and differential diagnosis are considered below.

Primary T wave abnormalities may occur with any form of myocarditis, coronary artery disease, hypothermia, malignant invasion of the myocardium, electrolyte imbalance, and a host of pharmacological agents. The T wave of coronary artery disease and the billowing leaflet syndrome will be considered in some detail.

THE T WAVE OF CORONARY ARTERY DISEASE

Various forms of T wave change are associated with coronary artery disease:

Two types of T wave abnormality may occur during the course of acute myocardial infarction:

(a) The T wave of the hyperacute early injury phase.

(b) The T wave of the fully evolved or subacute phase.

The T wave of the hyperacute injury phase is characterized by:

(a) An increase in the amplitude of the T wave.

(b) A widening of the T wave.

(c) The T wave is directed towards the surface of the injury.

(d) The associated S-T segment usually reflects slope or concave-upward elevation.

(e) The Q-Tc is normal or there may be some shortening.

These features are reflected in Electrocardiographic Studies 1, 2, 3, 4A, 5A, 6, 7, 12, 25A, 90 and 91.

The T wave of the fully evolved or subacute phase of myocardial infarction is pointed, symmetrical and inverted in leads orientated to the injured surface (Electrocardiographic Studies 12B, 14, 15, 17, 18, 19, 20, 21, 22, 23, 24 and 25B). The associated Q-T interval is usually *prolonged*.

The T wave of acute myocardial insufficiency, the classic form of angina pectoris, is an expression of acute subendocardial injury, and is consequently taller than normal in leads orientated to the epicardial surface (Electrocardiographic Studies 85 and 86). The associated S-T segment is commonly depressed, and the Q-T interval is frequently *shortened*. See also post-extrasystolic T wave change (p. 138).

ELECTROCARDIOGRAPHIC MANIFESTATIONS ASSOCIATED WITH THE BILLOWING POSTERIOR MITRAL LEAFLET

The syndrome of the posterior billowing leaflet of the mitral valve has recently received emphasis[B9, B50, H5, S130]. The T waves tend to be low to inverted in Standard leads II and III, and lead AVF, and the Q-Tc may be prolonged[B9, B50, E4, H5]. Similar changes have been reported with Marfan's syndrome[B72].

The mechanism of this phenomenon is unknown. Coronary angiograms in two patients with this syndrome were normal[S130]. It is possible that the changes are due to a localized dysfunction of the left ventricular myocardium[E4]. The mechanism may be similar to that which occurs in familial cardiomyopathy. It may also be due to prolonged repolarization within an abnormal left ventricular ridge which has been described in this syndrome[E4].

E THE POST-TACHYCARDIA SYNDROME

Paroxysmal tachycardia may be followed by inversion of the usually upright T wave[G39, K20, L15, L25]. The phenomenon occurs in about 20 per cent of cases, and may follow supraventricular tachycardia[K20], or ventricular tachycardia[G39]. The inversion may persist for hours or days. The manifestation persisted for 19 days after the termination of an attack in a 2-year-old individual with a normal coronary arteriogram[K20]. The T wave inversion is commonly associated with prolongation of the Q-T interval, suggesting the presence of a local prolongation of repolarization in the area of increased automaticity[K20]. The mechanism is unknown.

Chapter 16

The Electrocardiographic Exercise Test

A good history is usually sufficient to establish a diagnosis of angina pectoris or symptomatic coronary insufficiency. At times, however, the pain is atypical, the history doubtful, and the electrocardiogram recorded at rest, normal or equivocal. Furthermore, the response to amyl nitrate may also be equivocal; and it should be borne in mind that amyl nitrate may, at times, relieve pain that is not cardiac in origin. Under such circumstances, objective confirmation of the diagnosis becomes desirable, and the electrocardiographic changes seen in response to exercise may provide this confirmatory evidence.

The test can also be of value in the patient without symptoms of coronary insufficiency but who may have latent coronary artery disease *de novo* or as a result of manifest diabetes mellitus, familial hypercholesterolaemia or myxoedema. It has also been well documented that coronary artery disease may be present in apparently healthy and asymptomatic young men[F23, Y2]. This too may be revealed by the exercise test.

The test may also be used as a screening procedure as, for example, the screening of potential commercial pilots and applicants for insurance purposes.

THE BASIS OF THE EXERCISE TEST

The test is based on the premise that exercise increases the demands on the coronary blood supply, which may be adequate at rest but inadequate during exercise. The exercise thus results in a relative ischaemia and an inability of the coronary circulation to maintain the metabolic needs of the heart muscle.

THE HISTORY OF THE EXERCISE TEST

In 1908, Einthoven[E6] recorded the first electrocardiogram after exercise. He noted changes in the electrocardiogram of his old laboratory porter after he had climbed a few stairs. The following year Nicolai and Simons[N10] reported the changes after exercise in a patient who had angina pectoris. Changes occurring spontaneously during attacks of angina pectoris were recorded by Bousfield in 1918[B71], and Cowan and Ritchie in 1922[C50]. In those early days of electrocardiography, the changes after exercise were sometimes recorded fortuitously, since several flights of stairs had to be climbed to reach the electrocardiographic laboratory.

In 1931, Wood, Wolferth and Livezey[W63] first specifically used the test to provoke attacks of angina pectoris; they investigated the changes both in normal subjects and in patients with angina pectoris. Although no untoward occurrences took place, they considered it a dangerous procedure 'to induce anginal attacks indiscriminately'. It was in 1932 that Goldhammer and Scherf[G21] first recommended the use of moderate exercise followed by an electrocardiographic recording as an aid to the diagnosis of potential coronary insufficiency. Further observations were published by these authors in the following year[S50], and subsequently by many others.

The two-step procedure was first used for the electrocardiographic exercise test by Missal in 1938[M84]. In 1942, Master and his associates[M43] standardized the performance of the two-step test, which is now known as the Master two-step exercise test. Many further observations were published in subsequent years[M13, M31, M32, M35, M36, M37, M41, M42, M46, M48, M49, M50, M54, M55, M58, M67, N12, Y7].

THE PERFORMANCE OF THE EXERCISE TEST

Principles Governing the Performance of the Exercise Test

The test should be carried out in as near-constant and basal conditions as possible, and in a calm and unemotional atmosphere. The following principles should be observed:

1. The procedure must be fully explained to the patient before the commencement of the test.

2. The test must not be performed if the patient is reluctant to undergo the test.

3. The conventional 12-lead electrocardiogram is recorded at rest, and the QRS-T-U pattern must be normal or at most equivocal in respect of coronary artery disease [C49]. There may, for example, be borderline *T* wave and S-T segment changes, questionable horizontality of the S-T segment, and low *T* waves. There is little to be gained from the test if the electrocardiogram recorded at rest already shows clear-cut evidence of coronary insufficiency. For a possible exception to this statement, see the section on the performance of the exercise test after myocardial infarction on p. 166.

4. The patient must not be in pain. The history and physical examination must not suggest an impending myocardial infarction or acute pulmonary embolism. The patient must not be in congestive cardiac failure.

5. There must be no tachycardia.

6. The test may be performed according to the non-standardized or standardized method. The merits of these methods are discussed fully below.

7. The test is preferably performed before a meal or at least 1 hour after the ingestion of food or cold drink. This is because physiological variants are more likely to occur after a meal (see also Chapter 15, p. 148). If the patient gives a history of angina pectoris after meals, the test should then be performed before a meal and, if negative, repeated after a meal[S51].

8. The patient must not smoke for at least 1 hour before the performance of the test.

9. The exercise-induced electrocardiographic manifestations may be modified if the patient is on vasodilating drugs (for example, nitrates or aminophyllin)[F19, L25, L26, R66, R68, S51]. The patient must therefore not take any vasodilating drugs or beta receptor blocking agents for at least 24 hours before the performance of the test.

10. The test should not be performed for at least 3 weeks after the cessation of digitalis therapy.

11. The exercise test should not be performed within a week of a cold or other infection, since abnormal electrocardiographic manifestations after exercise have been observed in normal individuals during convalescence from infections[B36, L25, S51].

12. The test is best performed in a warm but not over-heated room.

13. When the patient gives a history of angina pectoris on exposure to cold, and the exercise test performed under basal conditions is normal, the test may be repeated with the patient holding a piece of ice wrapped in gauze in each hand[F20, L58].

14. The test is contra-indicated in the elderly patient over 65 years of age.

15. If pain, substernal discomfort, a feeling of faintness, or pallor develop during the performance of the test, the exercise *must* be stopped immediately. Exercise by intent to the point of pain is hazardous and unjustifiable.

16. The attendance of a physician experienced in the performance and interpretation of the electrocardiographic exercise test is mandatory.

17. The electrocardiogram is recorded immediately after the exercise and at 2-minute intervals for 6 minutes, or until such time as it returns to the resting configuration (see section on Technique below).

18. Since the hyperventilation which usually accompanies the exercise may of itself evoke *T* wave changes[L25, W12, Y9], it may be advisable (if so indicated) to record the electrocardiogram at rest and again after 30 seconds of hyperventilation before the actual exercise test is performed.

19. If the post-exercise test reflects *T* wave changes which suggest a physiological variant, the test may be repeated after the ingestion of potassium salts (see Chapter 15).

Note: It is not the patient's ability to perform the exercise of the test which is being tested, the exercise merely being used as a means to an end.

Methods of Exercise Performance

Electrocardiographic changes have been studied following the performance of various types of effort, for example, after maximal effort such as long-distance running[B23], strenuous marching[J15], rowing[C44], Olympic long distance skiing[H16], and other sports[B12, H37]. Many forms of exercise have also been used in the clinical laboratory, for example, the electrocardiogram has been studied after standardized exercise of a treadmill[S84, Y6], or a bicycle ergometer[B35, B45, S9].

Various forms of exercise have also been advocated for routine clinical use. These may be divided into two main groups: standardized methods and non-standardized methods. The merits of these procedures are considered below.

In most studies the electrocardiographic changes are recorded immediately after the exercise has been performed. In a few reports, the electrocardiographic changes have been recorded *during* the performance of the exercise[B35, B45, F21, R14, S9, Y5, Y7]. The introduction of the radio-electrocardiograph has facilitated this procedure[B26, B27, B28, D36, D37, H35, H36, P8, V3].

THE STANDARDIZED METHOD OF EXERCISE PERFORMANCE

Master and his associates[M43] standardized the test on the

TABLE 5. Standard Number of Ascents for Males

WEIGHT (lb.)	AGE IN YEARS												
	5–9	10–14	15–19	20–24	25–29	30–34	35–39	40–44	45–49	50–54	55–59	60–64	65–69
40–49													
50–59	33	35	32										
60–69	31	33	31										
70–79	28	32	30										
80–89	26	30	29	29	29	28	27	27	26	25	25	24	23
90–99	24	29	28	28	28	27	27	26	25	25	24	23	22
100–109	22	27	27	28	28	27	26	25	25	24	23	22	22
110–119	20	26	26	27	27	26	25	25	24	23	23	22	21
120–129	18	24	25	26	27	26	25	24	23	23	22	21	20
130–139	16	23	24	25	26	25	24	23	23	22	21	20	20
140–149		21	23	24	25	24	24	23	22	21	20	20	19
150–159		20	22	24	25	24	23	22	21	20	20	19	18
160–169		18	21	23	24	23	22	22	21	20	19	18	18
170–179			20	22	23	23	22	21	20	19	18	18	17
180–189			19	21	23	22	21	20	19	19	18	17	16
190–199			18	20	22	21	21	20	19	18	17	16	15
200–209				19	21	21	20	19	18	17	16	16	15
210–219				18	21	20	19	18	17	17	16	15	14
220–229				17	20	20	19	18	17	16	15	14	13

TABLE 6. Standard Number of Ascents for Females

WEIGHT (lb.)	AGE IN YEARS												
	5–9	10–14	15–19	20–24	25–29	30–34	35–39	40–44	45–49	50–54	55–59	60–64	65–69
40–49	35	35	33										
50–59	33	33	32										
60–69	31	32	30										
70–79	28	30	29										
80–89	26	28	28	28	28	27	26	24	23	22	21	21	20
90–99	24	27	26	27	26	25	24	23	22	22	21	20	19
100–109	22	25	25	26	26	25	24	23	22	21	20	19	18
110–119	20	23	23	25	25	24	23	22	21	20	19	18	18
120–129	18	22	22	24	24	23	22	21	20	19	19	18	17
130–139	16	20	20	23	23	22	21	20	19	19	18	17	16
140–149		18	19	22	22	21	20	19	19	18	17	16	16
150–159		17	17	21	20	20	19	19	18	17	16	16	15
160–169		15	16	20	19	19	18	18	17	16	16	15	14
170–179		13	14	19	18	18	17	17	16	16	15	14	13
180–189			13	18	17	17	17	16	16	15	14	14	13
190–199			12	17	16	16	16	15	15	14	13	13	12
200–209				16	15	15	15	14	14	13	13	12	11
210–219				15	14	14	14	13	13	13	12	11	11
220–229				14	13	13	13	13	12	12	11	11	10

basis of the patient's sex, weight and age. Using these parameters, tables were constructed based on the return of blood pressure and pulse rate to normal within 2 minutes after exercise (Tables 5 and 6). The exercise is performed on a special standardized two-step apparatus, each step being 9 inches high with a tread of 9 inches (Fig. 64). The patient is required to do a certain number of ascents and descents in 1½ minutes, prescribed from the Standard Tables which were evolved on the basis of the aforementioned parameters.

The principles governing the parameters upon which the Master two-step test is based may well be questioned, and has indeed been questioned[S49, S80, S84]. It has not, for example, been shown that coronary artery disease, once present, runs a course that is different in man or woman;

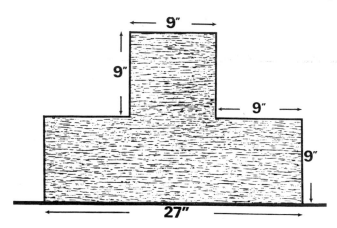

FIG. 64. Diagrammatic illustration of the Master Two-step apparatus.

nor has it been shown that electrocardiographic changes following exercise parallel those of pulse rate and blood pressure. Furthermore, although coronary artery disease is usually more prevalent and more marked in the older age groups, in the individual, as such, it may be very severe in a 40-year-old woman and not at all evident in a man of 80 years. According to Master's criteria, a man aged 50 years and weighing 160 pounds should do 20 ascents on the standardized apparatus in 1½ minutes, whereas a woman of the same age and weight is required to do only 16 ascents. This, despite the possibility that the coronary artery disease may be so advanced in the man that only a few steps may bring on an attack of angina pectoris, whereas the particular woman may be capable of undergoing much greater exercise and thus require far more than 16 ascents before either electrocardiographic changes or angina pectoris become manifest. In addition, other factors such as emotion and training may influence the outcome of the test, and must affect any attempt to standardize it.

In 1956, Simonson and Keys[S84] recommended a double

Master two-step exercise test: twice the number of ascents recommended for the single Master two-step test performed over twice the period. The diagnostic criteria remain the same. More recently, Master[M38] introduced the 'augmented' two-step exercise test: a 15 per cent increase in the number of trips prescribed for the regular double two-step test, to be performed in the same amount of time, namely 3 minutes. Such modifications further underline the difficulties and questionable physiological validity upon which this standardized procedure is based.

Nevertheless, although the validity of the criteria for standardization upon which the Masters two-step test is based may well be questioned, it should be stated that the Master two-step is recognized in numerous centres, and is commonly used as a routine procedure in many electrocardiographic laboratories.

A standardized procedure may, for purposes of uniform approach, be of some value, for example in the screening of asymptomatic air force personnel and in insurance practice. As such, the Master two-step test could well be used, since this standardization has become accepted as a well-known procedure. It must, however, be appreciated that the criteria for standardization are, vis-à-vis coronary artery disease, arbitrary and artificial.

THE NON-STANDARDIZED METHOD OF EXERCISE PERFORMANCE

Scherf (1933)[S50] originally recommended, and still recommends[S49], that the amount of exercise the patient is required to perform be adapted, 'tailored', to the needs of the particular individual. The patient is subjected to approximately the exertion that has been known to bring on an attack of angina pectoris. This does not mean that the patient is exercised indiscriminately until such time as he develops pain. If, for example, the patient has pain after only the slightest exertion, he may be asked to do a few knee-bends or sit up and down a few times; whereas a patient who has pain only after severe exertion may be asked to climb several flights of stairs rapidly. The form of exertion is unimportant, since the object of the test is to increase the demand for coronary blood flow where an inadequate flow is suspected. The induced coronary insufficiency and resultant inner-layer myocardial ischaemia or injury may precipitate electrocardiographic changes which are diagnostic. Indeed, if the two-step apparatus is available, it may well be used for the non-standardized procedure, the number of ascents being individualized.

If no changes are noted, and if the patient's condition warrants it, the exercise test may be repeated after a suitable interval (usually 1 hour) with a cautious increase in the amount of exercise.

The Dangers of the Exercise Test

If the aforementioned principles are strictly adhered to, the dangers of the test are infinitesimal and can, for all practical purposes, be ignored. Lepeschkin, Surawicz and Terrien (1959)[L31], in an analysis of 50,000 exercise tests reported in the literature, found that the occurrence of myocardial infarction in the day following the test occurred in only six instances, and in none of these were the aforementioned principles observed. Indeed, in most of these cases the electrocardiogram had returned to normal after the test and before the onset of the infarction.

The Technique of the Exercise Test

EQUIPMENT NECESSARY

1. Direct writing electrocardiograph with an instamatic switch.

2. A rectangular writing stylus. This usually results in better definition than a V-shaped stylus.

3. The following additional equipment is necessary if the test is performed according to the Master two-step standardization:

(a) Standard two-step apparatus (specifications in Fig. 64).

(b) Metronome or stop-watch.

(c) Table reflecting the appropriate number of ascents for the double two-step test (see p. 155, Tables 5 and 6).

THE TECHNIQUE OF THE TEST

1. The electrodes must be scrupulously clean.

2. The electrode jelly must be rubbed well into the skin.

3. The leg electrodes are best fastened just above the calf, with the cables inserted from *above*.

4. The arm electrodes are best fastened near the shoulder, with the cables inserted from *below*.

5. The precordial electrode positions are accurately determined and marked with a skin pencil.

6. The precordial electrodes are fastened in the V4, V5 and V6 positions by a special strap which can be secured around the shoulder in halter fashion.

7. The routine 12-lead electrocardiogram is recorded. Ideally, at least 6-second strips of each lead should be recorded.

8. When the electrocardiograph can record only one precordial lead at a time (as is the case with most electrocardiographs), rapid change from one electrode to the other can be facilitated by a special spring-type battery clamp.

9. The lead cable is unplugged from the electrocardiograph during the test.

10. The exercise may be performed according to a non-standardized or standardized procedure.

11. The subject holds the crotch of the cable in one hand and always turns towards the electrocardiograph after each ascent.

12. In the case of the Master two-step standardized procedure, the subject completes the number of ascents in the specified time. If he is going too slowly, he is encouraged to go faster, and vice versa.

13. Immediately after the exercise, strips of 6-second duration each are recorded in rapid succession of Standard lead II, Standard lead I and leads V4, V5 and V6, in that order. This is repeated at 2- 4-, and 6-minute intervals. If the electrocardiogram has not returned to normal at the time of the 6-minute recording, the procedure should be repeated at 8 and 10 minutes.

THE INTERPRETATION OF THE EXERCISE TEST

It must be stressed at the outset that the interpretation of the electrocardiographic changes evoked by the exercise test must always be interpreted in the light of the clinical presentation as a whole. Certainly, there are electrocardiographic manifestations which, if evoked, leave little doubt as to the presence of coronary artery disease, but there is also a broad twilight zone where the manifestations are difficult to interpret, and can only be made by an evaluation of *both* the electrocardiographic and clinical presentations.

The Muscle Region Most Affected by Exercise-induced Coronary Insufficiency

The region most affected by the exercise-induced coronary insufficiency is the apex of the left ventricle and the adjacent anteroseptal and anterolateral regions (Fig. 61). This involves the region of the heart with the major muscle mass.

It is usually the subendocardial region of the muscle mass which is dominantly affected by coronary insufficiency. This is because intramyocardial systolic pressure decreases progressively from endocardium to epicardium. Thus intramyocardial blood flow during systole will be more readily channelled to the subepicardial layers.

Leads in which the Exercise-induced Changes Are Best Seen

Since it is the major muscle mass which is involved, the changes are best seen in *leads with the tallest R waves*. These are usually the left lateral leads; leads V4–V6 (Electrocardiographic Study 94B) in the horizontal plane, especially lead V5; and Standard leads I and II and lead AVL in the frontal plane, especially Standard lead II. These leads will, in the ensuing discussion, be referred to as the left lateral leads.

The Electrocardiographic Manifestations of Exercise-induced Coronary Insufficiency

Exercise may cause changes involving any of the electrocardiographic deflections; the P wave, P-R interval, QRS complex, S-T segment, T wave, U wave and Q-T interval. Changes affecting the repolarization process, the S-T segment, T wave and U wave, are most commonly seen, and it is mainly on these parameters that the interpretation of the test is usually based. Exercise may also induce disturbances of cardiac rhythm.

CHANGES AFFECTING THE P WAVE

With exercise, the P wave vector tends to become more vertical, i.e. there is a slight right axis deviation of the frontal plane P wave vector[S51, V3]. Since the normal P wave vector is usually between $0°$ and $+60°$ on the frontal plane hexaxial reference system, it tends to deviate to the region of $+60°$. The P wave vector thus becomes aligned, more parallel, with the Standard lead II lead axis, and as a result tends to become taller in Standard lead II (Electrocardiographic Study 92). This is a normal physiological variant. The associated Ta deflection tends to become deeper and may possibly result in junctional S-T segment depression (see Chapter 14 pp. 130 and 137).

CHANGES AFFECTING THE P-R INTERVAL

The P-R interval shortens with exercise and tends to develop a downward slope. This is especially prone to occur in a lead which reflects a relatively tall P wave, such as Standard lead II. (See above, and $\frac{1}{2}$- and 2-minute tracings of Electrocardiographic Study 92.) This is due to the depressing effect of the Ta deflection, and may result in junctional S-T segment depression. This is especially likely to occur when the P-R interval is relatively short, for under these circumstances the Ta deflection tends to encroach more readily on the S-T segment (see p. 138).

CHANGES AFFECTING THE QRS COMPLEX

Exercise may precipitate an intraventricular conduction defect such as bundle branch block or a hemiblock.

Bundle Branch Block

Bundle branch block may occur whenever a critical rate is exceeded. Thus, the sinus tachycardia provoked by the exercise may result in a transient bundle branch block which regresses to normal intraventricular conduction with the ensuing cardiac slowing. This is an expression of phasic aberrant ventricular conduction (see Chapter 17). The aberration is usually of the right bundle branch block type, and when it occurs as an isolated phenomenon and in the absence of abnormal clinical manifestations, it has little diagnostic significance. When, however, it appears in conjunction with other electrocardiographic abnormalities of coronary insufficiency or a clinical presentation of coronary insufficiency, it constitutes corroborative evidence of the abnormality. Thus, Bauer (1964)[B14] noted the presence of coronary insufficiency in 13 out of 14 such cases.

Hemiblock

Transient hemiblock may also be precipitated by exercise. The manifestation is usually a left anterior hemiblock[K50], but may also occasionally be a left posterior hemiblock. Only a few cases have thus far been reported. The precipitation of a hemiblock by exercise most probably always connotes myocardial disease, and particularly coronary insufficiency. Further study, however, is needed.

CHANGES AFFECTING THE S-T SEGMENT

The commonest and most obvious electrocardiographic signs of exercise-induced coronary insufficiency are **deviation of, and a change in the shape of, the S-T segment**. The S-T segment may become depressed or, less commonly, elevated in leads orientated to the left lateral region of the heart. The depression or elevation is due to the presence of subendocardial or subepicardial electrical injury. The physiological principles governing these changes are discussed in Chapter 2.

THE S-T SEGMENT AND T WAVE DURING EXERCISE IN NORMAL SUBJECTS

It has recently been shown that when the electrocardiogram is recorded during and immediately after exercise in normal individuals, the following changes occur (Davies and associates 1971[D5]; Kitchin and Neilson 1972[K30]):

1   *Changes Recorded During Exercise*
   (a) The S-T segment becomes depressed.
   (b) The T wave becomes diminished in amplitude.

2 *Changes Recorded Immediately After Exercise*
(a) The S–T segment may become elevated.
(b) The *T* wave increases in magnitude. The increase in magnitude may be large and well above the values for the resting level.

An increase in the amplitude of the *T* wave during recovery from exercise had also been noted by Yu and Soffer (1952)[Y7], and Kahn and Simonson (1957)[K2].

Patients with severe ischaemic heart disease may reflect marked S–T segment depression with *T* wave flattening and inversion during both exercise and immediately after exercise.

DEPRESSION OF THE S–T SEGMENT: SUBENDOCARDIAL INJURY

Exercise-induced coronary insufficiency commonly results in subendocardial injury. This results in deviation of the S–T segment vector towards the subendocardial surface away from the left lateral leads (leads V5 and Standard lead II), and manifesting with S–T segment depression in these leads. It is the evaluation of this change which constitutes the major diagnostic challenge in the interpretation of the exercise test.

The S–T segment must be evaluated both *qualitatively and quantitatively*, i.e. both the *type* of the depression and the *degree* of the depression.

Qualitative Evaluation of S–T Segment Depression: The Type of S–T Segment Depression

Following exercise, the S–T segment may become more **horizontal** or **depressed**, and the depression may be **plane**, **sagging** or **junctional** in type.

Horizontal S–T Segment Depression

The normal S–T segment merges smoothly and gradually with the ascending limb of the *T* wave, so that a definite separation between the two is difficult or impossible to define (Electrocardiographic Study 93a, and Diagram A of Fig. 60). The earliest sign of S–T segment depression is the development of S–T segment horizontality resulting in a sharp angled ST-T junction. The S–T segment tends to hug the baseline for a relatively long period (see Chapter 15, p. 135). When this form of S–T segment configuration is precipitated by the exercise test, it should always be regarded with suspicion and is usually abnormal, even when associated with little or no S–T segment depression (Electrocardiographic Study 93, and Diagram E of Fig. 60). See also Chapter 15, p. 135. Measurement of the degree or duration of horizontality has been attempted by Lepeschkin and Surawicz[L30]. For details see Fig. 65.

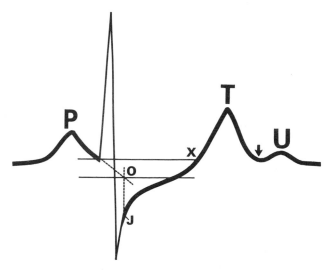

FIG. 65. Diagram illustrating methods of measuring (1), true and false S–T segment depression, and (2), the degree of horizontality of the S–T segment. (1) The line of the sloping P-R segment is continued until it meets, at point O, a vertical line drawn from the junction of the QRS complex and S–T segment. The distance O J indicates the true amount of S–T segment depression. (2) A horizontal line drawn from the beginning of the QRS deflection is continued till it meets the *T* wave at point X. The distance Q–X is expressed as a percentage of the Q-T interval (measured from the beginning of the QRS complex to the end of the *T* wave arrow). Q-X is greater than 50 per cent of Q-T in the majority of true positive tests.

Plane S–T Segment Depression

With the advent of plane depression of the S–T segment, the horizontality of the S–T segment and the sharp-angled ST-T junction are maintained in the depressed segment (Diagram F of Fig. 60; ½- and 2-minute tracings in Electrocardiographic Study 92, Electrocardiographic Studies 93 and 94). This is the usual form of S–T segment depression which occurs as an abnormal response to the exercise test.

Sagging S–T Segment Depression

At times the depressed S–T segment has a sagging concave-upward appearance. This form of response is relatively uncommon with the exercise test (Diagram G of Fig. 60).

Junctional S–T Segment Depression

Depression of the proximal or junctional part of the S–T segment may be physiological and rarely abnormal (Diagrams B and C of Fig. 60). The principles governing the interpretation are discussed in p. 138. See also comment in the section of prognosis (p. 166).

Quantitative Evaluation of S–T Segment Depression

The amount of S–T segment depression that is considered definitely abnormal is one of the most disputed points in the interpretation of the exercise test. The changes may range from a mere sharpening of the ST-T angle with or without minimal S-T segment depression (Electrocardiographic Study 93) to marked depression exceeding 2 mm (Electrocardiographic Study 94), and which may, at times be as much as 5 mm in depth. Master and associates[M43] originally considered that the depression of the S-T segment must exceed 0·5 mm in any lead (measured from the end of the P-R segment) to establish a diagnosis of an abnormal or positive exercise test. This degree of S-T segment depression was, however, also found in 6 per cent to 25 per cent of apparently normal individuals[F17, H38, L25, L30, M13, M24, M67, R66, S51, V7]. Figures in excess of 0·75 mm[L30], 1·0 mm[S94, U3, Y5], 1·5 mm[B46, G44, M63], and 2 mm[K31, S51, T16] depression in the precordial leads V4 and V5, have all been considered as definitely abnormal. The matter is further complicated by the fact that it is at times difficult to judge the position of the baseline as a reference point from which to measure the depression; and the depressing effect of the Ta deflection, which may encroach upon the S-T segment must also be taken into account (see Chapter 14 and pp. 130 and 137). The best baseline or isoelectric level for reference in the measurement of S-T segment depression is the U-P segment, but this often obscures the tachycardia which may accompany the exertion (see ½-minute recording in Electrocardiographic Study 92). In such cases, the baseline is measured from the junction of the P-R segment with the QRS complex. However, owing to the depressing effect of the Ta deflection, the P-R segment may have a downward slope and will, in turn, also have a depressing effect on the S-T segment.

To avoid inclusion of this false S-T segment depression and to allow for the physiological effect of the Ta deflection, the following procedure was proposed. The downward slope of the P-R segment is continued to meet a vertical line which extends from the junction (J) of the QRS complex with the S-T segment (Fig. 65)[L25, L30, S51]. This level is taken as the true baseline. Using this procedure, Lepeschkin and Surawicz (1958)[L30], in a well-controlled investigation, found that, with a criterion of 0·75 mm depression below this baseline, only 16 per cent false positives occurred, as compared with 26 per cent using the same procedure with Master's criterion of 0·5 mm depression. Nevertheless, 16 per cent is still a high percentage of false positives. Other reports have also shown that S-T segment depression of 1 mm or more may be found in normal individuals[S51, T7].

Note that the principle governing the downward projection of the P-R segment to determine true and false S-T segment depression is similar to the use of the hypothetical parabola, joining the P-R segment, S-T segment and proximal limb of the T wave, in such determination

(see p. 137 and Fig. 66). The unbroken, parabola indicates, in all probability, a normal physiological response. The broken parabola is a pointer to the presence of coronary insufficiency.

McConahay and associates (1971)[M65] correlated post-exercise electrocardiograms to coronary arteriograms and left ventricular end-diastolic pressure. The incidence and degree of post-exercise ischaemic S-T segment depression

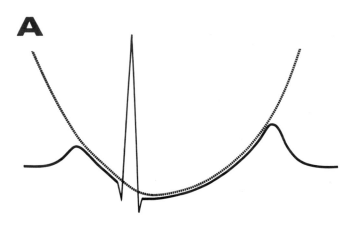

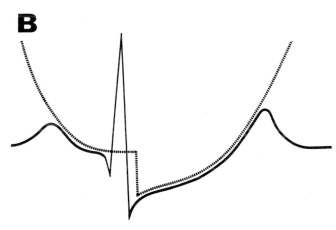

FIG. 66. Diagrams illustrating: A, the normal unbroken parabola of physiological junctional S-T segment depression; and B, the broken parabola of abnormal junctional S-T segment depression.

increased significantly with an increasing severity of coronary artery disease. S-T segment depression of 0·5 mm reflected a true positive response in 63 per cent of cases, and a true negative response (with due regard to the criteria examined) of 83 per cent. S-T segment depression of 1·0 mm or greater reflected 100 per cent specificity, but at the expense of reduced sensitivity, 35 per cent true positive response of the group as a whole. They also found that patients with S-T segment depression of 1 mm or more had significantly greater values for left ventricular end-diastolic pressure than patients with lesser degrees of S-T segment depression.

Scherf[S47, S49, S51] states that, since it is impossible to eliminate false negative tests, i.e. since a negative result or a normal electrocardiogram does not exclude cardiac disease, it becomes imperative to avoid false positive tests with consequent incorrect diagnoses and the induction of possible iatrogenic neurosis. He therefore deliberately sets extremely stringent criteria to avoid making incorrect diagnoses, so that a positive test should be based on incontestable standards. He therefore only considers the test diagnostically abnormal when the S-T segment depression in is 2 mm or more in the precordial leads, and 1·5 mm or more in the extremity leads. This approach will also mean that many cases of undoubted coronary artery disease will be missed or even passed as normal.

It is therefore necessary to adopt an approach that is not rigid, and where the electrocardiographic manifestations are used as a guide to the overall assessment.

The following is advocated. Minor S-T segment changes must be interpreted with caution. Nevertheless, the appearance of the following, however minimal, constitutes a *pointer* to the presence of coronary insufficiency:

1. The **broken parabola** between the *P* wave, the P-R segment and the S-T segment (see p. 160).

2. The presence of a **sharp angled ST-T junction**.

Any additional S-T segment depression strengthens the diagnostic accuracy. It must once again be stressed that both clinical and electrocardiographic factors must be taken into consideration for the final evaluation.

ELEVATION OF THE S-T SEGMENT: SUBEPICARDIAL INJURY

Acute exercise-induced coronary insufficiency may occasionally result in transient subepicardial injury resulting in elevation of the S-T segment in the left lateral leads (Electrocardiographic Study 91)[B90, F18, H21, K45, M26, M54, M55, S34]. The manifestation is usually accompanied by pain, and is part of the phenomenon known as the variant form of angina pectoris (synonyms: Prinzmetal's angina pectoris, atypical angina pectoris)[P28, P29, P30], and is discussed in greater detail in Chapter 15, p. 143. This manifestation usually indicates severe, near total, obstruction of a major coronary artery. Fortuin and Friesinger (1970)[F18] observed S-T segment elevation in 12 patients following exercise. In 8 patients the changes were notes in the anterior precordial leads, and 7 of these had total or near total occlusion of the left anterior descending coronary artery on coronary angiography. Four patients had S-T segment elevation in the inferiorly orientated leads,

Standard leads II and III and lead AVF, and in each of these total or near-total occlusion of the right coronary artery was demonstrated. Hegge and associates (1972)[H14] and (1973)[H15] determined the relationship between coronary arteriographic findings and S-T segment *elevation*. Post-exercise S-T segment elevation in the precordial leads was associated with severe coronary artery disease, particularly in the left anterior descending coronary artery. Post-exercise S-T segment elevation in Standard leads II and III and lead AVF was associated with severe coronary artery disease, but without predominant involvement of any specific artery.

The S-T segment elevation may occur as an isolated electrocardiographic manifestation, or it may, for example, occur in association with *U* wave inversion and ventricular extrasystoles[S34] (Electrocardiographic Studies 90 and 91).

Changes Affecting the T Wave

Exercise-induced coronary insufficiency may result in subendocardial or subepicardial ischaemia (see Chapter 2 for the definition of this term). This affects predominantly the apical and anteroseptal regions of the left ventricle, the region with the major muscle mass. The effects are consequently best reflected in leads which are orientated to this region, viz. leads V2–V6, and Standard leads II and I.

Myocardial ischaemia may result in changes in both the *configuration* and the *direction* of the *T* wave. The *T* wave vector is directed away from the surface of ischaemia and tends to become taller, symmetrical and arrow-head in appearance (see Chapter 2).

Exercise-induced Subendocardial Ischaemia: Tall Symmetrical T waves in the Left Lateral Leads

Subendocardial ischaemia is the common response to physical stress with a compromised coronary circulation. It results in a *T* wave vector that is directed away from the subendocardial surface, i.e. *towards* leads V4 and V5, and is consequently reflected by *tall* symmetrical arrow-head *T* waves in these and adjacent leads.

The increase in amplitude may exceed 5 mm or three times the resting value, but this was only observed in 10 per cent of cases with coronary artery disease[L30]. The change may appear as an isolated phenomenon, in which case its pathological significance should be interpreted with caution, since a slight increase in the *T* wave amplitude may reflect a physiological response (see above).

The manifestation is not infrequently associated with depressed S-T segments, an expression of subendocardial injury. The Q-Tc is, under these circumstances, frequently *shortened*. The change often occurs as a late phase in leads which previously reflected subendocardial electrical injury, viz., depressed S-T segments[L30].

Exercise-induced Subepicardial Ischaemia: Inverted T *Waves in Lateral Orientated Leads*

Subepicardial ischaemia results in a *T* wave vector that is directed *away* from the subepicardial surface, i.e. *away from* lead V4 and V5, and is consequently reflected by *inverted T* waves with a tendency to symmetrical and arrow-head configuration in these and adjacent leads.

These manifestations may occur as isolated phenomena, or they may be associated with changes of the other deflections reflecting the repolarization process, viz. S-T segment and *U* wave abnormalities. Furthermore, the *T* wave changes do not necessarily occur concomitantly with the S-T segment changes. It is also noteworthy that sub*endo*cardial injury, as manifested by depressed S-T segments in leads V4 and V5 for example, may be followed by sub*epi*cardial ischaemia, as manifested by inverted *T* waves in the same leads. The inverted *T* wave in lead V5, whether occurring as an isolated phenomenon or in association with S-T segment changes, not infrequently begins relatively late, a few minutes after the completion of the exercise[L25, L30], and may persist for relatively long periods, often as long as 40 minutes[L23]. It is not infrequently associated with a *prolonged* Q-Tc.

Exercise-induced *T* wave inversion in the left lateral leads (for example lead V5) may occur as an isolated phenomenon, and can be an expression of coronary insufficiency. The interpretation of an isolated *T* wave inversion may, however, be difficult since it may on occasion, though uncommonly, also occur as the expression of a normal physiological response (see below). The significance of an isolated *T* wave change is, however, considerably strengthened as an expression of coronary insufficiency when:

(a) the inverted *T* wave is sharply pointed and symmetrical, and the associated S-T segment tends to be iso-electric, i.e. it hugs the baseline for a relatively long period, 3 mm (0·12 sec) or more (see p. 135).

(b) the associated Q-T interval is prolonged.

(c) the *T* wave inversion after exercise is greater than in the electrocardiogram recorded after 30 seconds hyperventilation with the patient erect and at rest.

(d) the *T* wave inversion after exercise is associated with a relatively slow heart rate.

(e) the *T* wave inversion occurs in Standard lead I[L30]. This probably reflects a wide QRS-T angle since a negative *T* wave in Standard lead I represents a mean frontal plane *T* wave axis in the range of +91° clockwise to −91°, whereas the mean manifest frontal plane QRS axis is usually in the range of 0 to +60° (see p. 141).

Isolated *T* wave abnormality is at times the only response in patients with abnormal angiograms[A13, M27] and documented previous infarction[H21].

Abnormal *T* wave inversion may be associated with the S-T segment depression or elevation of myocardial injury. When it is associated with S-T segment depression, the expression of subendocardial injury, it usually *follows* the S-T segment depression chronologically appearing late after exercise when the S-T segment depression has already subsided or is subsiding[L25, L30].

Physiological T *Wave Inversion*

Isolated *T* wave inversion in the left lateral leads may at times, though rarely, be the expression of a normal physiological response to exercise. This normal or physiological *T* wave change is not associated with a symmetrical arrow-head appearance, a prolonged Q-T interval and a relatively prolonged isoelectric period, i.e. it is not baseline hugging S-T segment. The inverted *T* wave is less than 2 mm in depth[G8].

Physiological *T* wave inversion may be due to the following mechanisms:

1. **Hyperventilation**[W12].

2. **Increased sympathetic tone**[W26]: due to the secretion of adrenalin associated with the accompanying anxiety and stress of the test.

3. The effect of **tachycardia** on the myocardium[S51].

4. **Accentuation of a normal wide QRS-T angle.** When there is already a normal wide frontal plane QRS-T angle, the relatively tall *R* wave recorded at rest is associated with a relatively low *T* wave. The low *T* wave may become lower or inverted with exercise, especially during the phase of tachycardia. The ingestion of potassium salts may prevent this[G37]. This manifestation is especially prone to occur in the long, slender, aesthenic individual.

CHANGES AFFECTING THE U WAVE

The *U* wave is a small rounded deflection which occurs just after the *T* wave, and is normally in the same direction as the *T* wave (Diagrams A, B, C and E of Fig. 60, and Fig. 65). It is best seen in the precordial leads reflecting the transition zone, usually leads V2–V4 (see p. 139). The deflection may be so small as to make accurate recognition difficult. Furthermore, with exercise-induced tachycardia, the *U* wave may be superimposed upon the following *P* wave, making identification impossible (for example, ½-minute tracing in Electrocardiographic Study 92).

An inverted *U* wave, i.e. a *U* wave which is opposite in direction to the *T* wave, indicates the presence of cardiac disease. When the inversion develops after exercise, it always constitutes an abnormal response, and indicates the presence of coronary insufficiency. It is frequently associated with S-T segment depression[L30] (Electrocardiographic Study 92) or S-T segment elevation (Electrocardiographic Study 91). Occasionally it is the only abnormal finding.

CHANGES IN CARDIAC RHYTHM PRECIPITATED BY EXERCISE

The following disorders of cardiac rhythm may occur in response to the exercise test.

SINUS TACHYCARDIA

Sinus tachycardia is the normal response to exercise. It may occasionally precipitate rate-dependent left or right bundle branch block (see above, and Chapter 17, p. 184).

ECTOPIC VENTRICULAR RHYTHMS

Increased ectopic automaticity may be precipitated by exercise in a patient with coronary insufficiency. This includes unifocal or multifocal ventricular extrasystoles, ventricular extrasystoles in pairs (two or more consecutive ventricular extrasystoles), and extrasystolic ventricular tachycardia (three or more consecutive ventricular extrasystoles).

Significance
Occasional unifocal ventricular extrasystoles may occur in the apparently normal individual. They are less common in individuals without any other equivocal or overt electrocardiographic manifestations of coronary insufficiency than in patients with angina pectoris or other electrocardiographic signs of coronary insufficiency[L30]. Unifocal ventricular extrasystoles, however, have added significance when they are numerous, more than 1 in 6 sec, when they are precipitated in groups or in showers, when they occur in bigeminal rhythm, and when they are associated with marked sinus tachycardia.

Ventricular extrasystoles which are present at rest and which are increased by exercise, would appear to be particularly indicative of the presence of coronary insufficiency (Vedin and associates, 1972)[V6].

The appearance of ventricular extrasystoles in association with any other electrocardiographic sign of coronary insufficiency increases their significance *vis-à-vis* coronary artery disease, and also increases the adverse connotations of the interpretation of the electrocardiogram as a whole.

The precipitation of *multifocal* ventricular extrasystoles, ventricular extrasystoles in *pairs*, and *extrasystolic ventricular tachycardia* (Electrocardiographic Study 91) by exercise should be regarded as an indication of coronary insufficiency[V6].

When ventricular extrasystoles are present in the resting tracing, and disappear with exercise, they seem to have far less serious prognostic import than those ventricular extrasystoles precipitated by exercise, and may, in fact, be benign.

THE RELATIONSHIP OF EXERCISE-INDUCED ELECTROCARDIOGRAPHIC CHANGES TO THE DEVELOPMENT OF PAIN

While patients who develop pain on exercise usually develop abnormal electrocardiographic changes, this correlation is not invariable. Conversely, the appearance of abnormal electrocardiographic changes after exercise does not necessarily correlate with that of pain. Although the patient should not deliberately be exercised to the point of pain, when pain is precipitated by the exercise test, it may occur long after the appearance of abnormal changes and may disappear long before such changes have regressed. Furthermore, abnormal changes which cannot be reproduced by exercise may be found during an attack of spontaneous pain.

THE DURATION OF ELECTROCARDIOGRAPHIC ABNORMALITIES AFTER EXERCISE

Electrocardiographic changes reflecting coronary insufficiency, particularly S-T segment depression, tend to last longer than those caused by physiological variants. Although there are exceptions, normal variants or false positive changes usually last less than 2 minutes, whereas pathological or true positive changes may last five minutes or longer[L30]. For example, a depression of 0·5 mm in the precordial leads which is usually suggestive, though not definitely diagnostic, of coronary insufficiency is considerably strengthened as a criterion of abnormality when the change persists for 5 minutes or longer.

REPRODUCIBILITY OF ABNORMAL ELECTROCARDIOGRAPHIC CHANGES

When the exercise test is performed under the most basal conditions possible, any abnormal manifestation, for example S-T segment depression, can usually be reproduced quantitatively on the same or successive days[R66, R68]. Over a period of years, however the response is only reproducible in 40 per cent of cases[L26]. This would suggest the development of a collateral circulation.

INTERPRETATION OF EXERCISE-INDUCED S-T SEGMENT AND T WAVE CHANGES IN THE PRESENCE OF BUNDLE BRANCH BLOCK

The presence of bundle branch block does not necessarily connote the presence of coronary artery disease. Indeed, right bundle branch block may occur in the normal asymptomatic individual: in 1·5/1000 of the normal population under 40 years of age[J17], and in 2·9/1000 individuals of over 40 years of age[J17]. Bundle branch block is also associated with secondary S-T segment and *T* wave manifestations. These take the form of S-T segment and *T* waves that are opposite in direction to the QRS vector, particularly the terminal QRS vector; an upright terminal QRS vector is associated with a depressed S-T segment and *T* wave, and vice versa. The question may then be posed as to whether the effects of coronary insufficiency affecting the S-T segment and *T* wave may be recognized in the presence of these secondary S-T segment and *T* wave changes. The answer is that recognition may well be possible in the presence of right bundle branch block, but is very difficult, and may indeed be impossible, in the presence of left bundle branch block. This is because the primary S-T segment changes of coronary insufficiency are usually in the *same* direction and will consequently accentuate the secondary S-T segment and *T* wave manifestations of left bundle branch block, thereby making separation and recognition of the superimposed change extremely difficult. In right bundle branch block, however, the primary S-T segment changes of coronary insufficiency are usually *opposite* to that of the secondary S-T segment changes, thereby making recognition possible. This applies particularly to the left lateral leads, which are the most important in the interpretation of the exercise test. These principles are considered in greater detail below.

INTERPRETATION OF THE EXERCISE-INDUCED S-T SEGMENT AND T WAVE CHANGES IN THE PRESENCE OF RIGHT BUNDLE BRANCH BLOCK

In right bundle branch block the left lateral leads (leads V4–V6 and Standard leads I and II) usually reflect a QRS complex with a large terminal *S* wave. The terminal *S* wave is consequently associated with secondary S-T segment and *T* wave changes which manifest as a slight *elevation* of the S-T segment and an upright *T* wave which is asymmetrical (Diagram A of Fig. 67). The normal response to the exercise-induced tachycardia is a slight accentuation of these changes, i.e. the S-T segment may become a little more elevated and the *T* wave a little taller (Diagram B of Fig.

67). Exercise-induced coronary insufficiency may result in depression of the S-T segment (Diagram C of Fig. 67; Electrocardiographic Study 95). Thus, the physiological response to exercise, the slight increase in the elevation of the S-T segment, is opposite in direction, and tends to counteract the pathological response of coronary insufficiency, the depression of the S-T segment. Any depression of the S-T segment is therefore significant and probably indicates a greater degree of coronary insufficiency than would appear to be manifest.

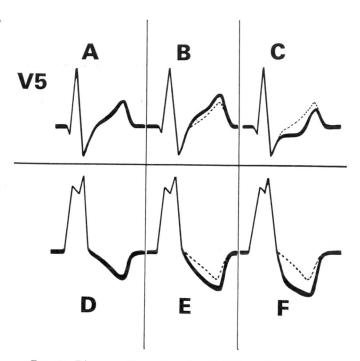

Fig. 67. Diagrams illustrating the QRS-T configuration in lead V5 of: A, right bundle branch block; B, the normal physiological response to exercise in right bundle branch block; C, the abnormal ischaemic response to exercise in right bundle branch block; D, left bundle branch block; E, the normal physiological response to exercise in left bundle branch block; and F, the abnormal ischaemic response to exercise in left bundle branch block.

INTERPRETATION OF EXERCISE-INDUCED S-T SEGMENT AND T WAVE CHANGES IN THE PRESENCE OF LEFT BUNDLE BRANCH BLOCK

In left bundle branch block the terminal QRS deflection is normally upright in the left lateral leads, leads V5 and V6, Standard lead I and lead AVL. Hence the secondary changes of repolarization, the S-T segment and *T* wave, are normally *downward*, i.e. the S-T segment is depressed and has a characteristic upward *convexity* which may be minimal, and the associated *T* wave is inverted (Diagram B of Fig. 37, and Diagram D of Fig. 67). Both the physiological response to tachycardia (Diagram E of Fig. 67) and the pathological response to coronary insufficiency (Diagram F of Fig. 67) will accentuate these secondary S-T segment and *T* wave changes. Thus, it may be difficult to interpret S-T segment depression in the left lateral leads in the presence of left bundle branch block. The following, however, are pointers to the presence of acute subendocardial injury of coronary insufficiency:

(a) The depressed S-T segment develops a *concave-upward* configuration.
(b) The S-T segment depression is very marked.
(c) The proximal as well as the distal angle of the S-T segment becomes more distinct (Diagram F of Fig. 67).
(d) The associated *T* wave, which is normally inverted, becomes upright.

An example of chronic coronary insufficiency with some of the aforementioned characteristics is illustrated in Electrocardiographic Study 57.

Exercise may also result in accentuation of the inverted *T* wave which, however, tends to become more symmetrical and arrow-head in appearance in the case of coronary insufficiency (Diagram D of Fig. 37). The manifestation is similar to that illustrated with chronic coronary insufficiency (Electrocardiographic Study 56).

INTERPRETATION OF EXERCISE-INDUCED S-T SEGMENT AND T WAVE CHANGES IN THE PRESENCE OF THE WOLFF-PARKINSON-WHITE SYNDROME

When the delta wave of the Wolff-Parkinson-White syndrome is upright in the left lateral precordial leads, the S-T segment is usually depressed and the *T* wave may become inverted. These are normal secondary S-T segment and *T* wave changes to the abnormal intraventricular conduction resulting from the pre-excitation (see Chapter 11). Exercise-induced tachycardia will exaggerate these secondary changes (compare left bundle branch block (see above)). It is thus difficult, if not impossible, to draw any conclusions from post-exercise S-T segment depression under these circumstances. If, however, the S-T segment is markedly depressed (2 mm or greater) following exercise, especially when it is virtually isoelectric in the tracing recorded at rest, the possibility of coronary insufficiency may be entertained. This manifestation requires further study.

INTERPRETATION OF EXERCISE-INDUCED S-T SEGMENT AND T WAVE CHANGES IN THE PRESENCE OF LEFT VENTRICULAR HYPERTROPHY AND STRAIN

Uncomplicated left ventricular hypertrophy manifests electrocardiographically with increased QRS voltage—tall *R* waves—in the left lateral leads. This is frequently accompanied by the appearance of the so-called left ventricular 'strain' pattern: depression of the S-T segment with *T* wave inversion. The S-T segment is usually slightly convex-upward, and the *T* wave limbs are asymmetrical with a relatively blunt apex (Electrocardiographic Study 87B).

The pattern of simple uncomplicated left ventricular hypertrophy—QRS changes only—can be transformed into one of left ventricular hypertrophy and strain (additional S-T segment and *T* wave changes) by exercise. This may be simply the result of the exercise-induced tachycardia, which causes the Q-T interval to shorten, and decreases the ventricular gradient[L25]. This does not necessarily connote coronary insufficiency. It is therefore very difficult to evaluate exercise-induced S-T segment depression under such circumstances, and many false positive results have been reported[L14]. Nevertheless, the presence of exercise-induced coronary insufficiency may be *suspected* even in association with left ventricular hypertrophy and strain when the following manifestations appear:

1. *Symmetrical arrow-head* inversion of the *T* wave.
2. Marked horizontal depression of the S-T segment.
3. If the *T* wave becomes *upright*, symmetrical and arrow-head in appearance.
4. If the *U* wave becomes inverted. In uncomplicated left ventricular hypertrophy and strain, the *U* wave usually becomes taller, more positive, after exercise[L26].
5. If the S-T segment becomes depressed in leads with a dominantly negative QRS complex as well as leads with the dominantly positive QRS complex.

THE EFFECT OF DIGITALIS ON THE EXERCISE TEST

The exercise test cannot be interpreted with confidence in the presence of digitalis effect. Digitalis itself may markedly influence the S-T segment. It usually results in a depressed S-T segment with a straight downward slope and a relatively sharp terminal rise, the mirror-image of a check or correction mark[S29]. The associated Q-Tc is shortened (Electrocardiographic Study 87C). Positive tests have been reported in patients taking digitalis in whom there was no evidence of coronary artery disease[H38, L25, L30, L51, V7, Z7].

It is usually necessary to allow a lapse of 3 weeks following the cessation of digitalis therapy before the exercise test can be interpreted with confidence.

POTASSIUM AND THE EXERCISE TEST

The exercise test cannot be interpreted in a patient with the electrocardiographic manifestations of hypokalaemia.

THE EXERCISE TEST AFTER MYOCARDIAL INFARCTION

It is perhaps a moot point whether the exercise test should ever be performed after a myocardial infarction, since the diagnosis of coronary insufficiency is already firmly established. The procedure has, however, been advocated and done in order to establish prognostic criteria and evidence of satisfactory resolution. This is discussed in greater detail in the section marked The prognostic implications of the exercise test (see below).

THE POOR MAN'S EXERCISE TEST

Harold Levine[L42] has facetiously styled the chance finding of post-extrasystolic *T* wave change in the control tracing as a 'poor man's exercise test', since it gives immediate evidence of abnormality and obviates the necessity for a further, more expensive, exercise test. The abnormality consists of a *T* wave change in the *first sinus beat following* an atrial or ventricular extrasystole (Electrocardiographic Study 96). The *T* wave usually becomes inverted, but may at times merely reflect a diminution in amplitude. The phenomenon is discussed in greater detail on p. 138.

Occasionally *U* wave inversion may also be observed in the first and possibly second sinus beats following an extra-systole[S19] (Electrocardiographic Study 97). The above signs are nearly always diagnostic of cardiac disease.

THE PROGNOSTIC IMPLICATIONS OF THE EXERCISE TEST

There can be little doubt that an unequivocally abnormal exercise test, even in the absence of clinical symptoms, connotes coronary insufficiency, and is associated with an increased morbidity and mortality. Since abnormalities affecting the S-T segment are the most striking of those precipitated by exercise-induced coronary insufficiency, and the easiest to quantitate, i.e. estimation of the amount of depression or elevation, most follow-up studies correlating the exercise test with morbidity and mortality are based on S-T segment changes.

THE PROGNOSTIC SIGNIFICANCE OF EXERCISE-INDUCED S-T SEGMENT DEPRESSION

ISCHAEMIC—PLANE OR SAGGING—S-T SEGMENT DEPRESSION

Several studies have reflected a clear association with ischaemic, plane or sagging, exercise-induced S-T segment depression and increased morbidity and mortality[B30, B52, D17, D24, K9, M57, R19, R20, R21, R23, R25, R64].

Furthermore, the degree of ischaemic S-T segment depression is roughly parallel or proportional to the increased mortality (Robb and Marks, 1964)[R20].

Thus:

1. **Slight S-T segment depression**, 0·1–0·9 mm depression, is associated with almost twice the Standard Mortality.

2. **Moderate S-T segment depression**, 1·0–1·9 mm depression, is associated with five times the Standard Mortality.

3. **Marked S-T segment depression**, 2 mm depression or more, is associated with about twenty times the Standard Mortality. A later study revealed a 15·8 times Standard Mortality Risk[R21].

A study by Kattus and associates (1971)[K9] demonstrated that near-maximal exercise in apparently normal, asymptomatic, individuals can occasionally unmask ischaemic electrocardiographic changes. Of 314 normal male insurance underwriters, 30 developed S-T segment depression during or after exercise which was not associated with pain. A 2½-year follow-up among the 30 ischaemic responders revealed 3 coronary deaths, 4 myocardial infarctions, 2 with angina pectoris, and 1 with multiple obstructions on coronary angiography.

Maximal stress on a bicycle in 510 asymptomatic males also revealed ischaemic changes in 61 subjects (12 per cent)[C55].

JUNCTIONAL S-T SEGMENT DEPRESSION

A significant finding by Robb and Marks, in their studies of 1960[R18], 1962[R19], and 1964[R20], was their observation that the junctional S-T segment depression was associated with an excellent prognosis; a very low morbidity, lower (better) than Standard Mortality. They concluded that this was a *normal* response to exercise, and connotes a better physiological response than the absence of any S-T segment change.

THE PROGNOSTIC SIGNIFICANCE OF EXERCISE-INDUCED S-T SEGMENT ELEVATION

Exercise-induced S-T segment elevation, an expression of

the variant, Prinzmetal's form of angina pectoris, is associated with a very adverse prognosis, and reflects a severe and unstable phase in the pathogenesis of coronary insufficiency. Myocardial infarction and/or death frequently occurs within 1 year[H6, J19, P23, P29, R25, S77].

THE PROGNOSTIC SIGNIFICANCE OF ISOLATED T WAVE INVERSION

While *T* wave inversion in the left lateral leads may occasionally appear in apparently normal individuals, it should always be interpreted with caution, especially when this occurs as the only abnormality. Such isolated *T* wave change has been found to be associated with a mortality that is 1·2 times higher than expected (Robb and Marks 1967)[R21].

It is the impression that the presence of *both* S-T segment and *T* wave abnormalities connotes a more severe degree of coronary insufficiency than the manifestation of either of these changes alone (Lepeschkin 1960[L23]).

THE PROGNOSTIC SIGNIFICANCE OF A NEGATIVE EXERCISE TEST

An exercise test that is normal after strenuous exercise, for example a double Master exercise test, indicates with great probability and for all practical purposes that there is no major impairment of coronary blood flow. The assumption is greatly strengthened if there are no symptoms of angina pectoris. It does not indicate the absolute absence of coronary artery disease, but any such disease, if present, is well compensated by an adequate collateral coronary circulation.

THE PROGNOSTIC IMPLICATIONS OF POST-MYOCARDIAL INFARCTION EXERCISE-INDUCED S-T SEGMENT CHANGES

As previously indicated, it is perhaps a moot point and debatable whether the exercise test should be performed at all after a myocardial infarction, since the diagnosis of coronary insufficiency or coronary artery disease is already clearly established. The test has, however, been performed under these circumstances in an attempt to assess the adequacy of healing and the efficacy of the collateral circulation, and to establish prognostic criteria. Such tests are usually performed at least 1 month after the infarction, provided there are no contra-indications or complications (for example, cardiac failure and arrhythmias)[A14, E7, L25]. These studies usually reflect an elevation of the S-T segment similar to that seen during the early post-myocardial infarction period, i.e. similar to those occurring in the acute attack of myocardial infarction[A14, E7, L23, L25]. Atterhög and associates (1971)[A14] studied 12 patients with anterior wall myocardial infarction, 3 weeks–18 months after the infarction, with serial electrocardiograms. Three weeks after the infarction, exercise induced an S-T segment elevation or an increase in the S-T segment elevation similar to that occurring during the acute phase. The change was no longer observed 2 months after the acute infarction. If the change persists, it would indicate the failure of the development of an adequate collateral circulation[A14, L23].

If typical S-T segment depression appears (as in angina pectoris without infarction), it may be concluded that there is still significant artery narrowing in addition to that scar of the infarction[L23, L25, S66].

Section 4 Abnormal Rhythms Associated with Acute Myocardial Infarction

Chapter 17

Abnormal Rhythms Associated with Acute Myocardial Infarction

This chapter is not a detailed presentation of the electro-cardiographic manifestations and mechanisms of the various arrhythmias. The purpose is rather to highlight the genesis, role and significance of certain arrhythmias with special reference to their relevance and occurrence in the context of acute myocardial infarction.

THE BASIC PRINCIPLES GOVERNING RHYTHM ANALYSIS

The analysis of abnormal rhythms involves three basic processes:

1. *The identification and analysis of the P waves.*
2. *The analysis of the QRS configuration.*
3. *The determination of the P:QRS relationship.*

The *P* waves are usually best seen and analysed in Standard lead II and Lead V1. The QRS configuration is best analysed in lead V1, since it is this lead which is most helpful in distinguishing the QRS complex of ventricular ectopy from the QRS complex of phasic aberrant ventricular conduction[M16, M17, M18, M19, S11]. Lead V1 is thus the best of the conventional leads for the analysis of the cardiac arrhythmias.

If a bipolar chest lead is used for monitoring, then the modified CL1 (MCL1) lead is most useful (Marriott and Fogg, 1970)[M18]. This lead is formed by placing the positive pole of a bipolar monitoring lead on the lead V1 position, and the negative pole on the left shoulder just under the outer end of the clavicle (Fig. 68).

In contrast to the usual monitoring bipolar lead placed on either side of the sternum, the MCL1 lead has the advantage that it does not interfere unduly with auscultation and other physical examination of the heart, it does not interfere with the administration of precordial electric shock, and it is less cumbersome for nursing the patient.

FACTORS PREDISPOSING TO THE DEVELOPMENT OF ABNORMAL RHYTHMS IN ACUTE MYOCARDIAL INFARCTION

Several factors associated with the acute myocardial infarction predisposes to the development of abnormal rhythm. These are as follows:

1. The infarction itself causes cellular ischaemia, injury or necrosis with possible oedema.

2. The myocardial infarction may be associated with an increase in the circulating catecholamines[R9]. The resulting positive chronotropic effect may facilitate the development of atrial and ventricular arrhythmias.

3. There is often an intense vagotonia[J4, J6, J7]. This may

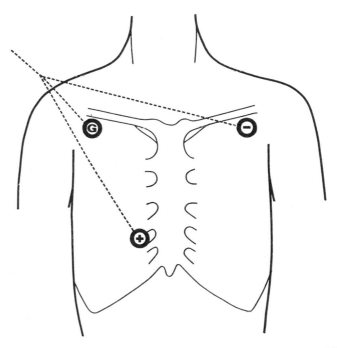

FIG. 68. Diagram illustrating the electrode placement of the MCL1 lead.

predispose to varying degrees of A-V block. The shortened repolarization of non-nodal atrial myocardium may also predispose to atrial fibrillation[A7].

4. The accumulation of metabolites, particularly potassium ions, may predispose to A-V block[J1].

5. Cardiac, and particularly atrial, *distention* due to cardiac failure, may predispose to various arrhythmias.

THE ABNORMAL RHYTHMS COMPLICATING MYOCARDIAL INFARCTION

Myocardial infarction may be associated with disorders of impulse formation and/or disorders of impulse conduction.

Disorders of Impulse Formation

ABNORMAL SINUS RHYTHMS

Damage to the S-A node in acute myocardial infarction is well described (James 1961)[J5]. The resulting abnormal function of the S-A node is of major import in the context of acute myocardial infarction. Not only does the disturbed sinus mechanism in itself constitute a significant hazard, but the potential bradyarrhythmias of sinus depression may, in addition, contribute to the genesis of ectopic rhythms such as ventricular extrasystoles and ventricular fibrillation. Furthermore, the artery to the S-A node is a major artery which also supplies a relatively large area of atrial myocardium. Hence, depression of the S-A node in acute myocardial infarction also constitutes an indirect sign that the blood supply to a significant part of the atrial myocardium has been compromised. Associated atrial infarction is, therefore, likely (see Chapter 14).

The abnormal sinus rhythm may take the form of:

Sinus bradycardia.
Sinus tachycardia.
Sinus arrest.

Sinus Bradycardia

Sinus bradycardia is reflected electrocardiographically by normal *P* waves which are inscribed at a rate of less than 50/min.

Mechanism. The sinus bradycardia complicating acute myocardial infarction may be due to two basic mechanisms, either or both of which may be operative:

1. **Intense vagal stimulation.** This is a common cause of sinus bradycardia and can usually be partially or totally reversed by the administration of atropine.

2. **Ischaemia of the S-A node.** Ischaemia may result in local tissue acidosis which depresses the S-A nodal automaticity. Ischaemia may also result in the liberation of adenosine (Imai and associates, 1964)[I1], which may have a significant negative chronotropic effect.

Complicating or associated arrhythmias. When sinus bradycardia occurs early during the course of acute myocardial infarction, it is associated with a high incidence of ventricular fibrillation (Adgey and Pantridge 1970)[A6]. There are two principal reasons for this:

1. Certain forms of ventricular extrasystoles tend to be precipitated by a relatively long preceding cycle, the expression of a slow rhythm. The phenomenon is known as the 'Rule of Bigeminy' (Langendorf and associates 1955)[L7] and is considered further on p. 176. The ventricular extrasystole so precipitated may initiate ventricular fibrillation.

2. The ventricular threshold is reduced with slower rates (Han and associates 1966)[H2].

The impulses of sinus bradycardia may be associated with normal S-A and A-V nodal conduction and may be complicated by S-A block and varying degrees of A-V block.

Incidence. Sinus bradycardia is the commonest of the sinus node arrhythmias complicating acute myocardial infarction. It is second only to ventricular extrasystoles in the overall incidence of arrhythmias complicating acute myocardial infarction[M78]. It is three times as common with posteroinferior infarction as with anterior infarction. *The arrhythmia is most likely to occur during the early hours of the attack.* This Adgey and associates (1968)[A5] noted that 40 per cent of cases with acute myocardial infarction are complicated by sinus bradycardia during the first few hours, whereas after 4 hours the incidence decreases to 9 per cent. The average incidence in coronary care units is 15 per cent (Meltzer and Kitchell 1966[M37]; Lown and associates 1967a)[L67].

Sinus Tachycardia

Sinus tachycardia is reflected electrocardiographically by normal *P* waves which are inscribed at a rate exceeding 100/min.

Etiology. The commonest cause is left ventricular failure, but contributing factors may be fever, pericarditis, pulmonary infection, pulmonary embolism and the ever present factor of anxiety. The association with left ventricular failure is reflected by the mortality. Thus, Julian and associates (1964)[J21] reported a mortality of 44 per cent, and Jewitt and associates (1967)[J14] a mortality of 52 per cent.

Furthermore, in both these series the sinus tachycardia was associated with extensive infarction.

Complicating arrythmias. Sinus tachycardia may be complicated by first, second or third degree A-V block and phasic aberrant ventricular conduction.

Incidence. Sinus tachycardia is a common manifestation, and occurs in 30 per cent of patients with acute myocardial infarction (Meltzer and Kitchell 1966[M79]; Lown and associates 1967[L67]; Jewitt and associates 1967[J14]).

SINUS ARREST

In sinus arrest the automaticity of the S-A node ceases for a few seconds or longer. No impulses are formed and no *P* waves are recorded. This results in a pause which is usually terminated by an A-V nodal or ventricular escape beat, and which, in the event of prolonged sinus arrest, may continue as an A-V nodal or ventricular escape rhythm.

It is important to appreciate that the advent of an A-V nodal (or ventricular) escape rhythm with retrograde conduction to the atria means that the potential automaticity of the S-A node is slower than that of the A-V node, and may even be completely absent, thereby reflecting sinus arrest. Indeed, if the relatively slow idionodal rhythm continues for a long period and there is no evidence of sinus activity, the presence of sinus arrest can be assumed. This principle has also been emphasized by Rokseth and Hatle (1971)[R32].

Differentiation from complete S-A block. Theoretically sinus arrest cannot be distinguished from complete S-A block. In both conditions there is an absence of *P* waves. Nevertheless, there is a pointer which may help in distinction. In cases of complete S-A block, the block is frequently and usually associated with atrial or A-V nodal escape rhythm, and possible atrial fusion, the rhythm manifesting as a 'wandering pacemaker'. In sinus arrest, the factors responsible for the arrest frequently have a depressing effect on the other potential atrial pacemakers, so that atrial escape is infrequent.

Sinus arrest must also be distinguished from *sino-ventricular conduction*; the conduction of sinus impulses to the A-V node (probably through the semi-preferential internodal atrial pathways) and ventricles without activation of the surrounding atrial myocardium. This is usually associated with hyperkalaemia because ordinary atrial myocardium is more sensitive to the effects of hyperkalaemia than the S-A node, the A-V node, the internodal pathways and the ventricular myocardium. Thus, ordinary atrial myocardium is depressed first, and this may occur while conduction from the S-A node to the A-V node through the internodal pathways and on to the ventricles is still possible. This, too, is associated with an absence of *P* waves and other atrial activity. The diagnosis is based on the concomitant manifestations of hyperkalaemia which affect the QRS complex.

Incidence. Sinus arrest is an uncommon arrhythmia. It was observed in only 1 of 100 consecutive patients (Julian and associates 1964)[J21]. No mention is made of the arrhythmia in a similar study of 273 patients by Day (1968)[D9], although 8 of these patients had nodal rhythm. Similarly, no mention is made of sinus arrest in the reports by Meltzer and Kitchell (1966)[M79], Stock and associates (1967)[S135], Jewitt and associates (1967)[J14], Lawrie and associates (1967)[L12], Lown and associates (1967)[L67]. Rokseth and Hatle (1971)[R32], in a prospective 4-year study of 1665 patients, encountered the arrhythmia in 32 patients, an incidence of just under 2 per cent. In 8 of these patients the rhythm was inferred from the presence of a slow idionodal rhythm. The arrhythmia was always observed in inferior wall myocardial infarction. Lippestad and Marten (1967)[L54] emphasized that the arrhythmia signified an occlusion of the proximal part of the right coronary artery. Mogenson (1970)[M86] encountered the arrhythmia in 5 per cent of cases. He also observed A-V nodal rhythm in 16 per cent of cases.

Complicating Arrhythmias. In 1961, James[J5] pointed out that injury to the S-A node is frequently associated with atrial fibrillation. This was also observed by Rokseth and Hatle (1971)[R32], who encountered atrial fibrillation in one third of their 32 patients with sinus arrest, the incidence being approximately the same as that which occurs in chronic sinus arrest (Rokseth and associates, 1970)[R33]. Rokseth and Hatle (1971)[R32] also observed a complicating A-V block.

ABNORMAL ATRIAL RHYTHMS

Atrial extrasystoles.
Extrasystolic atrial tachycardia.
Atrial flutter.
Atrial fibrillation.

ATRIAL EXTRASYSTOLES

An atrial extrasystole is the expression of an impulse which arises prematurely in an ectopic atrial focus. It is characterized electrocardiographically by a bizarre and premature *P'* wave (Electrocardiographic Study 113). These *P'* waves tend to have fixed or constant coupling intervals to the preceding sinus beats.

Mechanism. Atrial extrasystoles may be due to atrial ischaemia (atrial infarction) or due to atrial distension as a result of concomitant cardiac failure, the expression of an increased end-diastolic ventricular pressure. The most common mechanisms are probably a combination of ventricular failure (distension) with a diseased (infarcted) atria.

Incidence. Atrial extrasystoles are very common in acute myocardial infarction and the reported incidence ranges from 13–52 per cent (Julian 1969[J21]; Meltzer and Kitchell 1966[M79]; Lown and associates, 1967[L68]; Marshall and associates, 1968[M22]). If the atrial extrasystoles are numerous and multifocal, they frequently herald atrial fibrillation.

Extrasystolic Atrial Tachycardia: P.A.T.

Extrasystolic atrial tachycardia, 'P.A.T.' (paroxysmal atrial tachycardia), is a series of three or more consecutive atrial extrasystoles. It consequently has a sudden onset and termination, and is characterized by a series of bizarre and premature P' waves. The P' wave axis tends to be directed downwards and to the left, reflecting a cranio-caudal form of atrial activation. This contrasts with the usual caudo-cranial form of atrial activation in atrial flutter.

Complicating arrhythmias. The extrasystolic atrial tachycardia may be associated with (a) second degree A-V block with regular or irregular conduction ratios, and (b) phasic aberrant ventricular conduction, the transient, intermittent, abnormal intraventricular conduction of supraventricular impulses (discussed in greater detail below), which gives rise to a series of bizarre QRS complexes. This may simulate ventricular tachycardia, and is possibly a reason for the relatively low reported incidence.

Incidence. The rhythm was at one time thought to be very uncommon in acute myocardial infarction (Vazifdar and Levine 1966)[V5]. Yet recent reports would suggest that it is really not that rare. The arrhythmia has been observed in 3–17·7 per cent of cases (Meltzer and Kitchell 1966[M79]; Jewitt and associates 1967[J14]; Lown and associates 1967[L68]; Mogenson 1970[M86]).

Atrial Flutter

Atrial flutter is the expression of a very rapid form of atrial activation. It may be due to a circus movement; a continuous circulating activation wave front around the atria, particularly the vena cavae. It may also be due to the rapid discharge of an ectopic atrial focus. It is characterized electrocardiographically by wide bizarre P' or F, flutter, waves with an absence of an intervening isoelectric shelf,

giving rise to a saw-tooth or picket-fence appearance. This saw-tooth appearance is most frequently seen in Standard leads II and III, and lead AVF. An isoelectric shelf may be still present in other leads, particularly lead V1. The flutter waves are, in most cases, dominantly negative in Standard leads II and III and lead AVF, thus reflecting a superiorly directed F-wave axis, the expression of a caudo-cranial form of activation. This contrasts with the cranio-caudal form of activation usually associated with extrasystolic atrial tachycardia. The atrial rate is *characteristically about 300/min* with a range of 280–320 beats/min.

Complicating arrhythmias Atrial flutter is frequently associated with second degree A-V block, usually a 2:1 A-V block. This results in a *characteristic ventricular rate of 140–160 ventricular beats/minute*. The atrial flutter may also be complicated by phasic aberrant ventricular conduction, especially when associated with 1:1 conduction, resulting in bizarre QRS complexes which may mimic ventricular tachycardia. The differentiation from ventricular tachycardia is particularly difficult at the very rapid ventricular rates associated with 1:1 A-V conduction, for it is then difficult to identify the atrial activity and to establish a causal relationship to the QRS deflection. Recourse must then be made to analysis of the QRS complex (see p. 186). It is also evident that with 1:1 conduction, the resulting rapid ventricular rate will cause severe haemodynamic embarrassment.

Incidence. The arrhythmia appears to be uncommon in the context of acute myocardial infarction.

Most reports reflect an incidence of 1–2 per cent (Meltzer and Kitchell 1966[M79]; Julian and associates 1964[J21]; Jewitt and associates 1967[J14]; Marshall and associates 1968 [M22]). A possible reason for the relatively low reported incidence may be the difficulty of differentiating the arrhythmia when it is associated with phasic aberrant ventricular conduction from ventricular tachycardia. A higher incidence has been reported by Lown and associates, 1967[L68] (7 per cent), and Mogenson, 1970[M86] (10 per cent).

Atrial Fibrillation

Atrial fibrillation is the expression of the electrophysiological fragmentation of the atria into a mosaic of milling tissue islets in various stages of excitation and refractoriness. The arrhythmia is characterized by irregular, chaotic fibrillation f waves which completely distort the baseline (Electrocardiographic Studies 35, 43 and 113). The ventricular response is irregular due to a concomitant second degree A-V block, and in the untreated case is approximately 140 beats/min. The arrhythmia may be intermittent or sustained. It is commonly heralded and precipitated by frequent atrial extrasystoles (Electrocardiographic Study 113), particularly multifocal atrial extrasystoles. When the atrial fibrillation is episodic, it may fluctuate between normal sinus rhythm, atrial flutter or extrasystolic atrial tachycardia. The ƒ waves of atrial fibrillation may distort the QRS complexes and may, if superimposed on a QS complex, result in the simulation of an rS complex, particularly in the right precordial leads, and thereby masking the QS complex of myocardial infarction (Electrocardiographic Study 43).

Etiology. The atrial fibrillation may be due to distension of the atria secondary to cardiac failure, which occurs in combination with intrinsic atrial disease. It may also be due to involvement of the S-A nodal artery. Ischaemia of the S-A node frequently predisposes to atrial fibrillation (James 1961[J5]; see also section above on abnormal sinus rhythms), and which indicates, *inter alia*, the presence of atrial infarction.

Incidence. Atrial fibrillation as a complication of acute myocardial infarction has been reported with an incidence of 7 per cent (Meltzer and Kitchell 1966)[M79], 10–15 per cent (Julian and associates 1964[J21]; Jewitt and associates 1967[J14]; Stock and associates 1967[S135]; and 20 per cent (Mogenson 1970)[M86].

ABNORMAL A-V NODAL (JUNCTIONAL) RHYTHMS

A-V nodal extrasystoles.
Extrasystolic A-V nodal tachycardia.
Idionodal escape rhythm.
Idionodal tachycardia.

A-V NODAL EXTRASYSTOLES

An A-V nodal extrasystole is the expression of an impulse which arises prematurely in an A-V nodal focus. It is characterized by a normal or relatively normal QRS complex, resembling that of the conducted sinus impulse. The A-V nodal extrasystole may, because of its prematurity, also be complicated by phasic aberrant ventricular conduction, thereby resulting in an abnormal QRS complex. The extrasystole may then simulate a ventricular extrasystole. Differentiation under these circumstances must be based on careful analysis of the QRS configuration in lead V1 or lead MCL1. This is discussed in the section on phasic aberrant ventricular conduction (see p. 184).

The A-V nodal extrasystole may be dissociated from the near-synchronous sinus P wave, or its impulse may be conducted retrogradely to activate the atria in a caudocranial direction. This will result in a P' wave that is negative in Standard leads II, III and lead AVF, and is the expression of a mean frontal plane P' wave axis of −80° to −100°. The P' wave may precede, follow or be superimposed upon the associated QRS complex, depending upon the relative anterograde or retrograde conduction times.

Incidence. A-V nodal extrasystoles are very uncommon in the context of acute myocardial infarction, indeed, far less common than extrasystolic, A-V nodal, tachycardia which occurs with the very low incidence of 2 per cent (see below).

EXTRASYSTOLIC A-V NODAL TACHYCARDIA

Extrasystolic, paroxysmal, A-V nodal tachycardia is a series of three or more consecutive A-V nodal extrasystoles. It has an abrupt onset and termination. It has the electrocardiographic features of A-V nodal extrasystoles. It is relatively uncommon and probably does not occur in more than 2 per cent of patients with acute myocardial infarction[M78]. The rhythm may be associated with phasic aberrant ventricular conduction and may, therefore, present as a series of bizarre QRS complexes simulating extrasystolic ventricular tachycardia. The differential diagnosis is considered in the section on phasic aberrant ventricular conduction (see p. 185). The ectopic rate may be in the range of 120–180 beats/min.

Supraventricular tachycardia with rates greater than 200 beats/min in the adult, and which are not infrequently termed A-V nodal tachycardia, are most likely examples of reciprocating tachycardia.

IDIONODAL ESCAPE RHYTHM

Escape rhythms are not primary diagnoses, since they always occur secondary to other disturbances of impulse formation, e.g. sinus arrest or sinus bradycardia, or impulse conduction, e.g. S-A block or A-V block.

Idionodal escape rhythm is a not uncommon manifestation of myocardial infarction, particularly inferior wall myocardial infarction (Electrocardiographic Study 3). This is because inferior wall myocardial infarction is often associated with disorders of the S-A node, thereby leading to sinus arrest, sinus bradycardia or S-A block.

IDIONODAL TACHYCARDIA

Idionodal tachycardia, also termed non-paroxysmal A-V

nodal tachycardia to distinguish it from the paroxysmal form (Pick and Dominguez 1957)[P19], is the expression of an enhanced A-V nodal pacemaker, similar to the enhancement of a sinus pacemaker in sinus tachycardia. The rate is usually in the range of 70–100 beats/min, i.e. it is rather slower than the extrasystolic forms of A-V nodal tachycardia. Moreover, since it is in the same rate-range of the sinus rhythm, A-V dissociation is common and the rhythm frequently fluctuates between the sinus rhythm and the A-V nodal rhythm. The rhythm is characterized by the following electrocardiographic characteristics:

1. The QRS complex is normal or, if abnormal, has the same or similar configuration to that of the conducted sinus impulse.

2. The condition sequence of the idionodal tachycardia may take any of the forms associated with A-V nodal rhythm:

(a) There may be complete A-V dissociation between the QRS complexes of the idionodal rhythm and the sinus P waves.

(b) There may be retrograde conduction to the atria. The retrograde P' wave may precede, follow or be superimposed upon the QRS complex, depending upon relative anterograde and retrograde conduction times.

Mechanism. This is considered in the section dealing with the analogous rhythm of idioventricular tachycardia (see below, p. 178)

Incidence. Idionodal tachycardia is not infrequently associated with acute myocardial infarction, and has been reported with an incidence of 10 per cent (Konecke and Knoebel 1972)[K34].

ABNORMAL VENTRICULAR RHYTHMS

Ventricular extrasystoles.
Ventricular tachycardia.
Ventricular parasystole.
Ventricular asystole.

VENTRICULAR EXTRASYSTOLES

A ventricular extrasystole is an impulse which arises in an ectopic ventricular focus and is premature in relation to the prevailing rhythm. The extrasystole is further characterized by fixed or constant coupling; the interval between the extrasystole and the preceding sinus beat is constant for all ventricular extrasystoles arising from the same focus in the same tracing. This indicates that the extrasystole is in some way dependent upon, or precipitated by, the preceding

sinus beat. This contrasts with the manifestations of ventricular parasystole, an independent autonomous rhythm arising from an ectopic ventricular focus whose discharge is in some way *protected* from the impulses of the dominant sinus pacemaker. The independent nature of the ventricular parasystolic rhythm is reflected, in part, by the marked variation of the coupling intervals. The frequent lack of distinction between the two rhythms is due, in part, to the prevalent use of the non-definitive term 'premature ventricular conduction' (PVC) which applies to the manifest beats of *both* rhythms.

Electrocardiographic characteristics. The ventricular extrasystole is characterized electrocardiographically by a premature and bizarre QRS complex which is not preceded by a causally related *P* wave (Electrocardiographic Studies 66, 67, 90 and 91). The ventricular extrasystolic impulse may be conducted retrogradely to the atria, or it may be interfered with by the concomitant sinus impulse within the ventricles, resulting in ventricular fusion, within the A-V node, resulting in A-V nodal dissociation, within the atria, resulting in atrial fusion.

Ventricular extrasystoles arising in the right ventricle tend to have a left bundle branch block-like pattern, whereas those arising in the left ventricle tend to have a right bundle branch-like pattern. The ventricular extrasystoles may be multifocal in origin, manifesting with multiform QRS complexes.

Distributional patterns. The ventricular extrasystoles may occur occasionally in haphazard distribution. They may alternate with conducted sinus beats, resulting in bigeminal rhythm (Electrocardiographic Study 90). They may occur consecutively in pairs (Electrocardiographic Study 91). Three or more consecutive ventricular extrasystoles constitute an ectopic ventricular tachycardia. (Electrocardiographic Study 91).

The Rule of Bigeminy. The precipitation of certain types of ventricular extrasystoles is favoured by a long preceding cycle length, a long preceding R-R interval. The phenomenon is best demonstrated in cases where the basic rhythm is markedly irregular as in atrial fibrillation. When this occurs, a relatively long pause may favour the precipitation of a subsequent ventricular extrasystole. The compensatory pause which follows the ventricular extrasystole constitutes another long pause, which favours the precipitation of another ventricular extrasystole. Thus, extrasystolic bigeminal rhythm tends to be perpetuated. Langendorf, Pick and Winternitz (1955)[L7] consequently termed the phenomenon 'The Rule of Bigeminy'. The precipitation of these ventricular extrasystoles is thus favoured by a slow or relatively slow rhythm, since slow or relatively slow rhythms are characterized by long R-R intervals. The phenomenon is thus important in the context of acute myocardial infarction, for when the basic rhythm is a sinus bradycardia thereby resulting in long or relatively long R-R intervals, it favours the precipitation of those ventricular extrasystoles which are dependent upon the Rule of Bigeminy. The abolition of such extrasystoles may be achieved by shortening the prevailing cycle lengths, i.e. by accelerating the basic rhythm, for example by the administration of atropine. It must, however, be stressed that not all ventricular extrasystoles are dependent upon the Rule of Bigeminy. Ventricular extrasystoles that do not obey the rule have been termed *primary extrasystoles*, and those that do obey the rule *secondary extrasystoles* (Schamroth 1965)[S20]. The precipitating mechanism in the two forms are different (Schamroth 1965[S21]; Schamroth 1965[S22]; Schamroth 1969[S28]).

Ventricular extrasystoles with very short coupling intervals: The R on T phenomenon. Ventricular extrasystoles which complicate acute myocardial infarction may manifest with very short though constant coupling intervals, reflecting a marked degree of prematurity. When this occurs, the QRS complex of the ventricular extrasystole may be superimposed upon the distal limb of the apex of the preceding *T* wave. This is termed the '*R on T*' phenomenon. It reflects an ominous situation, for a ventricular extrasystole with this degree of prematurity occurs in the vulnerable phase of ventricular recovery, and the precipitation of extrasystolic ventricular tachycardia, ventricular flutter or ventricular fibrillation is likely (Electrocardiographic Study 111; Dolara 1967[D19]; Gutierrez 1968[G49]; Wiggers and Wegria 1940[W38]; Smirk and Palmer 1960[S93]; Palmer 1962[P2]). Ventricular extrasystoles with the R on T phenomenon have been observed in 7–9 per cent of patients in coronary care units (Julian and associates, 1964[J21]; Lawrie, 1966[L11]). The overall incidence of the R on T phenomenon in myocardial infarction is probably higher since the first such ventricular extrasystole may, in fact, precipitate the fatal ventricular fibrillation.

The precipitation of ventricular fibrillation by an extrasystole with a short coupling interval has two implications [S26, S27]:

1. It indicates that the myocardium is then in an out-of-phase state.

2. The mere fact that an extrasystole with a short coupling interval can manifest indicates that there has been a shortening of the refractory period, and this shortening affects at least part of the myocardium. For, although an ectopic ventricular focus may in the absence of significant heart disease discharge during, or towards the end of, the ventricular refractory period, it cannot become manifest if the surrounding myocardium is refractory. This is evident from cases of ventricular parasystole (see below), where calculation reveals that the ectopic discharge may occur during *all* phases of the cardiac cycle, yet only those with *relatively* long coupling intervals become manifest. Ectopic discharges that occur with shorter coupling intervals encounter a refractory myocardium and are thus confined to the ectopic focus, being unable to invade the surrounding myocardium. Indeed, parasystolic rhythm with very short coupling intervals are not seen, for if this should occur, precipitation of ventricular fibrillation would be very likely, and the opportunity for recording such parasystolic rhythms would then be minimal. Thus, a ventricular ectopic beat that *manifests* with a short coupling interval clearly implies a shortening of the refractory period, and it is this shortening together with the ectopic impulses generated by the extrasystole that predisposes to the precipitation of ventricular fibrillation. The significance of this is not often appreciated. It is usually thought that the ventricular extrasystole is the only villain of the peace. Yet, its mere occurrence with a short coupling interval should alert one to the presence of a potentially ominous state of the co-villain, the out-of-phase underlying myocardium.

The significance of the ectopic site. Ventricular extrasystoles which arise in the left ventricle are potentially more dangerous than ventricular extrasystoles arising in the right ventricle, since they are more likely to precipitate ventricular fibrillation[B81]. This is probably because myocardial infarctions occur predominantly or exclusively in the left ventricle, and hence a ventricular extrasystole arising in the left ventricle occurs within or near the diseased area; the diseased out-of-phase state of the ventricular myocardium. It is consequently, under this circumstance, especially likely to occur during the vulnerable phase. Right ventricular extrasystoles are relatively remote from the infarction, and the time taken for the extrasystolic impulse to reach the left ventricle may be sufficient to enable recovery and hence an equalization or stabilization of the terminal out-of-phase state.

The relationship to the site of infarction. There does not appear to be any relationship between the site of infarction (for example anterior or inferior) and the frequency of the arrhythmia (Mogenson 1970[M86]; Meltzer and Cohen 1972[M78]).

Incidence. When the entire spectrum and evolution of acute myocardial infarction is considered, the incidence of ventricular extrasystoles is probably 100 per cent, one or more ventricular extrasystoles invariably occurring during some stage of the disease. The incidence of ventricular extrasystoles during the first few days in coronary care units have been reported as high as 80 per cent (Lown 1967[L68]; Lawrie and associates 1968[L12]). Moss and associates 1971[M89] noted that 73 per cent of patients with acute myocardial infarction had ventricular extrasystoles as late as 3 weeks after admission to hospital.

Clinical significance. Any ventricular extrasystole which occurs during the course of acute myocardial infarction must be viewed as potentially ominous. The hazard increases with the following manifestations:

1. Frequent ventricular extrasystoles.
2. Ventricular extrasystoles which occur in salvos.
3. Ventricular extrasystoles which occur in bigeminal rhythms.
4. Ventricular extrasystoles which occur in pairs; consecutive ventricular extrasystoles.
5. Multiform ventricular extrasystoles.
6. Ventricular extrasystoles with short coupling intervals, the R on T phenomenon.
7. Ventricular extrasystoles which originate in the left ventricle.

It is my *impression* that ventricular extrasystoles with small amplitude QRS complexes are more ominous than those with large amplitude QRS complexes. This requires further study and confirmation.

VENTRICULAR TACHYCARDIA

Ventricular tachycardia may be defined as a series of three or more consecutive ectopic ventricular beats which are inscribed at a rate of faster than the prevailing normal sinus rhythm. There are three forms: *extrasystolic ventricular tachycardia, idioventricular tachycardia* and *parasystolic ventricular tachycardia*[S27, S28]. The first two are the most important in the context of acute myocardial infarction, and will be considered here. Parasystolic ventricular tachycardia is briefly presented in the section on ventricular parasystole (see below).

It is difficult to evaluate the incidence of the arrhythmia from the literature, since most reports do not reflect a separation between the various forms. Moreover, the definition varies. For example, some authors consider six consecutive ventricular ectopic beats as a ventricular tachycardia, whereas others only consider ventricular tachycardia present when there are three or more consecutive ventricular ectopic beats.

Extrasystolic Ventricular Tachycardia

Extrasystolic ventricular tachycardia is a series of three or more consecutive ventricular extrasystoles and, as such, it has an abrupt onset and termination (Electrocardiographic Studies 91 and 112). The basic electrocardiographic features are essentially those of the ventricular extrasystole (see above). The arrhythmia must be distinguished from supraventricular tachyarrhythmias such as extrasystolic atrial tachycardia and atrial flutter which are conducted with phasic aberrant ventricular conduction. The differentiation is considered on p. 186.

The arrhythmia is frequently heralded by sporadic ventricular extrasystoles. The extrasystolic ventricular tachycardia is especially likely to be precipitated by a ventricular extrasystole with the R on T phenomenon (see above). When this occurs, the rhythm not infrequently transforms into ventricular fibrillation. This again emphasizes that the shortened Q-T interval of at least part of the ventricular myocardium is as much the villain of the peace as the ventricular extrasystole itself.

Ventricular Flutter

It is debatable whether the rhythm of ventricular flutter represents a definite separate dysrhythmic entity. The features are essentially those of an extrasystolic ventricular tachycardia, a series of consecutive ventricular extrasystoles. In the case of ventricular flutter, however, intraventricular conduction of the extrasystolic impulse is markedly abnormal and is reflected electrocardiographically by very *widened and bizarre QRS complexes associated with widened and bizarre T waves* (Electrocardiographic Study 111). These blend with each other in the form of a continuous sine-like wave so that it is difficult to separate the QRS complex, the S-T segment and the T wave. The rhythm reflects an ominous *clinical* state. The manifestation is usually associated with a fall in cardiac output, and syncope is frequent (Smirk and associates 1964)[S92]. It is difficult to establish the incidence, since most reports do not distinguish between the condition and extrasystolic ventricular tachycardia. The arrhythmia may also be simulated by atrial flutter conducted with phasic aberrant ventricular conduction.

Idioventricular Tachycardia

Idioventricular tachycardia is particularly important in the context of acute myocardial infarction. It occurs relatively frequently and is usually benign. The mechanism and significance has only recently received emphasis. It will consequently be considered in some detail.

The heart has many potential pacemaking cells which are situated in the sinoatrial node, the atria, the A-V node, and the ventricles. Only one of these pacemaking cells, however, is in control of the heart. This is the pacemaker with the highest automaticity or discharge rate, since its impulses reach the potential slower subsidiary pacemakers and abolish or discharge their immature impulses before they have the time or opportunity to reach maturity and 'fire' (Diagram A of Fig. 69). The subsidiary pacemaking centres thus enjoy *no protection* from the impulses of the fastest pacemaker, and it is this which ensures that only one pacemaker is normally in control of the heart. The sinus pacemaker has the fastest inherent automaticity (70–80 beats/min), and is therefore normally in control of the

A-V nodal pacemaker, for example, is approximately 50–60 beats/min, while the inherent rate of a ventricular pacemaker is approximately 30–40 beats/min.

This inherent automaticity of the S-A node and potential subsidiary pacemakers may, under certain circumstances, become enhanced. When the automaticity of the sinus pacemaker is enhanced so that its rate exceeds 100 beats/min, the rhythm is well recognized as *sinus tachycardia*. The inherent rate of an A-V nodal pacemaker, the idionodal rhythm, may be similarly enhanced, and if the enhanced A-V nodal rate exceeds the sinus rate, the A-V nodal rhythm, or idionodal rhythm, becomes manifest. This accelerated idionodal rhythm is known as *idionodal tachycardia*[S22, S27, S28]. An inherent idioventricular rhythm may be similarly enhanced, resulting in an *idioventricular tachycardia* (Diagram C of Fig. 69, and Fig. 70)[S25, S27].

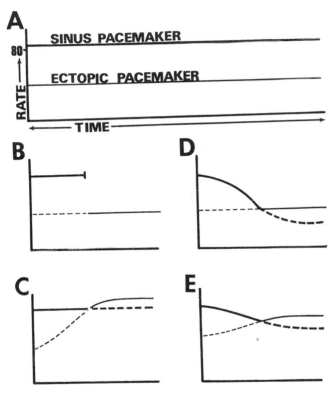

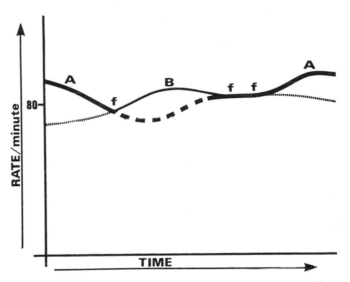

FIG. 70. Diagram illustrating the interplay of sinus rhythm (A) and an idioventricular tachycardia (B). See text.

FIG. 69. Diagrams illustrating the mechanisms of escape rhythms and idiofocal (idionodal and idioventricular) tachycardia. See text.

heart. The other potential pacemakers have slower inherent rates and can only become manifest, as escape beats or escape rhythms, when there is slowing of the sinus pacemaker (Diagram D of Fig. 69), or a failure of sinus impulse conduction, i.e. as a result of sinoatrial or atrioventricular block (Diagram B of Fig. 69). Teleologically, the escape rhythm may be viewed as a safety or rescue mechanism which enables the atria, the A-V node, or the ventricular myocardium to initiate its own inherent rhythm whenever the sinus impulse fails or defaults. The more distal a subsidiary pacemaker is situated from the S-A node, the slower is its inherent automaticity. The inherent rate of an

Idioventricular Tachycardia

Idioventricular tachycardia is the expression of an accelerated idioventricular rhythm, an enhancement of the inherent automaticity of a latent or potential idioventricular pacemaker. The rhythm becomes manifest when its rate exceeds that of the sinus pacemaker. It therefore reflects the presence of *differential enhancement*, the rate of the idioventricular pacemaker being accelerated to a greater degree than that of the sinus pacemaker.

Diagnosis and Electrocardiographic Manifestations

The diagnosis of idioventricular tachycardia is based on the following criteria[S25]:

1. criteria for the establishment of ventricular origin.

2. the presence of an enhanced idioventricular rate, a relatively rapid idioventricular rate.

3. an increased propensity to A-V dissociation and ventricular capture beats.

4. the *absence of protection*.

These are illustrated in Electrocardiographic Study 68 and considered further below.

1. The establishment of ventricular origin. The establishment of ventricular origin is inferred from the abnormal or bizarre QRS complex, and is further substantiated by:

(a) the presence of ventricular fusion complexes, incomplete capture beats, resulting from the simultaneous invasion of the ventricles by both supreventricular and ventricular impulses, each contributing to the activation of the ventricles, and

(b) the relatively normal QRS contour of the capture beat, a contour that differs markedly from the QRS complex of the ectopic beats, and which resembles the QRS contour during sinus rhythm. See also section below on phasic aberrant ventricular conduction.

2. The Idioventricular Rate. The rate of idioventricular tachycardia is but moderately increased when compared to the usual rates of extrasystolic ventricular tachycardia. The normal unenhanced idioventricular rhythm rarely exceeds 40 beats/min, so that an idioventricular tachycardia could in fact be defined as an idioventricular rhythm whose rate exceeds 40 beats/min. Allowing for a measure of overlap, however, the rhythm has been arbitrarily defined as an idioventricular rate that is greater than 55 beats/min[S24]. The rates of the idioventricular tachycardias in the series reported by Schamroth (1969)[S24] varied from 55–108 beats/min, the most frequent rate being in the range of 75–80 beats/min. The rate of an idioventricular tachycardia may fluctuate slightly, but this fluctuation does not usually exceed 10 beats/min. Nevertheless, the fluctuation may on rare occasions be very marked (Schamroth 1968)[S24].

3. The propensity to A-V dissociation and capture beats. Since idioventricular tachycardia usually manifests with a rate approximately the same as that of the sinus rhythm, the two rhythms commonly discharge synchronously or near synchronously and *A-V dissociation is, therefore, a common occurrence* (Fig. 70). Furthermore, capture beats, complete and incomplete (ventricular fusion), are very common in idioventricular tachycardia (Electrocardiographic Study 68). This too is due to the relatively slow rate of the idioventricular tachycardia. The relatively long cycle permits adequate recovery time, and thereby a greater opportunity for capture. With very fast ectopic rates, as in extrasystolic tachycardia, the refractory period occupies the whole, or practically the whole, ensuing cycle, and the opportunity for capture is consequently minimal or absent.

Since idioventricular tachycardia becomes manifest when its rate equals the sinus rate, the ectopic rhythm usually begins with several consecutive fusion beats, incomplete captures (Fig. 70, and Electrocardiographic Study 68A). And since the two rhythms tend to fluctuate within the same narrow range, the ectopic rhythm tends to terminate with several successive fusion complexes. *It is, therefore, very common for idioventricular tachycardia to begin and end with fusion complexes.*

4. The absence of pacemaker protection. The *absence* of protection of the ectopic pacemaking focus is evident from the dislocation of the ectopic rhythm, the resetting of the ectopic cycle, by the capture beat.

Review
Idioventricular tachycardia was described by Harris in 1950[H7] who observed the rhythm in experimental myocardial infarction. He noted that '*it appeared that a ventricular focus with a frequency of impulse formation almost equal to that of the S-A node was alternately gaining and losing dominance of the cardiac rhythm*'. The arrhythmia has aroused considerable interest during recent years[B13, G7, K29, R56, R57, R59, R60, S21, S22, S24, S123]. This is probably due, in part, to the advent of constant electrocardiographic monitoring in coronary care units, for the arrhythmia is frequently associated with myocardial infarction, particularly inferior myocardial infarction[C10, D26, G7, K29, L61, P19, R56, R57, R58, R60, S24, S25, S123]. Spann and associates (1964)[S123] described the arrhythmia in 15 of 30 monitored patients. Rothfield and associates (1968)[R60] noted the arrhythmia in 30 of 100 consecutive cases of acute myocardial infarction. Several comments appeared in the Symposium on Intensive Coronary Care which took place in Philadelphia in July 1966[G7, K29].

Further cases were reported, and clinical spectrum and nomenclature reviewed, by Schamroth (1969)[S24, S25]. Castellanos and associates (1969)[C10] also observed its frequent association with clinical myocardial infarction, and stressed its automatic non-parasystolic intermittent character. Logic and associates (1969)[L61] observed the arrhythmia in experimental myocardial infarction and noted the absence of haemodynamic deterioration. They further stressed that it did not predispose to ventricular fibrillation.

Management of Idioventricular Tachycardia
The arrhythmic disturbance of idioventricular tachycardia may be viewed in the same light as sinus tachycardia, an

expression of an underlying condition in which the rhythm itself does not require active treatment since it rarely causes haemodynamic embarrassment. If the loss of atrial drive becomes significant, the ectopic ventricular rhythm may be overdriven by accelerating the sinus rate with atropine. It is doubtful whether it is ever necessary to resort to electrical overdriving or the use of cardiosup-pressive drugs such as lignocaine, a principle that was stressed by Rothfield and associates[R60].

INCIDENCE OF IDIOVENTRICULAR TACHYCARDIA

The arrhythmia is common in the context of acute myocardial infarction. Rothfield and associates[R60] noted the disorder in 36 of 100 consecutive cases with acute myocardial infarction. Norris and associates (1970)[N17] observed the rhythm in 8 per cent of 737 patients, while Marriott (1972)[M17] noted it in 70 of 500 cases (an incidence of 14 per cent), an inferior location of the infarction being the commonest association.

VENTRICULAR PARASYSTOLE

The heart has many pacemaking cells which are situated in the sinoatrial node, the atria, the atrioventricular node, and the ventricles. Only one such pacemaking cell is, however, in control of the heart. This is the pacemaker with the fastest inherent discharge rate. Its impulses reach the slower subsidiary pacemakers before they have the opportunity to 'fire' and abolish their immature impulses prematurely. This ensures that there is only one pacemaker in control of the heart. At times, however, a subsidiary and slower ectopic pacemaking cell develops a protective mechanism which is situated in the immediate vicinity of the ectopic pacemaking cell and is operative throughout its entire cycle. This enables the slower ectopic pacemaker to co-exist with the more rapid supraventricular pacemaker, a condition known as parasystole. Though the sinus impulse cannot penetrate into the ectopic pacemaking focus, the ectopic impulse can leave the ectopic focus and activate the surrounding myocardium, when it is responsive consequent to activation by the supraventricular impulses. The ectopic impulses, therefore, manifest intermittently when the myocardium is responsive.

The independence of the regular ectopic ventricular parasystolic rhythm is evident from the following features (Electrocardiographic Study 110):

1. **Varying coupling intervals.** The interval between the ectopic beat and its preceding sinus beat is different for each ectopic beat. This contrasts with the extrasystolic mechanism which is associated with constant coupling

intervals, and which therefore indicates a causal relationship between the extrasystole and the preceding sinus beat.

2. **Mathematically related interectopic intervals.** The long interectopic intervals are in simple multiples of the shorter interectopic intervals. This reflects a *regular* ectopic discharge. The ectopic focus discharges uninterruptedly but some of its impulses are unable to activate the myocardium due to refractoriness from prior activation by the sinus impulse.

3. **Ventricular fusion beats.** These are due to co-incidental activation of the ventricles by the sinus and ectopic impulses, resulting in a QRS complex with a configuration in between that of the pure sinus beat and the pure ectopic beat.

Incidence of Ventricular Parasystole in Acute Myocardial Infarction

It is very difficult to estimate the incidence of ventricular parasystole in acute myocardial infarction. Indeed, most reports on ectopic ventricular rhythms during infarction do not even separate extrasystolic and parasystolic rhythms, the enhanced automaticity being referred to by the very unsatisfactory term *PVC*, premature ventricular contraction. The true incidence of parasystole in myocardial infarction must, however, be exceptionally rare. If indeed it did occur with a potentially short coupling interval (as is likely in acute myocardial infarction), it would discharge within the vulnerable period very soon after the onset of the arrhythmia, for the independence of the ectopic rhythm means that its impulse falls during all phases of the sinus cycle. Consequently ventricular fibrillation would most likely be precipitated very early, and it would therefore be very difficult to record the rhythm. Salazar and McKendrick (1970)[S4] reported its occurrence in 11 out of 630 cases (an incidence of 1·74 per cent).

Parasystolic Ventricular Tachycardia

Parasystolic ventricular tachycardia is the rhythm resulting from the rapid discharge of an ectopic ventricular focus that is completely protected from the concomitant sinus rhythm. The rhythm is usually enhanced to the same rate-range as an idioventricular tachycardia. Unlike idioventricular tachycardia, however, the pacemaker is completely protected and continues to discharge at all times. At times, the manifest rhythm disappears, but this disappearance is due to an *exit block*. The continuous discharge of the ectopic focus during the period of exit block is evident from the fact that the long interectopic interval between the paroxysms of tachycardia is in a simple multiple of the ectopic cycle length. In other words, the parasystolic rhythm continues during the apparent intermission, but is not manifest due to the presence of exit block. The arrhythmia is very rare, especially so in acute myocardial infarction; no convincing case has yet been reported. Its importance in the context of acute myocardial infarction is that it is not uncommonly mistaken for idioventricular tachycardia, a common manifestation during myocardial infarction. The distinction is based on the following. In parasystolic ventricular tachycardia, the apparent intermissions are in exact multiples of the ectopic cycle length, thereby indicating that the ectopic rhythm continues during the apparent intermission; whereas in idioventricular tachycardia, the intermission bears no such relationship, and merely reflects that the sinus rhythm has become momentarily faster than the ectopic rhythm, and has consequently usurped the ectopic rhythm once again.

Ventricular Asystole

Ventricular asystole, ventricular standstill, refers to complete failure of ventricular pacemaker activity. It is usually associated with complete A-V block, particularly bilateral bundle branch block. It is, in fact, the electrocardiographic expression of a Stokes Adams attack, no QRS complexes are recorded. Its occurrence in acute myocardial infarction has been reported with an incidence of 2 per cent (Julian and associates 1964)[J21], 10 per cent (Meltzer and Kitchell 1966)[M79], 1 per cent (Lown and associates 1967)[L68], 3 per cent (Lawrie and associates 1967)[L13], 7 per cent (Mogenson 1970)[M86], and 14 per cent (Sloman and associates 1971)[S91]. The prognosis is very adverse, with the mortality approaching 100 per cent.

Disturbances of Impulse Conduction

A-V block.
Phasic aberrant ventricular conduction.

A-V BLOCK

It must be stated at the outset that any appraisal of A-V block must take into account the rate of the sinus or supraventricular impulses which are delayed or blocked. For example, the unqualified diagnosis of 2:1 A-V block has very little meaning unless the supraventricular rate is stated. This is because a 2:1 A-V block complicating an atrial flutter at 300/min is physiological and merely indicates that the rapidity of the discharge causes alternate impulses to fall in the absolute refractory period; whereas a 2:1 A-V block complicating sinus rhythm with a rate of 60/min indicates a true inherent increase in A-V nodal refractoriness.

This is of special significance in acute myocardial infarction, for it has been shown that the rate at which a particular degree of A-V block develops is lower during

the acute phase of myocardial infarction. Thus, Danzig and associates (1969)[D1], in a study of A-V block due to myocardial infarction, showed that increasing degrees of A-V block developed with either a spontaneous increase in rate, or with an increase in rate due to the administration of atropine or isoproterenol, or by an increase in rate effected by atrial pacing. During convalescence, atrial rates 20–40 per cent higher were necessary to cause the same degree (second degree) of A-V block.

There are several factors which are pertinent to the genesis of A-V block in the context of acute myocardial infarction. These are:

1. The blood supply of the A-V node in man is supplied in 90 per cent of cases by the right coronary artery, and in 10 per cent of cases by the left circumflex artery (James 1968)[J8]. Consequently, acute A-V block is usually a complication of inferior or posterior wall myocardial infarction. This has been recognized for a long time (Rosenbaum and Levine 1941[R40]; Kay 1948[K15]; James 1961[J6]).

2. Acute myocardial infarction is commonly associated with a most marked vagotonia (James 1960[J4]; James 1961[J6]). The anatomic basis for this excessive vagal discharge is the presence of vagal neuroreceptors in the region of the coronary sinus (Juhasz-Nagy and Szentivanyi 1961)[J20].

3. Acute A-V block is usually due to ischaemia. Lev and associates (1970)[L34] showed that acute A-V block in the context of coronary artery disease was due to ischaemia, whereas chronic A-V block was due to the combination of an ischaemic factor with a mechanical factor such as fibrosis or calcification of the summit of the interventricular septum.

4. It has also been demonstrated experimentally that the A-V node is less resistant to ischaemia than other parts of the conducting system (Stuckey and Hoffman 1961)[S140]. When A-V block is associated with acute myocardial infarction, it is usually due to ischaemia of the A-V node, although necrosis or oedema has occasionally been observed at autopsy[B55, B56]. While ischaemia is certainly the basic factor in many cases of A-V block in acute myocardial infarction, it certainly cannot be the only factor. If it were, the incidence of A-V block in acute myocardial infarction would be very much higher. Furthermore, the onset of A-V block is usually delayed for 24–36 hours following the onset of myocardial ischaemia, as reflected by chest pain. This suggests that other factors may be involved. One such postulate is that there is an accumulation of metabolites. Jackrell and associates (1967)[J1] demonstrated an increase in potassium ions in the conducting system of the dog following septal artery ligation. Those dogs with normal potassium content remained in uncomplicated sinus rhythm, whereas those with increased

potassium content developed A-V block. They concluded that the A-V block was related to potassium levels and not to oedema, necrosis or inflammatory cell infiltration. When, however, A-V block is associated with anterior wall myocardial infarction, there is usually widespread damage to the septum with marked and significant lesions of the bundle branch system[B55, B56, D6, F28].

First Degree A-V Block

This is reflected electrocardiographically by a prolonged P-R (P-Q) interval; an interval greater than 0·20 sec with normal sinus rates in the adult (Electrocardiographic Studies 7, 29 and 34). In most cases this is due to a delay within the A-V node. It may be due to increased vagal activity, or to ischaemia of the A-V node. A *slight* increase in A-V conduction time may, at times, also be an expression of bilateral bundle branch conduction delay, but this is uncommon in the context of acute myocardial infarction. First degree A-V block occurs with an incidence of 4–14 per cent in coronary care units (Julian and associates 1964[J21]; Lown 1966[L66]; Day 1968[D9]; Mogenson 1970[M86]).

First degree A-V block frequently progresses to second and third degree A-V block. This is especially prone to occur with postero-inferior infarctions. Thus, Norris (1970)[N15] observed that of 64 patients with acute postero-inferior infarction, 75 per cent developed second degree A-V block and 41 per cent progressed to third degree A-V block.

A high incidence of first degree A-V block has been noted with coronary artery disease[C3].

The Type I Second Degree A-V Block

Type I second degree A-V block (synonyms: The Wenckebach Phenomenon, the Mobitz Type I second degree A-V block) is reflected by increasing A-V conduction times—increasing P-R intervals—until conduction fails. This failure manifests with a dropped beat, a *P* wave that is not followed by a QRS complex. The block permits recovery of the conducting tissues and the sequence is then repeated (Electrocardiographic Study 9). The manifestation may be an expression of intense vagal activity, or ischaemia of the A-V node. The rhythm tends to be transient, and is most frequently associated with postero-inferior infarction. It occurs in 4–10 per cent of patients admitted to coronary care units (Lown and associates 1967[L67]; Day 1968[D9]; Lawrie and associates 1968[L11]).

The Type II Second Degree A-V Block

Type II second degree A-V block (synonym: Mobitz Type II second degree A-V block) is an intermittent interruption of A-V conduction which occurs during rhythm which otherwise shows absolutely constant A-V conduction times. The rhythm is, with few exceptions, due to an interruption of A-V conduction *below* the bundle of His, and consequently an expression of bilateral bundle branch block (Narula and Samet 1970)[N3].

It is most often associated with anterior myocardial infarction, but is nevertheless distinctly uncommon in the context of acute myocardial infarction, having one-tenth the incidence of the Type I second degree A-V block[M78].

Third Degree—Complete—A-V Block

This is characterized by a complete and prolonged failure of A-V transmission. None of the supraventricular impulses are conducted to the ventricles which are paced by its own pacemakers. Complete A-V block may be due to complete A-V nodal block or complete bilateral bundle branch block. In the case of complete A-V nodal block, the pacemaker is usually sited in the A-V node just below the block, resulting in idionodal rhythm. In the case of bilateral bundle branch block, the pacemaker is sited peripherally in the ventricles—an idioventricular pacemaker—resulting in idioventricular rhythm. There is no relationship between the *P* waves of the sinus rhythm and the QRS complexes of the pacemaker governing the ventricles, i.e. there is complete A-V dissociation. In the case of a subsidiary A-V nodal pacemaker, the QRS complexes will have a normal configuration or may have the features of *classic* right or left bundle branch block. The rate, under these circumstances, is usually between 40 and 50 beats/min. In the case of an idioventricular pacemaker, the QRS complexes will be bizarre (Electrocardiographic Study 8), and will not be characteristic of either left or right bundle branch block. The rate is usually between 30 and 35 beats/min, or even lower.

Most cases of complete A-V block complicating acute myocardial infarction are intranodal in origin, and are thus associated with a subsidiary idionodal rhythm. This is particularly so in the case of posteroinferior infarction.

Complete A-V block may be complicated by ventricular standstill, failure of the subsidiary ventricular pacemaker, which results in a Stokes Adams syncopal attack or death (see above; Electrocardiographic Study 8). This is more likely to occur with an idioventricular pacemaker, i.e. with a peripheral pacemaker, than with an idionodal pacemaker. Thus, the average mortality associated with complete intranodal block is about 25 per cent (Epstein and associates 1966[E12]; Friedberg and associates 1968[F26]; Beregovich and associates 1969[B37]). In contrast, the average mortality of complete bilateral bundle branch block is near 80 per cent (Lasser and Julian 1968[L10]; Chatterjee and associates 1969[C21]; Kostuk and Beanlands 1970[K43]). It must be emphasized, however, that complete bilateral bundle branch block is far less common than intranodal A-V block in the context of acute myocardial infarction. Bilateral bundle branch block is usually an expression of:

(a) chronic coronary artery disease,
(b) Lenegre's disease[L18, L19] idiopathic degeneration of the conducting system, or
(c) Lev's disease[L33], an encroachment on the conducting system by calcification or fibrosis from neighbouring structures.

In the context of coronary artery disease it is of interest to recapitulate the observations of Lev and associates (1970)[L34] that acute A-V block is related to ischaemia, whereas chronic A-V block is due to the combination of ischaemia with a mechanical factor, such as fibrosis or calcification of the interventricular septum.

It is also worthwhile recapitulating the aphorism of Rosenbaum (1970)[R45] that *the A-V node is the weak point in the context of the acute insult to the heart, whereas the bundle branches are the weak point in the context of the chronic insult to the heart*.

The Characteristics of Complete A-V Block Complicating Acute Posteroinferior Wall Myocardial Infarction

When A-V block complicates acute posterior or inferior wall myocardial infarction, it is usually associated with the following features:

(a) Since there is no significant necrosis of the conducting tissue, the block is frequently transient and reversable. There may be some residual first degree A-V block[S136].
(b) The clinical cause is usually benign[F27, S136].
(c) The third degree A-V block usually develops from an increasing first degree A-V block through a second degree A-V block of the Wenckebach type, Type I[N14, S136]. The Type II second degree A-V block is exceptionally rare. It is indeed very doubtful whether it ever occurs in uncomplicated posteroinferior wall myocardial infarction. The development and regression are usually gradual[F1].
(d) The subsidiary ventricular pacemaker is usually subnodal or junctional, and the QRS complexes are consequently narrow and normal or near normal.
(e) The ventricular rate is relatively high and stable.
(f) Ventricular standstill or asystole is rare.
(g) The prognosis is good, and the patients do not usually require artificial pacing.

The Characteristics of Complete A-V Block Complicating Acute Anterior Wall Myocardial Infarction

The mechanism of the A-V block complicating acute anterior wall myocardial infarction is controversial. According to James (1961)[J5], (1961)[J6], (1968)[J8], the manifestation implies that there is not only an occlusion of the anterior descending artery but also an old or recent occlusion of the posterior descending artery. While this is certainly the case in some instances, the manifestation may, nevertheless, apparently occur in association with an occlusion of the anterior descending artery only. Thus, Davies (1971)[D6], in an autopsy study of 24 patients who developed A-V block during the course of acute myocardial infarction, found a combined anterior and posterior infarction in 9, the remaining 15 being associated with anteroseptal infarction and occlusion of the anterior descending coronary artery only. This caused a destruction of both bundle branches.

The A-V block has the following features:

(a) The prognosis is poor[N14], far worse than the A-V block associated with posterior infarction, and the mortality is high[S136].
(b) The block, once present, tends to remain for long periods, and is usually permanent[S136].
(c) The A-V block tends to occur early, and may reach advanced degrees suddenly.
(d) The block is frequently preceded by progressive bundle branch block[L53], thereby indicating that the final stage of complete A-V block is probably a bilateral bundle branch block.
(e) The subsidiary ventricular pacemaker must, under these circumstances, be located distally in the ventricular myocardium, and the QRS complexes are consequently wide and bizarre, and do not resemble the classic forms of either left or right bundle branch block.
(f) Previous Type II second degree A-V block—the Mobitz Type II second degree A-V block—is common[L6, S136].
(g) Ventricular asystole—ventricular standstill—is a common complication.

PHASIC ABERRANT VENTRICULAR CONDUCTION

Phasic aberrant conduction refers to the transient, intermittent, abnormal intraventricular conduction of a supraventricular impulse. This results in a transient bundle branch block pattern which occurs during rhythm that otherwise reflects normal intraventricular conduction. The appearance of bizarre, bundle branch block, complexes during rhythm with normal intraventricular conduction may mimic ventricular ectopy, for example ventricular extrasystoles and ventricular tachycardia.

The phenomenon is due to unequal refractoriness of the

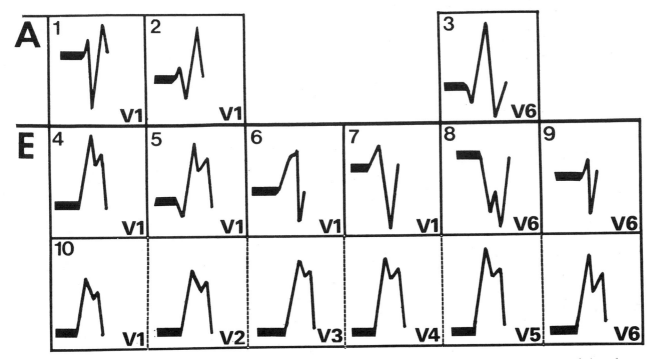

FIG. 71. Diagrams illustrating various presentations of phasic aberrant ventricular conduction (Diagrams 1, 2 and 3), and various presentations of ventricular ectopy (Diagrams 4–10). See text.

bundle branches, so that an early or relatively early impulse may encounter one bundle branch that is responsive while the other is still refractory[S33]. The impulse is consequently conducted down one bundle branch only, resulting in the bizarre QRS pattern of bundle branch block. The differentiation of phasic aberrant ventricular conduction from ventricular ectopy constitutes one of the major diagnostic challenges in electrocardiology, since it may affect both treatment and prognosis (Electrocardiographic Study 113). It is particularly important in the context of continuous monitoring in a coronary care unit, for aberration occurs in no less than 8 per cent of patients admitted with myocardial infarction[M19].

Atrial fibrillation, for example, may be associated with phasic aberrant ventricular conduction, the relatively early impulses will be conducted with a bundle branch block pattern, whereas relatively late impulses will be associated with normal intraventricular conduction. If, under these circumstances, the abnormal QRS complexes are diagnosed as ventricular extrasystoles, digitalis may be withheld, whereas its administration is clearly indicated to slow the ventricular response (Electrocardiographic Study 113).

Much of the following account in the differentiation between phasic aberrant ventricular conduction and ventricular ectopy is based on the elegant clinical studies of Marriott and his associates[M16, M17, M18, M19, S11].

THE DIAGNOSIS OF PHASIC ABERRANT VENTRICULAR CONDUCTION AND ITS DIFFERENTIATION FROM VENTRICULAR ECTOPY

The differentiation of phasic aberrant ventricular conduction from ventricular ectopy is dependent upon the establishment of the P:QRS relationship, and the recognition of the characteristic features from the QRS complex which tend to connote either aberration or ectopy (Fig. 71).

The Significance of the Preceding Atrial Event

Phasic aberrant ventricular conduction reflects the abnormal intraventricular conduction of a supraventricular impulse, and is thus usually preceded by an atrial event, a P or P' wave. For example, a bizarre QRS complex preceded by a premature and bizarre P' wave usually represents an atrial extrasystole conducted with phasic aberrant ventricular conduction (Electrocardiographic Study 113), whereas a bizarre QRS complex that is not preceded by a related P wave usually connotes ventricular ectopy. However, preceding and related atrial activity may not always be evident electrocardiographically. There is, for example, no related preceding recognizable atrial activity in cases of atrial fibrillation (Electrocardiographic Study 113). And it may be very difficult to identify the atrial deflections in a series of rapidly inscribed bizarre QRS complexes of a tachycardia (Electrocardiographic Study 112). Furthermore, even if the P waves and the QRS complexes in a tachycarrhythmia are identified, the relationship of the P' wave to an ensuing bizarre QRS complex may not be clear unless the beginning of the tachycarrhythmia is observed. For example, the P' wave may, during a tachycarrhythmia, represent an ectopic atrial origin, or it may reflect the retrograde conduction from a ventricular or A-V nodal impulse. It may consequently be difficult to establish whether the P' wave is related to the preceding or the ensuing QRS complex. When this occurs, the characteristics of the QRS complex itself may help in the differentiation. These are considered below.

The significance of the QRS configuration

The features are best observed in lead V1 or lead MCL1 (Marriott and Fogg 1970)[M18].

The significance of the initial vector. Most examples of phasic aberrant ventricular conduction reflect a right bundle branch block pattern. Right bundle branch block does not alter the initial vector of the QRS deflection (see Chapter 9). Hence the initial vectors of the QRS complex will tend to be the same during both normal intraventricular conduction and phasic aberrant ventricular conduction (Electrocardiographic Study 113). In ventricular ectopy, however, the initial vectors are usually markedly different (Electrocardiographic Study 113).

The significance of the triphasic configuration. The QRS complex of right bundle branch block characteristically has a triphasic configuration, an rsR variant in lead V1 (Diagrams 1 and 2 of Fig. 71). The initial vectors (the rS deflection in right ventricular leads, and the qR deflection in left ventricular leads) are essentially unchanged. The right bundle branch merely results in the addition of a terminal deflection, an anterior and rightward directed vector (see also Fig. 35). Hence, phasic aberrant ventricular conduction is usually associated with a triphasic configuration in lead V1 (Diagrams 1 and 2 of Fig. 71). Similarly, a qRs complex in lead V6 is also an expression of right bundle branch block, and favours phasic aberrant ventricular conduction (Diagram 3 of Fig. 71). Ventricular ectopy, however, tends to have a monophasic or diphasic configuration in leads V1 or V6, a wide and bizarre dominantly upward or dominantly negative deflection with a notched apex or nadir (Diagrams 4–9 of Fig. 71). Furthermore, the QRS complex of ventricular ectopy is completely bizarre, and does not resemble either the classic forms of either right or left bundle branch block (Electrocardiographic Studies 68 and 112).

The significance of the relative amplitude of the R and R' deflections: the significance of the QRS 'Rabbit Ears'. When lead V1 reflects a bizarre, dominantly upright QRS complex with a notched apex, and the initial deflection of the QRS complex, the R wave, is taller than the second deflection of the QRS complex, the R' wave, ventricular ectopy is the most likely diagnosis[M16, M17] (Diagrams 4 and 5 of Fig. 71; Electrocardiographic Study 68). The notched upright QRS complex has been likened to a pair of rabbit ears[M16, M17], and when the first or left rabbit ear (viewing the rabbit from behind) of the QRS configuration is taller than the second rabbit ear, ventricular ectopy is the likely diagnosis. This may occasionally be preceded by a small initial q wave (Diagram 5 of Fig. 71; Electrocardiographic Study 68).

The significance of the concordant pattern. If the electrocardiogram presents with a series of bizarre QRS complexes which are dominantly positive in *all* the precordial leads, ventricular ectopy is the most likely diagnosis (Diagram 10 of Fig. 71; Electrocardiographic Study 112). The only other condition with a similar presentation is the Type *A* Wolff-Parkinson-White syndrome with atrial fibrillation, in which case the rhythm will be markedly irregular.

The significance of an rS or RS complex in lead V1. An rS or RS complex in lead V1 with a rather broad initial r or R wave usually indicates right ventricular ectopy (Diagram 7 of Fig. 71).

The significance of an rS complex in leads V5 and V6. An rS complex in leads V5 and V6 is usually due to ventricular ectopy (Diagram 9 of Fig. 71). It may also be due to:

(a) right bundle branch block with left anterior hemiblock.
(b) marked right ventricular dominance.
(c) mirror-image dextrocardia.

Thus, when the features of the latter three conditions can be excluded (and this does not usually present any great difficulty), the presence of an rS complex in leads V5 and V6 connotes ventricular ectopy.

The significance of the mean frontal plane QRS axis. Phasic aberrant ventricular conduction is usually associated with a normal or near normal frontal plane QRS axis, for example, in the range of 0 to +90° or 100°, whereas ventricular ectopy is commonly associated with a bizarre QRS axis, for example −150° (Electrocardiographic Study 112).

The significance of a QS complex in lead V6. A QS complex in lead V6 usually connotes ventricular ectopy (Diagram 8 of Fig. 71). It may also occur with extensive transmural anterior wall myocardial infarction, but this differentiation does not cause any great difficulty.

The significance of the compensatory pause. When phasic aberrant ventricular conduction complicates atrial fibrillation, the bizarre QRS complex of the aberration is not usually nor necessarily followed by a compensatory pause, or an attempt at a compensatory pause (Electrocardiographic Study 113). When, however, a ventricular extrasystole, for example, complicates atrial fibrillation, the bizarre QRS complex is usually followed by a long or relatively long pause. This is due to concealed retrograde conduction of the extrasystolic impulse into the A-V node, thereby rendering it refractory to the immediately ensuing fibrillation impulses (Electrocardiographic Study 113).

The significance of ventricular fusion complexes. One of the best signs of ectopic ventricular origin is the presence of a ventricular fusion complex. This complex results from fortuitous concomitant activation of the ventricles by a supraventricular impulse and a ventricular impulse. The resulting QRS complex thus has a configuration that is inbetween that of the pure ectopic beat and the pure conducted supraventricular beat (Electrocardiographic Study 68). Examples of all three complexes must be present in the same tracing before the diagnosis can be established.

PART TWO

1

Acute Inferior Wall Myocardial Infarction

The electrocardiogram shows the early hyperacute injury phase of inferior wall myocardial infarction. This is reflected by the marked slope-elevation of the S-T segments, and the increased amplitude of the T waves in Standard leads II and III and lead AVF. Reciprocal S-T segment depression occurs in Standard leads I, lead AVF and leads V4–V6.

The ventricular activation time of 0·04 sec in Standard leads II and III and lead AVF may indicate the presence of injury block.

COMMENT

The electrocardiogram only reflects the parameters of acute inferior wall injury. The parameters of necrosis have not yet developed.

2

Acute Anterior and Inferior Wall Myocardial Infarction

The electrocardiogram shows the early hyperacute injury phase of anterior and inferior wall myocardial infarction. This is reflected by the marked slope-elevation of the S-T segments, and the increased amplitude of the T waves, in Standard leads II and III, and lead AVF, which reflect the inferior infarction, and in leads V1–V6 which reflect the anterior infarction.

Leads V3 and V4 reflect QS complexes. This represents the development of anteroseptal necrosis particularly low-septal necrosis. Prominent Q waves are also present in Standard leads II and III and lead AVF, reflecting the early development of inferior wall necrosis. Very small initial r waves are still present in leads V1 and V2, and small initial q waves are still present in leads V5 and V6. This reflects sparing of the midseptum of the effects of necrosis.

The ventricular activation time is prolonged to 0·05 sec, for example, in Standard lead II, lead AVF, and leads V4 and V5. This indicates the presence of injury block.

COMMENT

The early hyperacute injury phase reflects an ominous state in the evolution of myocardial infarction. This patient died half an hour after this electrocardiogram was recorded, from ventricular fibrillation.

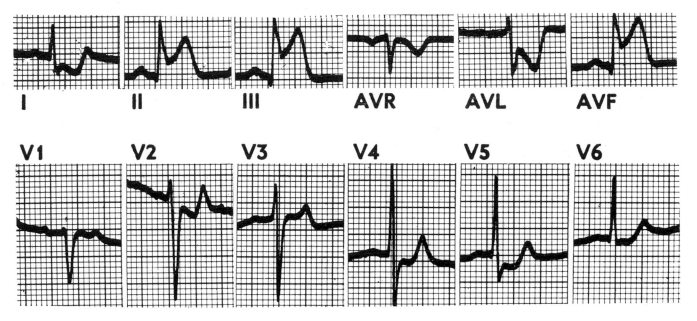

STUDY I

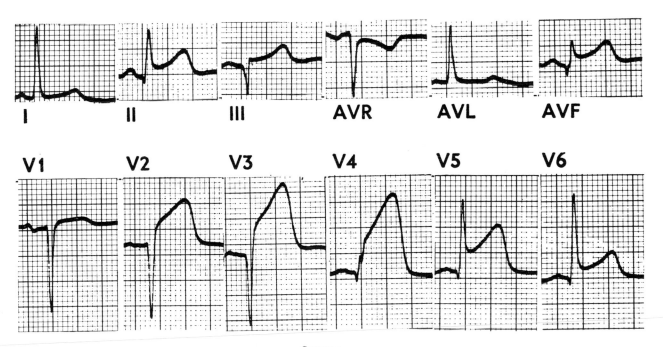

STUDY 2

3

Acute Inferior Wall Myocardial Infarction Associated with Idionodal Rhythm

The electrocardiogram shows the early hyperacute injury phase of inferior wall myocardial infarction. This is reflected by the slope-elevation of the S-T segments and the increased magnitude of the T waves in Standard leads II and III and lead AVF.

There is reciprocal depression of the S-T segments in Standard lead I and lead AVL.

There is *no* injury block since the ventricular activation time is normal.

The parameters of necrosis, pathological Q waves or diminution in the amplitude of the R wave, have not yet developed.

The idionodal rhythm is reflected by the inverted P' waves in Standard leads II and III and lead AVF, an expression of a frontal plane P' wave axis of $-85°$.

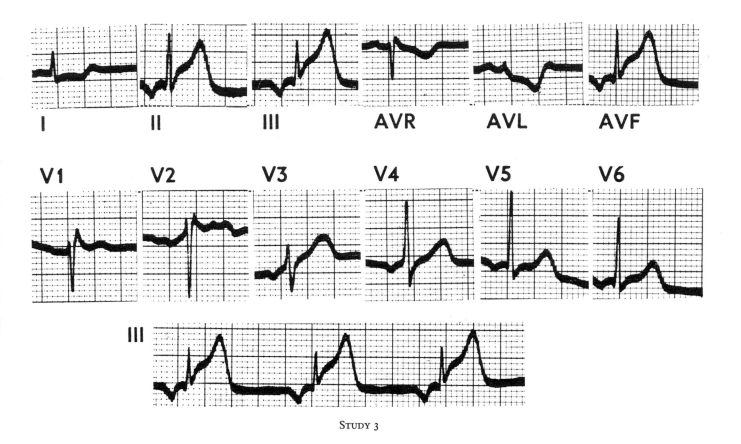

I II III AVR AVL AVF

V1 V2 V3 V4 V5 V6

III

4

Acute Inferior Wall Myocardial Infarction with Apparent Normalization during Evolution

(Courtesy of Dr Houghton)

Electrocardiogram A was recorded within a few hours of the onset of an acute attack of myocardial infarction and shows the hyperacute early injury phase of inferior wall myocardial infarction. This is reflected by the slope-elevation of the S-T segments and the increased amplitude of the *T* waves in Standard leads II and III and lead AVF.

Injury block is also present, as evidenced by the increased ventricular activation time of 0·05 sec in these leads.

There is reciprocal depression in leads VI–V6, Standard lead I and lead AVL.

Electrocardiogram B was recorded on the following day, and shows an apparent normalization of the various abnormalities outlined in Electrocardiogram A. The elevated and depressed S-T segments have become isoelectric and the *T* wave amplitude has diminished to normal. The S-T segments in Standard lead II, leads AVF and V5 and V6 are rather horizontal with sharp angled ST-T junctions, suggesting the presence of coronary insufficiency. In addition, there are no *U* waves in leads V4 and V5, but rather a shallow depression.

Electrocardiogram C was recorded 5 days after Electrocardiogram B, and shows the fully evolved phase of inferior wall myocardial infarction. This is reflected by the presence of pathological Q waves, coved and slightly elevated S-T segments and inverted *T* waves in Standard leads II and III and lead AVF. The low, isoelectric, *T* waves in leads V5 and V6 represent lateral or apical extension of the parameter of ischaemia. The *T* waves in leads V2–V4 tend to be rather tall and symmetrical. This is a reciprocal effect.

COMMENT

It is evident that progression from the hyperacute early injury phase to the fully evolved phase may be characterized by apparent normalization of the electrocardiographic abnormalities.

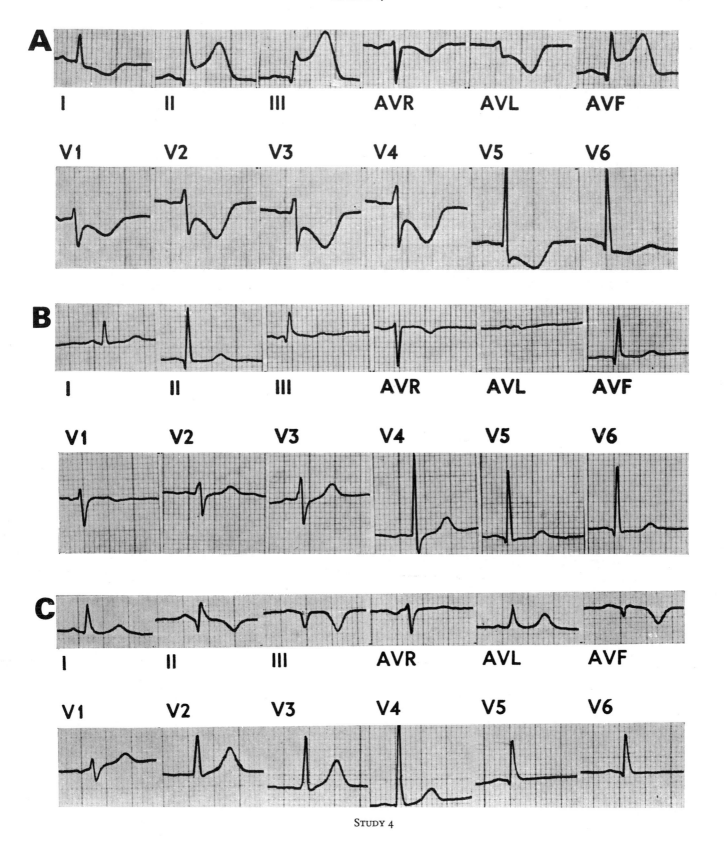

5

Anteroseptal and High Lateral Myocardial Infarction: Septolateral Infarction

Electrocardiogram A was recorded on admission of the patient to a coronary care unit, and reflects the hyperacute early injury phase of anteroseptal and high-lateral myocardial infarction. This is reflected by the widening and increased amplitude of the *T* wave in Standard lead I and lead AVL, the expression of the high-lateral myocardial infarction, and in leads V2–V4, the expression of the anteroseptal myocardial infarction. A tendency to slope-elevation of the S-T segments in Standard lead I, lead AVL and lead V2 is also evident. There is reciprocal depression of the S-T segments in Standard leads II and III and leads AVF, V5 and V6. Standard lead III and lead AVF also reflect inverted *T* waves. These two leads show the true mirror-image reciprocal effect of the anterior myocardial infarction.

Note: The slope-elevation is not as obvious or as evident as, for example, in Electrocardiographic Studies 1, 2, 3, 4, 7, 25 and 34A. This electrocardiogram, however, illustrates the early, less protean manifestation of acute anterior myocardial infarction.

Electrocardiogram B was recorded the day after Electrocardiogram A, and shows the fully evolved phase of anteroseptal and high anterolateral myocardial infarction. The anteroseptal myocardial infarction is reflected by the QS complex in lead V2 and the coved elevated S-T segments and inverted *T* waves in leads V1–V4. The high anterolateral myocardial infarction is reflected by the QS complex in lead AVL, the pathological Q wave of the QR complex in Standard lead I, and the coved elevated S-T segments and inverted *T* waves in these leads.

COMMENT

(a) Although lead V2 reflects a QS complex, initial *r* waves are present in leads V1, V3 and V4. This indicates that the brunt of the anteroseptal necrosis occurred in the lower part of the midseptal region.

(b) The low *T* waves in leads V5 and V6 indicate lateral—apical—extension of the ischaemia.

(c) The combination of anteroseptal infarction with high lateral infarction and relative sparing of the apex, may be termed septolateral infarction.

6

The Very Early Hyperacute Phase of Anteroseptal Myocardial Infarction

The electrocardiograms show complexes from a monitor lead with a positive electrode in approximately the lead V2 position. They were recorded from a hospital orderly who developed the pain of acute myocardial infarction while working in the hospital.

Electrocardiogram A was recorded on admission to the coronary care unit approximately 20 minutes after the onset of severe chest pain. It is abnormal as reflected by the relatively tall and symmetrical *T* wave.

Electrocardiogram B was recorded 3 hours later, and shows a straightening of the S-T segment. Note how the S-T segment has, in effect, been incorporated within the proximal limb of the *T* wave which has become widened.

The patient died soon after the electrocardiogram B was recorded.

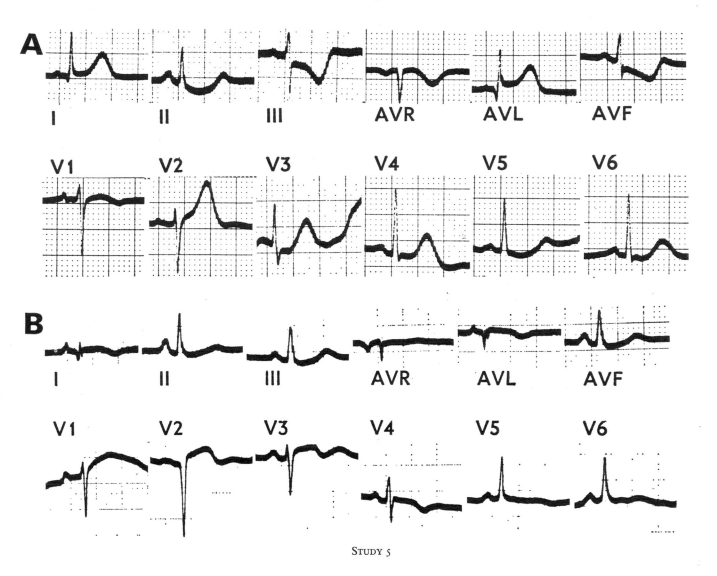

I   II   III   AVR   AVL   AVF

V1   V2   V3   V4   V5   V6

I   II   III   AVR   AVL   AVF

V1   V2   V3   V4   V5   V6

STUDY 5

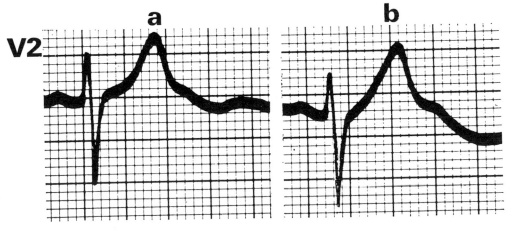

V2   a   b

STUDY 6

7

8

Acute Inferior Wall Myocardial Infarction. Acute Atrial Infarction
(Courtesy of Dr H.D.Friedberg)

Electrocardiogram A shows the hyperacute early injury phase of acute inferior wall myocardial infarction. This is reflected by the slope-elevation of the S-T segments and the increased amplitude of the *T* wave in Standard leads II and III and lead AVF. Reciprocal depression of the S-T segments and inversion of the *T* wave is evident in Standard lead I, leads AVL, V1, V2, V5 and V6. Standard leads II and III and lead AVF also reflect injury block. This is evident from the increased ventricular activation time of 0·05 sec, particularly well seen in Standard lead III.

The acute atrial myocardial infarction is evident from the elevated P-R segment in Standard leads II and III and lead AVF. An enlargement of lead AVF is shown in Electrocardiogram B.

COMMENT

(a) The presence of atrial myocardial infarction was confirmed at autopsy.

(b) There is a first degree A-V block, as is evident from the prolonged P-R interval of 0·34 sec. This is not an infrequent complication of inferior wall myocardial infarction.

Acute Inferior Wall Myocardial Infarction and Acute Atrial Infarction Complicated by Complete A-V Block

The electrocardiogram was recorded from a 53-year-old man with a typical clinical and biochemical (enzyme) presentation of acute myocardial infarction.

The complete A-V block is reflected in Electrocardiogram A by:

(a) the complete dissociation between *P* waves and QRS complexes, and

(b) the very slow idioventricular escape rhythm of 33 beats/min.

The presence of the acute myocardial infarction is indicated by the QS complexes and the coved and elevated S-T segments with inverted *T* waves. Accurate localization is difficult with an idioventricular pacemaker. However, the elevated S-T segment and inverted *T* wave in Standard lead II suggest an inferior infarction.

The presence of acute atrial infarction is reflected by the elevated P-Ta segment, a coved elevation immediately following the *P* wave. An enlargement of one such complex is shown in Electrocardiogram B.

COMMENT

1. The P-Ta segment is normally opposite in direction to the *P* wave. Its deviation in the same direction as the *P* wave is abnormal.

2. The A-V nodal artery arises from the right coronary artery in 90 per cent of cases. The right coronary artery also supplies the major part of the atria. It is therefore not uncommon for inferior infarction to be associated with disturbances of A-V conduction and atrial infarction.

3. The presence of an atrial infarction and an inferior wall myocardial infarction was confirmed at autopsy.

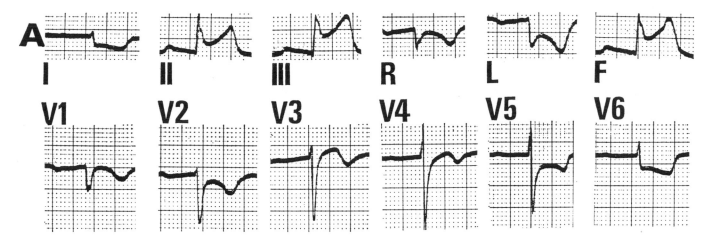

STUDY 7A

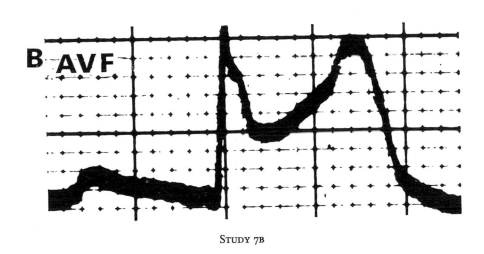

STUDY 7B

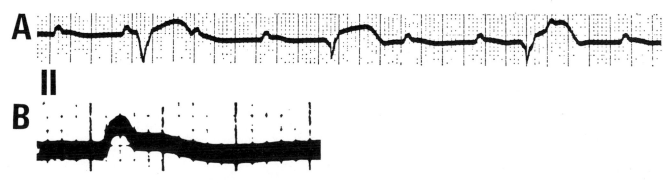

STUDY 8

9

Acute Inferior Wall Myocardial Infarction. Acute Atrial Myocardial Infarction. 3:2 Second Degree A-V Block Showing the Wenckebach Phenomenon

The acute inferior wall myocardial infarction is evident from the rather prominent Q wave, elevated and coved S-T segment, and the inverted *T* wave in Standard lead II. The manifestation of a prominent terminal 0·04 sec positive QRS deflection suggests the presence of diaphragmatic peri-infarction block. This would, however, require confirmation of a terminal right and inferior QRS vector from other leads.

The acute atrial infarction is strongly suggested by the presence of the marked depression of the P-R segments. No pathological confirmation was obtained since the patient's relatives refused autopsy.

The first P-R interval measures 0·21 sec. The second P-R interval measures 0·25 sec. Accurate measurement is difficult because the *P* wave is superimposed upon, and somewhat obscured by, the S-T segment. The third *P* wave is also superimposed upon the S-T segment and is not followed by a QRS complex. This reflects a 3:2 second degree A-V block of the Wenckebach type.

COMMENT

Second degree A-V block, particularly of the Wenckebach type, is a not uncommon complication of acute inferior wall myocardial infarction.

10

Acute Extensive Anterior Wall Myocardial Infarction

The electrocardiogram shows the fully evolved phase of acute extensive anterior wall myocardial infarction.

1. The necrosis is reflected by the QS complexes in leads V1–V6 and the pathological Q waves of the Qr complexes in Standard lead I and lead AVL.

2. The injury and ischaemia are reflected by the coved, elevated S-T segments and the inverted *T* waves in leads V1–V6, Standard lead I and lead AVL. Standard lead II and lead AVF reflect reciprocal S-T segment depression.

COMMENT

The rather sharp angle between the *P* wave and the P-R segment in Standard leads I and III, leads AVR, AVF and V1 are suggestive, but not diagnostic, of atrial infarction.

11

Acute Extensive Anterior Wall Myocardial Infarction. Left Posterior Hemiblock

The electrocardiogram shows the fully evolved phase of acute extensive anterior wall myocardial infarction. This is reflected by:

(a) the QS complexes in leads V1–V6, Standard lead I and lead AVL.

(b) the coved, elevated S-T segments and inverted symmetrical *T* waves in leads V2–V6, Standard lead I and lead AVL.

The mean manifest frontal plane QRS axis is directed at +130°, reflecting a right axis deviation. This could theoretically be due to the anterolateral infarction itself and/or a complicating left posterior hemiblock. The absence of a terminal *r* or *R* wave in Standard lead I or lead AVL, however, suggests the presence of a complicating left posterior hemiblock. See Chapter 12 and Electrocardiographic Study 12.

STD. 2

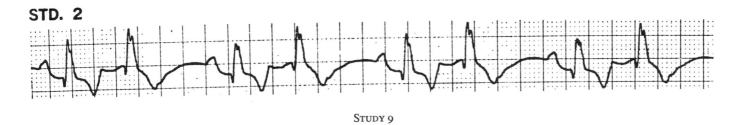

STUDY 9

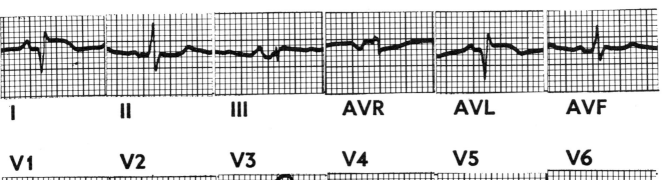

| I | II | III | AVR | AVL | AVF |

| V1 | V2 | V3 | V4 | V5 | V6 |

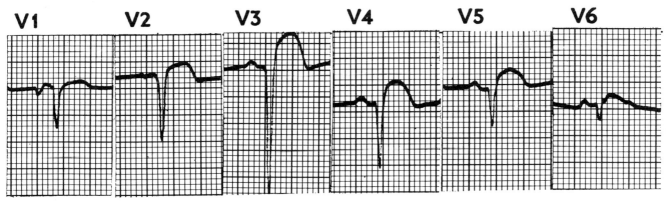

STUDY 10

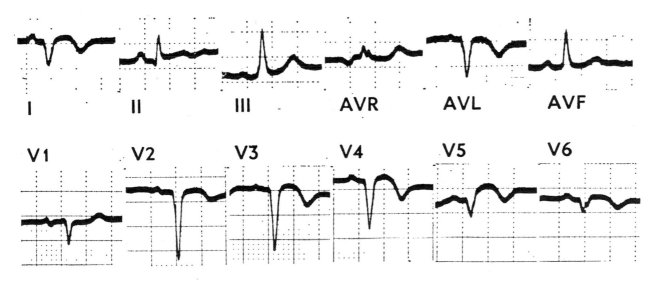

| I | II | III | AVR | AVL | AVF |

| V1 | V2 | V3 | V4 | V5 | V6 |

STUDY 11

12

Acute Extensive Anterior Wall Myocardial Infarction. Left Posterior Hemiblock

Electrocardiogram A shows the very early hyperacute phase of acute anterior wall myocardial infarction. This is reflected by the very tall T waves in leads V2–V6, Standard lead I and lead AVL. There is also a degree of slope-elevation of the S-T segments in leads V2–V4 and lead AVL.

Standard leads II and III and lead AVF reflect reciprocal depression of the S-T segments. This is the mirror-image pattern of the S-T segment slope-elevation and the inverted T waves.

The QS complexes of myocardial necrosis are present in leads V2 and V3, reflecting a loss of the initial positivity. Note that the initial small r wave is still present in lead V1, but has disappeared in leads V2 and V3.

Note: Very tall and wide T waves are, at times, the earliest and most striking manifestations of acute myocardial infarction.

Electrocardiogram B shows the fully evolved phase of the acute extensive anterior wall myocardial infarction. The parameters of myocardial necrosis is reflected by the QS complexes in leads V1–V5, Standard lead I and lead AVL, and the pathological Q wave of the Qr complex in lead V6. The parameters of myocardial injury and ischaemia are reflected by the coved and elevated S-T segments and inverted, symmetrical T waves in leads V2–V6, Standard lead I and lead AVL.

COMMENT

1. Note that, although there has been a minor degree of apical sparing, as reflected by the presence of a small initial r wave in lead V6, the normal positivity in this lead has been markedly reduced. This indicates a subendocardial extension of the necrosis to the apex with a relatively small amount of overlying viable epicardial tissue.

2. The mean manifest frontal plane QRS axis is directed at +110°, reflecting a right axis deviation. This could be due to the anterolateral infarction itself and/or a complicating left posterior hemiblock. The absence of a terminal r or R wave in Standard lead I and lead AVL, however, suggests the presence of a complicating left posterior hemiblock. See Chapter 12 and Electrocardiographic Study 11.

13

Evolving Anterior Wall Myocardial Infarction. Old Inferior Wall Myocardial Infarction

The evolving anterior wall myocardial infarction is evident from the following:

(a) The parameters of necrosis are reflected by the QS complexes in lead V2 and V3, the rather prominent Q waves of the QR complexes in leads V4–V6, Standard lead I and lead AVL.

(b) The parameters of myocardial injury and ischaemia are reflected by the elevated and coved S-T segments and inverted symmetrical T waves in leads V2–V6, Standard leads I and II, and lead AVL. The parameters of ischaemia, the inverted T wave, is also evident in lead AVF.

The old inferior wall myocardial infarction is evident from the prominent initial q wave in Standard lead II, the small initial rs, a Q equivalent, which precedes the dominant rS in Standard leads III and lead AVF.

COMMENT

Note that the q wave in lead V4 is more prominent than the q wave in lead V6. The normal initial q wave should become progressively deeper from lead V4–V6.

The parameters of injury and ischaemia are not evident in Standard lead III. Their minimal manifestations in Standard lead II and lead AVF represent an infero-apical extension of the acute anterior wall myocardial infarction.

The presence of an initial r wave in lead V1 indicates that the upper part of the midseptum has been spared.

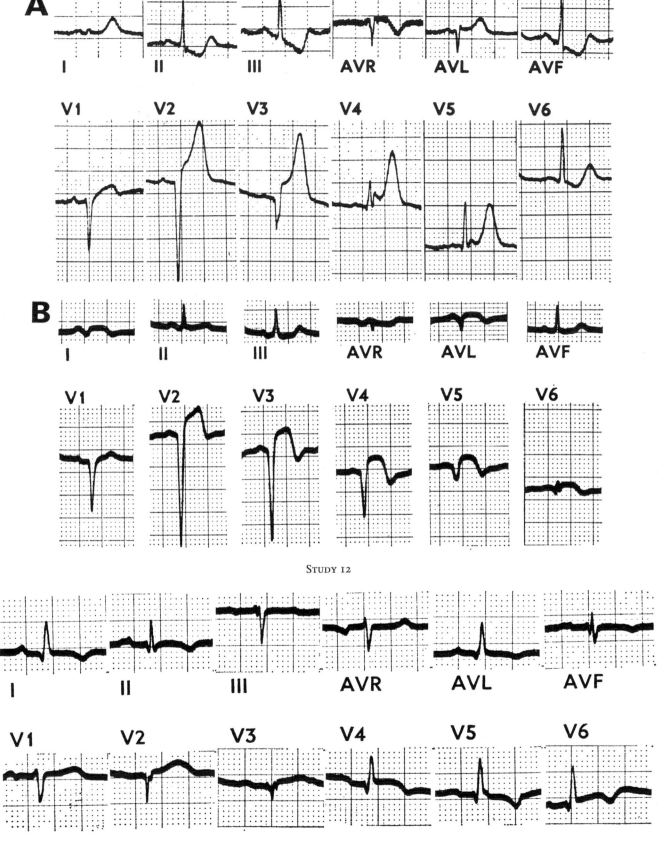

STUDY 12

STUDY 13

14

Acute Extensive Anterior Wall Myocardial Infarction Associated with Sinus Bradycardia

The electrocardiogram shows the fully evolved phase of acute extensive anterior wall myocardial infarction.

The myocardial necrosis is evident from the following:

(a) The QS complexes in leads V1–V3.

(b) The diminution in the amplitude of the R waves in lead V6, Standard lead I and lead AVL.

(c) The loss of the initial small q wave in lead V6, the loss of the midseptal vector.

The myocardial injury and ischaemia is evident from the coved, elevated S-T segments and inverted T waves in leads V1–V6, Standard lead I and lead AVL.

The rate is 40/min, representing a marked sinus bradycardia.

COMMENT

1. The myocardial necrosis is mainly anteroseptal, as evidenced by the QS complexes in leads V1–V3, and extends laterally.

2. The Q-Tc is prolonged.

15

Acute Anterior Wall and Inferior Wall Myocardial Infarction

The electrocardiogram shows the fully evolved phase of acute anterior and inferior wall myocardial infarction.

The myocardial necrosis involves chiefly the lower part of the midseptal region, and the lowseptal region, as reflected by the QS complexes in leads V2 and V3. Note that the initial small r wave is still present in lead V1, and the initial small q wave is still present in leads V5 and V6, thereby indicating that the upper part of the midseptum has been spared.

The amplitude of the R wave is diminished in lead V6, thereby suggesting some lateral extension.

The myocardial injury and ischaemia is evidenced by the elevated, coved S-T segments in leads V2–V6, Standard leads I, II and III, and lead AVF. The myocardial injury and ischaemia is thus more widespread than the myocardial necrosis, and involves the anterior and inferior myocardial walls. These parameters are absent in lead AVL, thereby indicating that the high-lateral region of the heart has been spared.

The Q-Tc is prolonged.

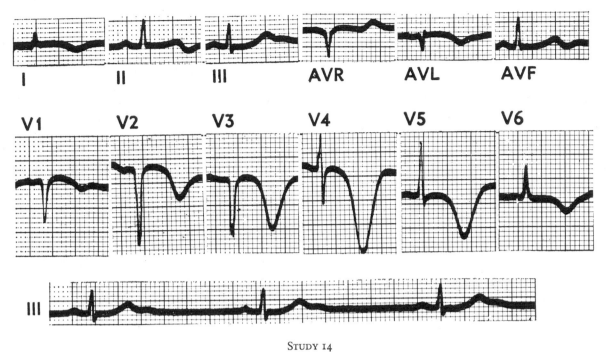

I   II   III   AVR   AVL   AVF

V1   V2   V3   V4   V5   V6

III

STUDY 14

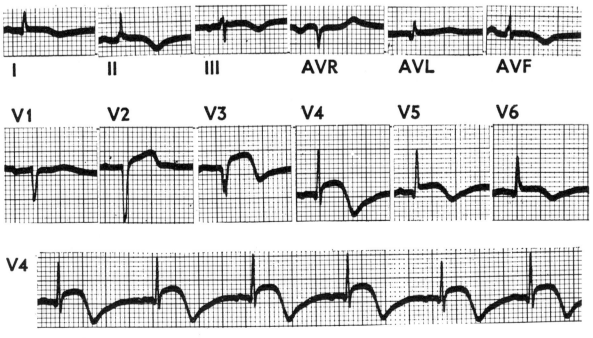

I   II   III   AVR   AVL   AVF

V1   V2   V3   V4   V5   V6

V4

STUDY 15

16

Acute Subendocardial Infarction with Recurrent Episodes of Subendocardial Ischaemia

The electrocardiograms were recorded from a 59-year-old woman with a typical presentation of acute myocardial infarction.

The electrocardiogram recorded on the second day after the onset of the chest pain, 27 June, revealed:

(a) depressed S-T segments,
(b) deeply inverted and widened T waves, and
(c) prolonged Q-T interval, Q-Tc of 170 per cent, in leads V3–V6, Standard leads I and II and lead AVF.

Tracing A shows representative strips from Standard lead II and lead V4. There were no pathological Q waves, and the diagnosis of a diffuse subendocardial infarction affecting principally the apical region of the left ventricle was made.

Six days later, 3 July, the patient had a recurrence of severe chest pain which lasted for 1 hour, and the electro-cardiogram (Tracing B) now revealed upright T waves, slightly elevated S-T segments in the aforementioned leads. The Q-Tc shortened to 100 per cent.

A tracing recorded the next day, 4 July, (Tracing C) shows a reversion to the pattern depicted in Tracing A.

Two days later, 6 July, she experienced another episode of severe chest pain. The electrocardiogram (Tracing D) was now similar to that of Tracing B on 3 July.

COMMENT

Subacute ischaemia is associated with a prolonged Q-T interval. Acute ischaemia is associated with a normal or shortened Q-T interval.

17

Acute Extensive Anterior Wall Myocardial Infarction

The electrocardiogram shows the fully evolved phase of acute extensive anterior wall myocardial infarction.

The myocardial necrosis is evident from the following:

(a) The presence of the QS complexes in leads V1–V4, indicating involvement of the mid and lower septal regions.

(b) The presence of prominent initial Q waves, of QR complexes, in Standard lead I and lead AVL, indicating high lateral extension.

Note that the R waves in leads V5 and V6, Standard lead I and lead AVL are diminished in amplitude, and probably also reflect a loss of viable, mainly subendocardial, tissue.

The myocardial injury and ischaemia are evident from the coved, elevated S-T segments, and the symmetrical inverted T waves in leads V2–V6, Standard lead I and lead AVL.

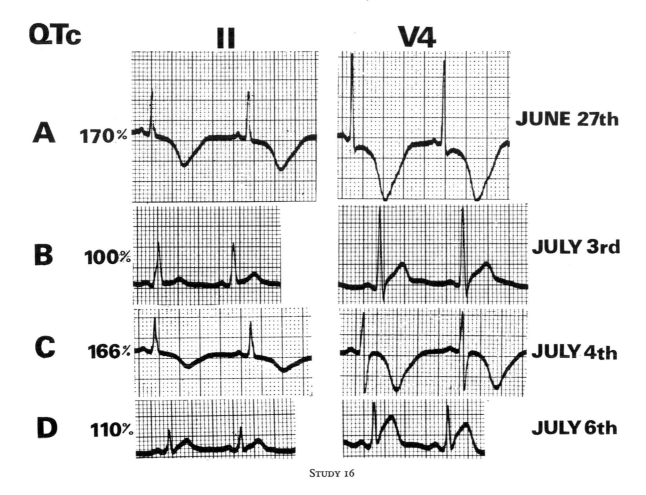

STUDY 16

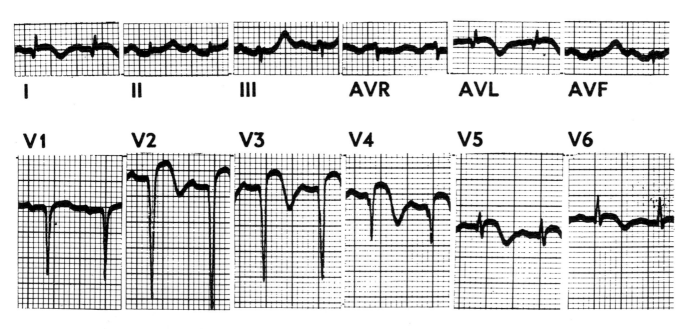

STUDY 17

18

Acute Extensive Anterior Wall Myocardial Infarction. Old Inferior Wall Myocardial Infarction

The electrocardiogram shows the fully evolved phase of acute anterior wall myocardial infarction. The myocardial necrosis is evident from the following:

(a) the QS complexes in leads V2–V4.

(b) the deep, wide pathological Q waves of the QR complexes in leads V5 and V6 and Standard lead I.

(c) the diminution in the R wave amplitude in leads V5 and V6, indicating some degree of subendocardial apical extension.

The myocardial injury and ischaemia are evident from the coved, elevated S-T segments, and the inverted T waves in leads V2–V6, Standard lead I and lead AVL.

The old inferior wall myocardial infarction is evident from the small initial rs deflections, Q wave equivalents, which precede the dominant rS deflection in Standard leads II and III, and lead AVF.

COMMENT

The initial normal r wave in lead V1 indicates that the upper part of the midseptal region has been spared.

19

Acute Anteroseptal Myocardial Infarction. Old Inferior Wall Myocardial Infarction

The electrocardiogram shows the fully evolved phase of acute anteroseptal myocardial infarction.

The myocardial necrosis is evident from:

(a) The QS complexes in leads V1–V4.

(b) The loss of the initial normal q wave in leads V5 and V6 (due to loss of the midseptal vector).

(c) The tendency to a relatively low R wave in leads V5 and V6.

The myocardial injury and ischaemia are reflected by the coved, elevated S-T segments and inverted T waves in leads V1–V6, Standard lead I and lead AVL.

COMMENT

The brunt of the necrosis is anteroseptal, as reflected by the localization of the QS complexes to leads V1 and V2.

The electrocardiogram also shows old inferior wall myocardial infarction. This is evident from the small initial q wave in Standard lead II and the slurred and thickened initial deflection of the proximal limb of the QS deflection in Standard lead III and lead AVF. This results in the formation of a ledge on the proximal limb.

These initial QRS abnormalities represent pathological Q wave equivalents.

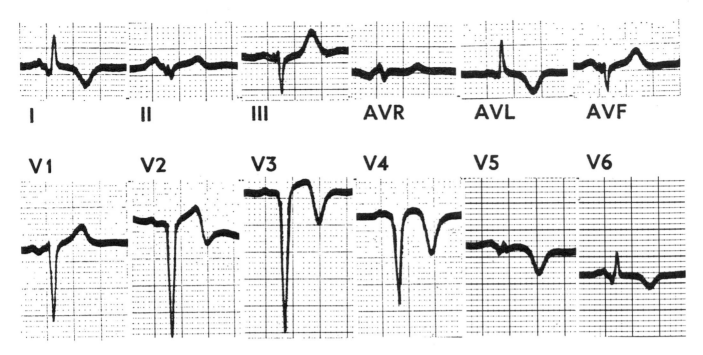

STUDY 18

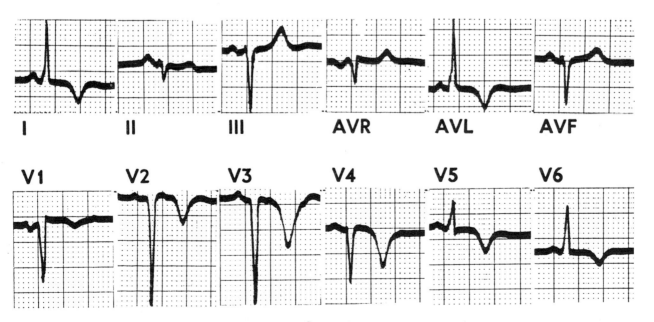

STUDY 19

20

Acute Anteroseptal Myocardial Infarction

The electrocardiogram shows the fully evolved phase of acute anteroseptal myocardial infarction.

The myocardial necrosis is reflected by:

(a) the QS complexes in leads V1–V3.

(b) the loss of the normal initial *q* wave in leads V5 and V6.

(c) the rather low amplitude of the *R* wave in leads V5 and V6, indicating some apical subepicardial extension.

The myocardial injury is reflected by the coved, elevated S-T segments and the symmetrical inverted *T* waves in leads V1–V3, Standard lead I and lead AVL.

The Q-Tc is prolonged to +130 per cent.

COMMENT

The brunt of the infarction is anteroseptal. The necrosis involves predominantly the midseptal region and the upper part of the lower septal region. The elevated S-T segments and inverted *T* waves in Standard lead I and lead AVL indicate that the injury and ischaemia have extended to the high lateral region of the heart, a septolateral infarction. The apical region has been largely spared.

There is a reciprocal depression of the S-T segment in Standard leads II and III, and lead AVF.

21

Acute Extensive Anterior Wall—Dominantly Anteroseptal—Myocardial Infarction. Left Anterior Hemiblock

The electrocardiogram shows the fully evolved phase of the anterior wall myocardial infarction.

The myocardial necrosis is reflected by the following:

(a) There are QS complexes in leads V1–V3. The loss of the normal initial *r* waves reflects a loss of the mid-septal and right paraseptal vectors.

(b) There is an appreciable loss of positive deflection in lead V4 which reflects but a small initial *r* wave.

(c) There is a loss of the normal initial *q* waves in leads V5 and V6, also indicating a loss of the midseptal vector.

(d) There is a relative diminution of the *R* wave in leads V5 and V6.

The myocardial injury and ischaemia are reflected by the elevated, coved S-T segments and the deeply inverted symmetrical *T* waves in leads V1–V6, Standard lead I and lead AVL.

COMMENT

The parameters of injury and ischaemia are widespread, reflecting an extensive anterior wall myocardial infarction, whereas the parameters of the necrosis are dominantly anteroseptal.

Left anterior hemiblock is present, as reflected by the presence of the negative QRS deflections in Standard leads II and III and lead AVF, and the tall *R* waves in Standard lead I and lead AVL, representing a mean manifest frontal plane QRS axis of −40°.

22

Acute Anteroseptal Myocardial Infarction

The parameters of anteroseptal necrosis, injury and ischaemia are reflected as follows:

1. *The necrosis* is reflected by:

(a) the QS complexes in leads V1 and V2.

(b) the rather prominent Q waves in leads V3 and AVL, and

(c) the absent initial *q* waves in leads V5 and V6.

2. *The injury* is reflected by the coved and elevated S-T segments in leads V1–V4.

3. *The ischaemia* is reflected by the inverted symmetrical *T* waves in leads V1–V4, and lead AVL, and the rather low *T* wave in Standard lead I.

COMMENT

The dominant region of the infarction is anteroseptal, as reflected by the manifestations in leads V1–V4. The manifestations of necrosis in leads V1 and V2 reflect midseptal involvement. The manifestation of necrosis in lead V3 reflects involvement of the proximal upper part of the lower septum. The infarction extends to the superior or lateral surface, as reflected by the abnormalities in lead AVL. The apical region is largely spared, as reflected by the relative normality of the deflections in leads V5 and V6 and Standard lead II, and the minimal involvement of Standard lead I. Lead V6, however, has a relatively low *R* wave which may reflect some anterolateral epicardial extension.

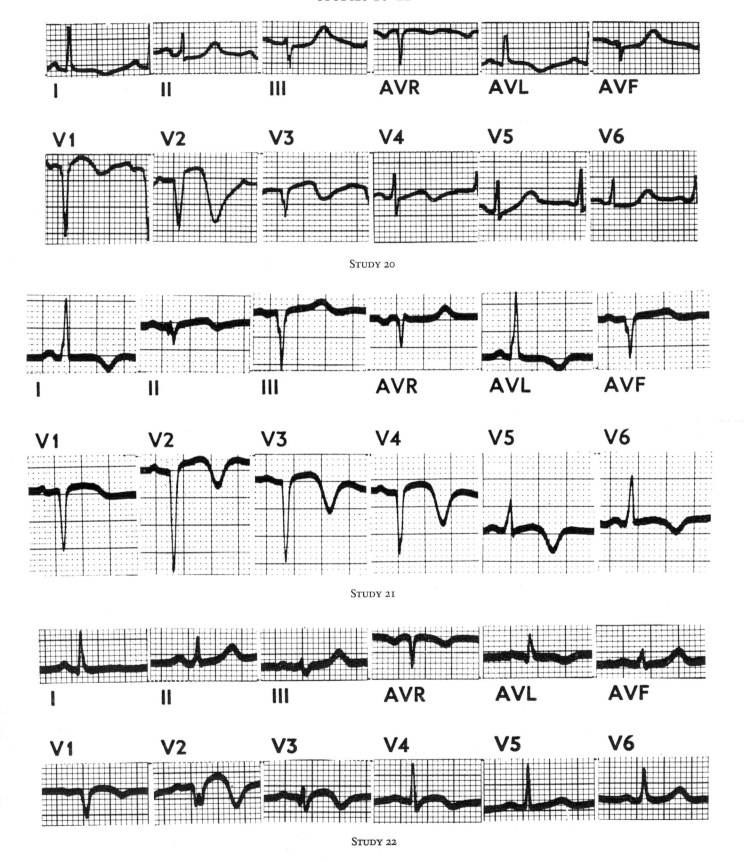

I　II　III　AVR　AVL　AVF

V1　V2　V3　V4　V5　V6

STUDY 20

I　II　III　AVR　AVL　AVF

V1　V2　V3　V4　V5　V6

STUDY 21

I　II　III　AVR　AVL　AVF

V1　V2　V3　V4　V5　V6

STUDY 22

23

Acute Anterolateral and Acute Inferior Myocardial Infarction

The electrocardiogram shows the fully evolved phase of acute anterolateral (lowseptal and apical) myocardial infarction.

The myocardial necrosis is reflected by the rather prominent Q waves in leads V4–V6. Note that the q wave is deeper in lead V4 than V6.

The myocardial injury and ischaemia is reflected by the elevated coved S-T segments and the inverted T waves in leads V3–V6 and Standard lead I.

The fully evolved phase of the inferior myocardial infarction is reflected by the rather prominent q waves in Standard lead II and lead AVF, the small initial rs deflection in Standard lead III (a Q wave equivalent), and the coved, elevated S-T segments and inverted T waves in Standard leads II and III, and lead AVF.

COMMENT

(a) The initial r wave is still present in lead V1, thereby indicating that the upper part of the midseptum has been spared. The brunt of the necrosis affects the lower septum as reflected by the relatively deep q wave in lead V4.

(b) The parameters of myocardial injury and ischaemia are more marked and widespread than those of myocardial necrosis.

24

Acute Anterolateral Wall Myocardial Infarction. Possible Old Inferior Wall Myocardial Infarction

The electrocardiogram shows the fully evolved phase of anterolateral myocardial infarction.

The myocardial necrosis is reflected by the following features:

(a) There is a lack of progression in the amplitude of the initial r wave from lead V1 to lead V4.

(b) Lead V3 shows a very small initial rs deflection which is inscribed before the dominant S wave. This is, in effect, a Q wave equivalent.

(c) Leads V4 and V5 show marked notched dominantly negative deflections.

(d) Lead V6 shows a marked notched dominantly positive deflection.

COMMENTS

(a) The necrosis is, in effect, reflected by the failure of significant positive QRS development in leads V2–V5.

(b) The marked notching and slurring of the QRS complexes in leads V3–V6 reflect a significant degree of intra-infarction block.

The myocardial injury and ischaemia is reflected by the coved, elevated S-T segments, and the inverted T waves in leads V3–V6, the coving being most marked in leads V5 and V6. Note how the T wave vector has deviated from the left to the right in the horizontal plane, and is consequently upright and prominent in leads V1 and V2.

The old inferior wall myocardial infarction is suggested by the slurred initial rs ledge in Standard lead III and lead AVF. These are Q wave 'equivalents'. The q wave in Standard lead II is also rather prominent.

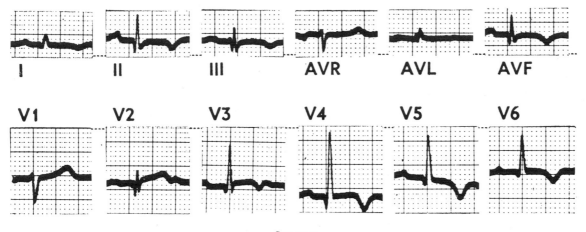

I   II   III   AVR   AVL   AVF

V1   V2   V3   V4   V5   V6

STUDY 23

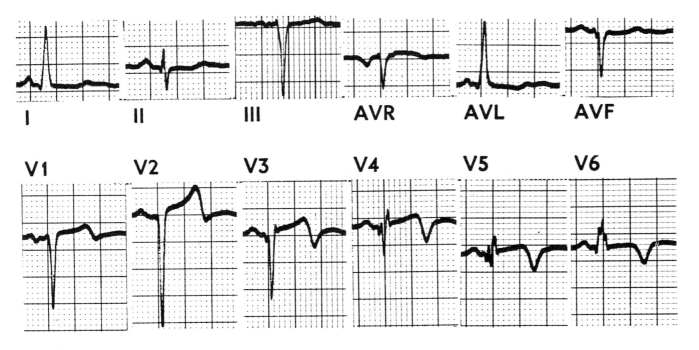

I   II   III   AVR   AVL   AVF

V1   V2   V3   V4   V5   V6

STUDY 24

25

Acute Anteroseptal Myocardial Infarction. Old—Chronic—Inferior Wall Myocardial Infarction. Left Anterior Hemiblock

Electrocardiogram A reflects the hyperacute early injury phase of acute anterior wall myocardial infarction, as evidenced by the S-T segment slope-elevation and tall widened T waves in leads V2–V5.

Electrocardiogram B was recorded on the following day, and shows the fully evolved phase of acute anterior wall myocardial infarction. This is evidenced by the following:

1. The parameters of myocardial necrosis are reflected by the QS complexes in leads V1 and V2. This indicates that the brunt of the infarction is midseptal. The amplitude of the R waves is diminished in leads V5 and V6, thereby indicating some lateral extension.

2. The parameters of myocardial injury and ischaemia are more extensive and are reflected by the coved and elevated S-T segments and the inverted T waves in leads V1–V6.

Both Electrocardiograms A and B show evidence of old, chronic, inferior wall myocardial infarction, as reflected by initial small rs deflections in Standard leads II and III, and lead AVF (best seen in Electrocardiogram A).

The mean manifest frontal plane QRS axis is directed at $-60°$. The left axis deviation is due to a complicating left anterior hemiblock and not merely the result of the inferior wall myocardial infarction. This is because Standard lead II does not reflect a terminal r wave, i.e. a qR or qr complex (see Chapter 12).

26

Regressing Inferolateral Wall Myocardial Infarction

The electrocardiogram was recorded 3 weeks after the onset of acute myocardial infarction.

The myocardial necrosis of the inferior wall myocardial infarction as reflected by the slurred initial rs ledge in lead AVF, and the slurred initial negative ledge on the downstroke of the negative deflection in Standard lead III. These ledges are, in effect, Q wave equivalents. The q wave in Standard lead II is also rather prominent.

The myocardial injury and ischaemia are reflected by the slightly elevated and coved S-T segments, and the inverted T waves in Standard leads II and III, and lead AVF.

The lateral, mainly apical, extension is reflected by:

(a) the slightly coved and elevated S-T segment in leads V4–V6,

(b) the inverted T waves in leads V4–V6, and

(c) the diminution of the R wave in lead V6.

COMMENT

Note how the T wave vector has deviated from the left to the right in the horizontal plane, and is consequently upright, tall and symmetrical in leads V1 and V2.

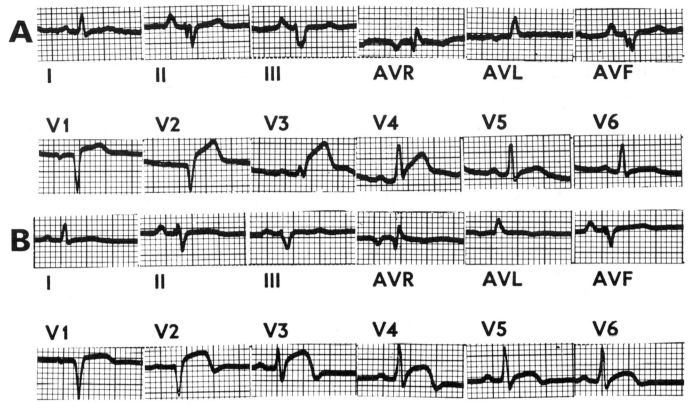

STUDY 25

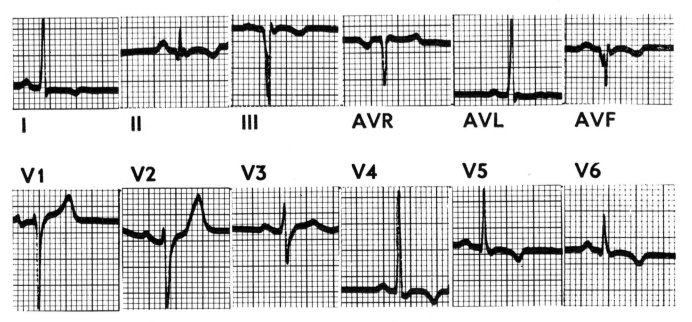

STUDY 26

27

Acute Inferior Wall Myocardial Infarction. Possible True Posterior Myocardial Infarction

The electrocardiogram shows the fully evolved phase of acute inferior wall myocardial infarction.

The myocardial necrosis is reflected by the QS complexes in Standard lead III and lead AVF, and the prominent and relatively deep pathological Q wave of the QR complex in Standard lead II. The diminution of the R wave in lead V6 indicates some apical extension.

The myocardial injury and ischaemia are reflected by the elevated, coved S-T segments in Standard leads II and III and lead AVF. The low T waves in leads V5 and V6 indicate an apical extension of the myocardial ischaemia.

The true posterior wall myocardial infarction is suggested by the relatively tall R waves and the associated tall and widened T waves in leads V2 and V3.

28

Acute Inferolateral Myocardial Infarction. Possible True Posterior Extension

The electrocardiogram shows the fully evolved phase of acute inferolateral myocardial infarction. The necrosis of the inferior infarction is reflected by the pathological Q wave of the Qr complex in Standard lead II, and the QS complexes in Standard lead III and lead AVF. The injury and ischaemia of the inferior infarction is reflected by the elevated, coved S-T segments and symmetrical, sharply pointed inverted T waves in Standard leads II and III and lead AVF. The lateral extension is reflected by:

(a) the pathological Q waves of the QR complexes in leads V5 and V6,

(b) the diminution of the R waves in leads V5 and V6, and

(c) the coved, elevated S-T segments in leads V5 and V6.

The rather tall R wave with the tall symmetrical T wave in lead V2 suggests a true posterior extension.

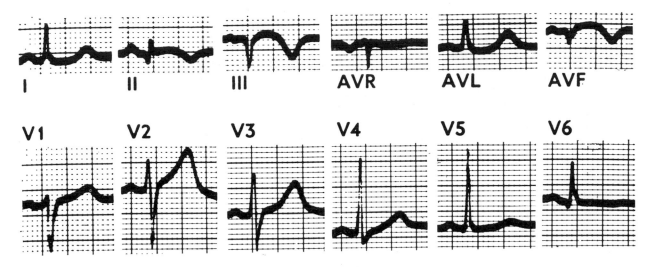

STUDY 27

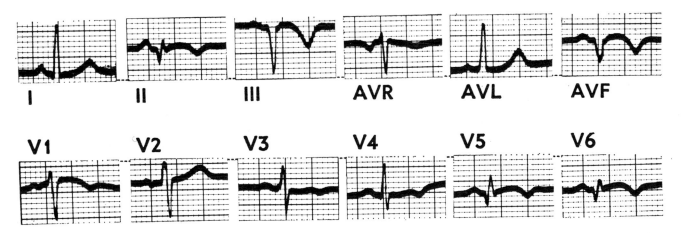

STUDY 28

29

Acute Inferior and Posterior Wall Myocardial Infarction. Possible Left Anterior Hemiblock. First Degree A-V Block

The electrocardiogram shows the fully evolved phase of acute inferior wall myocardial infarction. This is reflected by the QS complexes, elevated S-T segments, and low to inverted T waves in Standard leads II and III and lead AVF. Standard lead I and lead AVL reflect reciprocal S-T segment depression. The true posterior wall myocardial infarction is reflected by:

(a) the rather tall R waves in leads V1–V3, particularly in leads V2 and V3,

(b) the depressed S-T segment in lead V2, and

(c) the relatively tall and symmetrical T waves in leads V1–V3.

The mean manifest frontal plane QRS axis is in the region of -30–$-40°$, reflecting a left anterior hemiblock.

The P-R interval is prolonged to 0·25 sec, reflecting first degree A-V block.

It is unusual for Standard lead II to reflect a pure QS complex in the fully evolved phase of acute inferior wall myocardial infarction. This lead usually shows a pathological Q wave followed by a terminal R wave, a QR complex. If Standard lead II does reflect a QS complex it may be due to lateral extension of the infarct to involve:

(a) the posterior part of the inferior wall, and/or

(b) the lower part of the lateral or superior wall, in which case Standard lead I and possibly lead AVL may show prominent or pathological Q waves. The latter is clearly not evident in this tracing. Another possible cause of a QS complex in Standard lead II in cases of inferior wall myocardial infarction is the presence of a complicating left anterior hemiblock. This interpretation is strongly suggested by the tall R waves in Standard lead I and lead AVL, the expression of left axis deviation, and the small, normal initial q waves in these leads. If there is a complicating left anterior hemiblock, it would further indicate that the whole of the inferior wall has been infarcted, since there are no initial small r waves in Standard lead III and lead AVF.

It is possible that Standard lead II reflects a small terminal positivity, a small terminal r wave. If so, the diagnosis of left anterior hemiblock is questionable. However, it appears more likely that the positivity occurs *within* the QS complex and represents an expression of intrainfarction block.

30

Acute Inferior Wall Myocardial Infarction Complicated by Complete A-V Block

The electrocardiogram shows the fully evolved phase of acute inferior wall myocardial infarction. This necrosis is reflected by the QS pattern in Standard lead III and lead AVF, and the qr pattern in Standard lead II which also shows a general loss of QRS amplitude. The injury and ischaemia are reflected by the coved and elevated S-T segments and the inverted T waves in Standard leads II and III and lead AVF. Precordial leads V1–V6 reflect reciprocal tall, symmetrical and widened T waves. Precordial leads V2–V5 show reciprocal S-T segment depression.

The complete A-V block is reflected by the complete dissociation between P waves and QRS complexes in the long strip of lead V1. The relative normality of the QRS complexes reflect a lower junctional pacemaker.

COMMENT

When complete A-V block complicates myocardial infarction it commonly occurs in association with inferior wall myocardial infarction.

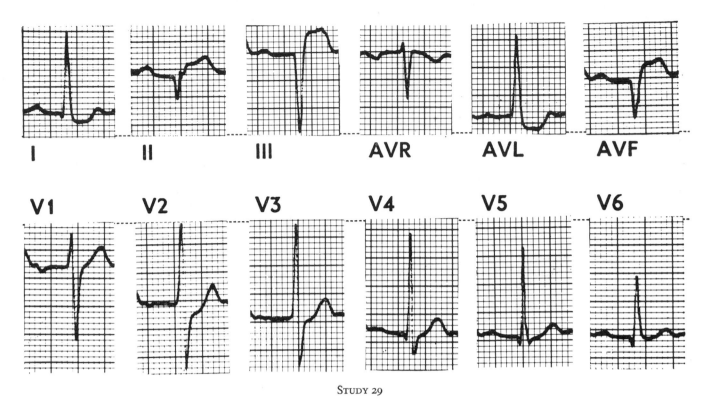

STUDY 29

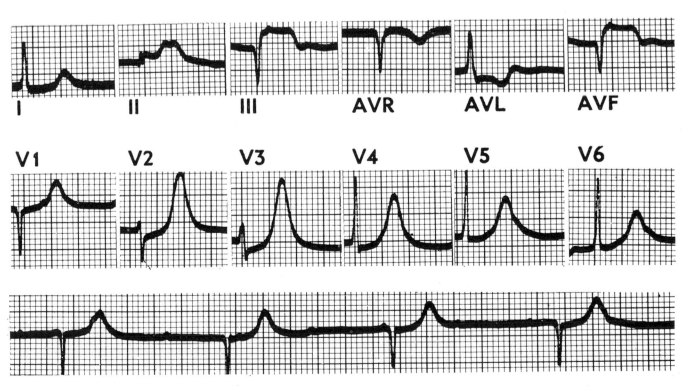

STUDY 30

31

Acute Inferolateral Wall Myocardial Infarction. Acute True Posterior Wall Myocardial Infarction[S38]

The electrocardiogram shows the fully evolved phase of acute inferolateral wall myocardial infarction. The myocardial necrosis is revealed by the following:

(a) There is a loss of positive deflection in Standard lead III. This lead reflects but a very small initial r wave, the deflection being virtually a QS complex.

(b) There are prominent Q waves (of QR complexes) in Standard lead II and lead AVF.

The myocardial injury and ischaemia are reflected by the elevated, coved S-T segments, and the inverted T waves in Standard leads II and III, and lead AVF.

The lateral, apical, extension is reflected by the elevated, coved S-T segment and inverted T waves in leads V5 and V6. The initial q wave in lead V6 is also rather prominent and there is a diminution in the height of the R wave in lead V6.

The true posterior wall myocardial infarction is reflected by the tall R waves and the associated tall symmetrical T waves in leads V1–V4.

32

Acute Inferolateral Myocardial Infarction with True Posterior Extension. The S1 S2 S3 Syndrome

Electrocardiogram A shows the features of acute inferior wall myocardial infarction, as evidenced by pathological Q waves, coved and elevated S-T segments, and inverted T waves in Standard leads II and III and lead AVF. The lateral, apical, extension is reflected by:

(a) the rather prominent q wave in lead V6,

(b) the rather low R waves in leads V5 and V6,

(c) the coved, elevated S-T segments and inverted T waves in leads V5 and V6.

The true posterior infarction is reflected by:

(a) the tall and wide R waves in leads V1–V4, and

(b) the tall, wide and sharply pointed T waves in leads V1–V4.

The electrocardiogram also reflects the S1 S2 S3 syndrome: terminal S waves in Standard leads I, II and III.

COMMENT

1. The tall, wide R wave and tall, wide, symmetrical T wave in the right precordial leads, e.g. lead V2, is the mirror-image of the pathological Q wave and deeply inverted T wave in a lead which would be reflected to the epicardial surface of the acute myocardial infarction. (Electrocardiogram B).

2. The parameters of the true posterior infarction were noted 5 years later, whereas the parameters of the infero lateral infarction had largely regressed.

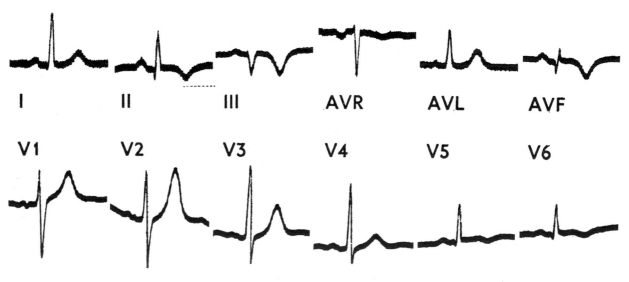

STUDY 31

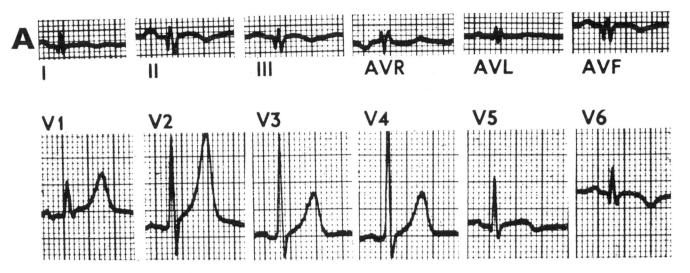

STUDY 32A

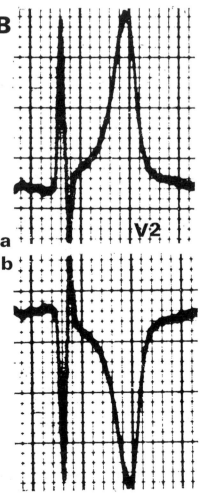

STUDY 32B

33

Acute Inferolateral and True Posterior Wall Myocardial Infarction. The S1 S2 S3 Syndrome

The electrocardiogram shows the fully evolved phase of inferolateral myocardial infarction.

The myocardial necrosis is reflected by the deep and wide pathological Q waves in Standard leads II and III, and lead AVF.

The myocardial injury and ischaemia are reflected by the coved and elevated S-T segments, and the inverted symmetrical T waves in Standard leads II and III and lead AVF, the inferior wall infarction, and in leads V5 and V6, the lateral, apical, extension.

The true posterior wall infarction is reflected by the tall R waves and the tall and wide symmetrical T waves in leads V1–V3.

COMMENT

The electrocardiogram also shows the S1 S2 S3 syndrome: prominent S waves in Standard leads I, II and III.

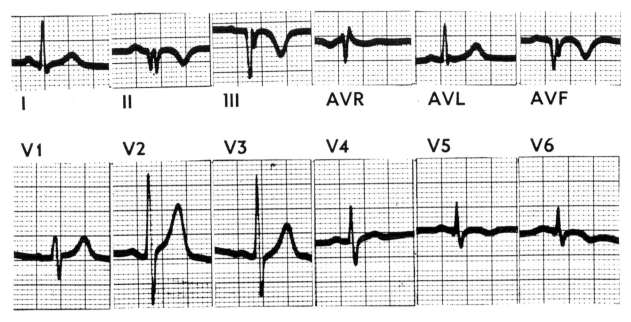

I   II   III   AVR   AVL   AVF

V1   V2   V3   V4   V5   V6

34

Acute Inferior Wall Myocardial Infarction
(Courtesy of Dr J.deKock)

The electrocardiograms were recorded from a 53-year-old man with a classic clinical and biochemical presentation of acute myocardial infarction.

Electrocardiogram A was recorded on admission to the coronary care unit, and shows the hyperacute early injury phase of acute inferior wall myocardial infarction. This is reflected by the following:

(a) There is marked slope-elevation of the S-T segments in Standard leads II and III, and lead AVF.

(b) There is an increase in the amplitude of the R wave in Standard leads II and III, and lead AVF (compare with Electrocardiogram B and C).

(c) There is an increase in ventricular activation time, as reflected by a *delay* in the inscription of the intrinsicoid deflection to 0·06 sec in Standard lead III and lead AVF.

(d) There is a reciprocal depression of the S-T segment in leads VI–V5, Standard lead I and lead AVL.

(e) The single ventricular extrasystole in lead V6 reflects a primary S-T segment change. This is reflected by the upward coving of the S-T segment instead of the straight or minimally concave-upward secondary S-T segment change of uncomplicated ventricular extrasystole.

(f) The low to inverted T waves in leads V5 and V6 reflect a lateral extension of the myocardial ischaemia.

(g) There is first degree A-V block, the P-R interval measures 0·24 sec.

Electrocardiogram B was recorded on the following day when the patient no longer had any chest pain, and shows the fully evolved phase of acute inferior wall myocardial infarction. This is reflected by the following:

(a) The S-T segments are coved and elevated, and the T waves are inverted, sharply pointed and arrow-head in appearance in Standard leads II and III, and lead AVF.

(b) Standard lead III has a pathological Q wave.

(c) The T waves are low to inverted in leads V5 and V6, representing some lateral, apical, extension of the myocardial ischaemia.

(d) Standard lead I, lead AVL and leads VI–V3 reflect reciprocal, symmetrical and widened T waves.

(e) There is first degree A-V block, the P-R interval measures 0·24 sec.

Electrocardiogram C was recorded 4 days later, when the patient experienced a further episode of chest pain which lasted for half an hour. The features are the same as those shown in Electrocardiogram B except that (a) the S-T segments are now depressed and concave upward in leads V5 and V6, and (b) the T waves have become upright in leads V5 and V6. This represents apical subendocardial injury and ischaemia as occurs in angina pectoris. These additional features were temporary, and the electrocardiogram regressed half an hour later to that shown in Electrocardiogram B.

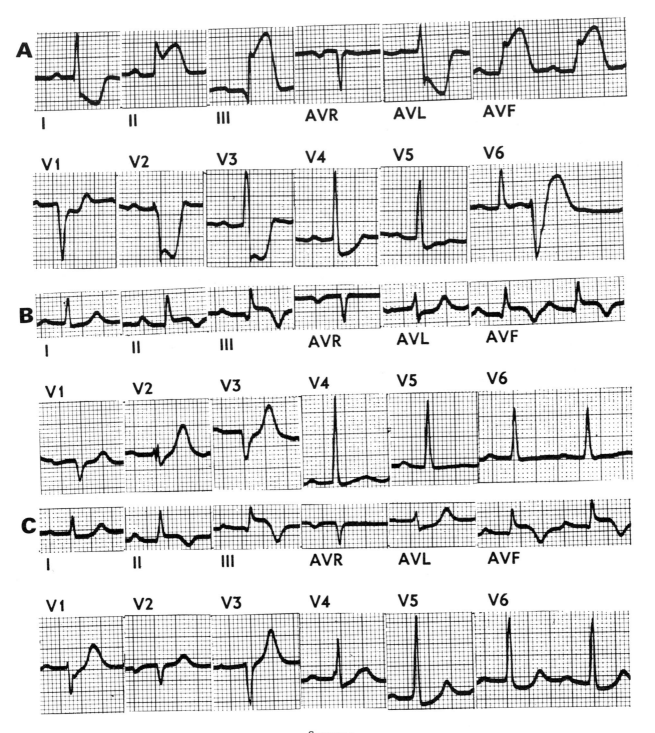

35

Old Inferior Wall Myocardial Infarction. Old Anteroseptal Myocardial Infarction. Possible Ventricular Aneurysm. Atrial Fibrillation

The electrocardiogram shows the fully stabilized phase of old inferior wall myocardial infarction. The scar of the old myocardial necrosis is reflected by the deep, wide, pathological Q waves in Standard lead II and lead AVF, and the QS complex in Standard lead III. The S-T segments and T waves of these leads do *not* reflect the manifestations of acute myocardial injury and ischaemia.

The old anteroseptal infarction is reflected by the QS complexes in leads V3 and V4. Note that small initial r waves are present in leads V1 and V2, but these fail to progress. The S-T segments are coved and elevated and the T waves inverted in leads V1–V4. These manifestations were stable for 2 years, and suggest the possible presence of a ventricular aneurysm.

The atrial fibrillation is reflected by the absent P waves and the slightly irregular baseline.

36

Old Inferior Wall Myocardial Infarction. The S1 S2 S3 Syndrome

The electrocardiogram shows the chronic stabilized phase of an old inferior wall myocardial infarction. This is reflected by the deep and wide pathological Q waves in Standard leads II and III, and lead AVF. The coved, elevated S-T segments and inverted T waves of acute myocardial injury and ischaemia are absent.

The presence of chronic coronary insufficiency is also evident from anterior wall subendocardial injury, the plane S-T segment depression with sharp angled ST-T junction in leads V3, V4 and V5.

COMMENT

The electrocardiogram also shows the S1 S2 S3 syndrome: prominent S waves in all the three Standard leads.

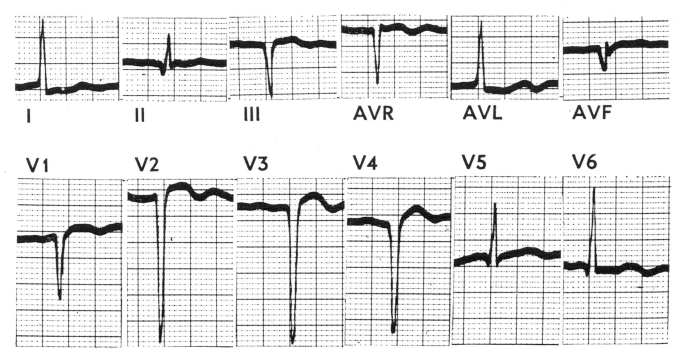

STUDY 35

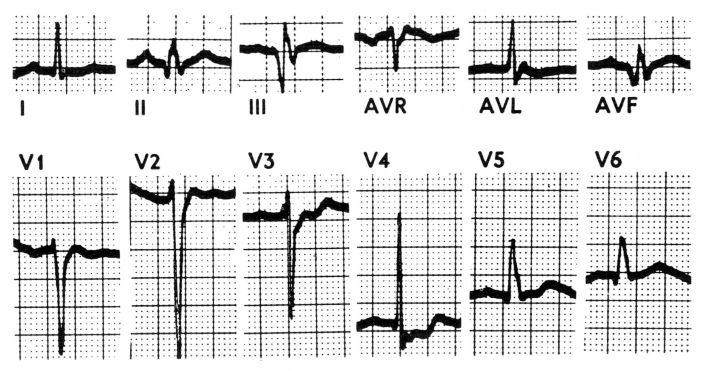

STUDY 36

37

Old Inferior Wall Myocardial Infarction. Chronic Coronary Insufficiency. Left Anterior Hemiblock

Electrocardiogram A shows the *old stabilized phase of inferior wall myocardial infarction*, as evidenced by the following:

(a) Standard lead II reflects a small initial rs deflection before the dominant major rS complex. An enlargement of this complex is shown in Electrocardiogram B.

(b) Lead AVF also shows small initial rs deflection which slurs and distorts the proximal limb of the major deflection. An enlargement of this complex is shown in Electrocardiogram B. These small initial rs deflections are pathological Q wave equivalents.

(c) The rather prominent initial q wave in lead V6 (though within normal limits) suggests a possible lateral, apical, extension.

The presence of *chronic coronary insufficiency* is evidenced from the following:

(a) The presence of S-T segment horizontality and a tendency to sharp angled ST-T junction in Standard lead I and lead AVF.

(b) The presence of left axis deviation, the left anterior hemiblock. The mean manifest frontal plane QRS axis is deviated to $-40°$.

(c) The wide angle of 115 degrees between the mean manifest frontal plane QRS axis ($-40°$) and the mean manifest frontal plane T wave axis of $+75°$.

(d) The wide angle between the horizontal plane QRS and T wave axes. The QRS axis is directed to the left, as reflected by the dominantly positive QRS deflections in the left precordial leads, whereas the T wave axis tends to be directed to the right, as reflected by the dominantly positive T waves in the right precordial leads. This is an example of the TV1 greater than TV6 manifestation.

(e) The T waves tend to be symmetrical in Standard leads II and III and leads AVF, V2 and V3.

38

Old Inferior, Anterolateral and True Posterior Myocardial Infarction

The electrocardiogram shows the chronic stabilized phase of inferior, anterolateral and true posterior myocardial infarction.

The necrotic scar of the old inferior wall myocardial infarction is reflected by the deep and wide pathological Q waves in Standard leads II and III, and lead AVF.

The necrotic scar of the old anterolateral, mainly apical, myocardial infarction is reflected by the deep, wide, pathological Q waves in leads V4–V6. Note that the Q wave in lead V4 is deeper than the Q wave in lead V6.

The true posterior wall myocardial infarction is reflected by the tall R waves in leads V1 and V2, and the tall symmetrical T waves in leads V1–V3.

The T waves are inverted in Standard leads II and III and leads AVF, V5 and V6, and reflect the presence of chronic coronary insufficiency.

COMMENT

(a) There are *no* signs of acute myocardial infarction, i.e. coved, elevated S-T segments and deeply inverted T waves.

(b) There is residual intrainfarction block as reflected by the marked notching and irregularity of the QRS complexes in Standard leads II and III, and leads AVF, V2, V4, V5 and V6.

(c) The T wave changes of acute true posterior infarction do not usually regress, and tend to remain permanently.

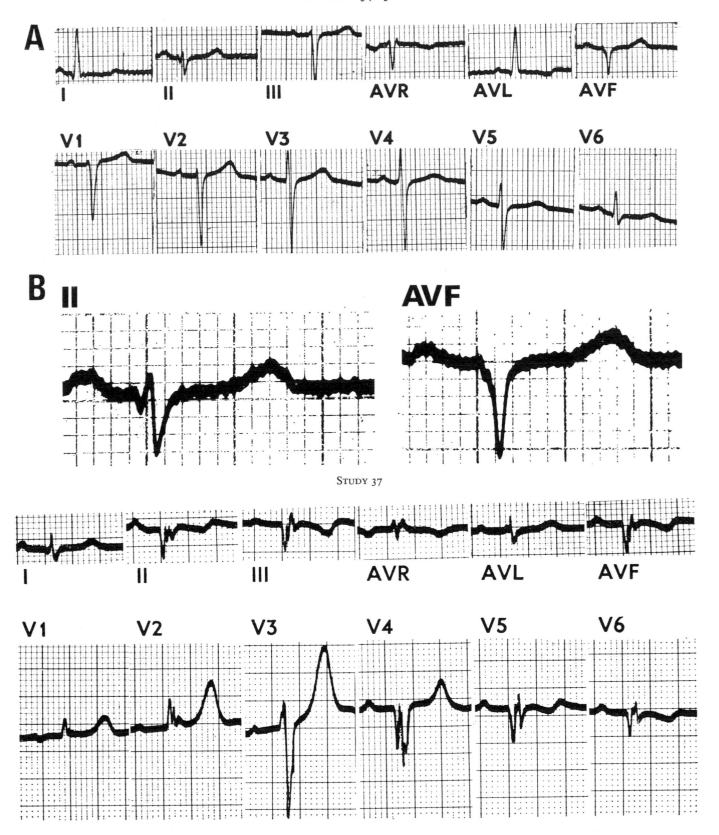

A

I   II   III   AVR   AVL   AVF

V1   V2   V3   V4   V5   V6

B   **II**   **AVF**

STUDY 37

I   II   III   AVR   AVL   AVF

V1   V2   V3   V4   V5   V6

STUDY 38

39

Old—Chronic—Extensive Anterior and Inferior Wall Myocardial Infarctions

The electrocardiogram shows the old, chronic, stabilized phase of multiple infarctions. This is evidenced by the following:

(a) There is a generalized low QRS voltage in the frontal plane leads. The QRS deflections are less than 5 mm in amplitude in all the frontal plane leads. Standard leads I, II and III, and leads AVR, AVL and AVF.

(b) There is a lack of positive QRS deflection in the horizontal plane leads, leads V1–V6.

(c) There is a deep, wide, pathological Q wave of the QR complex in lead V6 and the QR complex of lead AVL. This reflects the scarring of old necrosis.

(d) There is a prominent, though not pathological, q wave in Standard lead I.

(e) There is a QS complex in lead V2, and a lack of an increasing r wave amplitude progression from lead V1–V5. Note that lead V1 shows a very small initial r wave. This is absent in lead V2 and present again in leads V3–V5. However, this initial r wave shows no evidence of a progressive increase in amplitude from leads V3–V5.

(f) The T waves are low to inverted in all the leads.

(g) The S-T segment is depressed in lead V6 and minimally elevated in leads V1–V4. This reflects the presence of chronic subendocardial apical injury.

COMMENT

(a) This presentation is the classic end-result of multiple infarctions and long-standing coronary insufficiency.

(b) The extensive reduction in viable tissue is reflected by the loss of positive deflections in virtually all the leads.

40

Extensive Old Anterior Infarction, Old Masked Inferior Wall Infarction—Evident in a Complicating Ventricular Extrasystole. Associated Right Bundle Branch Block with Left Anterior Hemiblock

The right bundle branch block is evident from the rightward and anteriorly directed terminal QRS vectors, as reflected by the deep, wide S waves in the left lateral leads, and the R′ deflection in lead V1.

The extensive old anterior wall infarction is revealed by the presence of prominent pathological Q waves in leads V1–V6. The absence of S-T segment change indicates an old, non-acute, phase. The inverted T waves in leads V1–V5 reflect residual chronic anterior wall epicardial myocardial ischaemia.

The left anterior hemiblock is reflected by the deep S waves and the prominent initial r waves in Standard leads II and III, and lead AVF.

The old inferior wall infarction is reflected by the initial q wave of the complicating ventricular extrasystole in Standard lead III.

COMMENT

(a) The old inferior wall infarction is masked by the prominent initial inferiorly-directed vector, the prominent r waves in Standard lead II and III, and lead AVF, of the left anterior divisional hemiblock. This indicates that the posterior region of the inferior wall is not involved by the infarction.

(b) The inferior infarction is revealed by the single ventricular extrasystole. This is dominantly positive and, consequently, should not be preceded by an initial Q wave.

(c) The right bundle branch block does not obscure the diagnostic initial abnormal QRS vectors of the old anterior wall infarction.

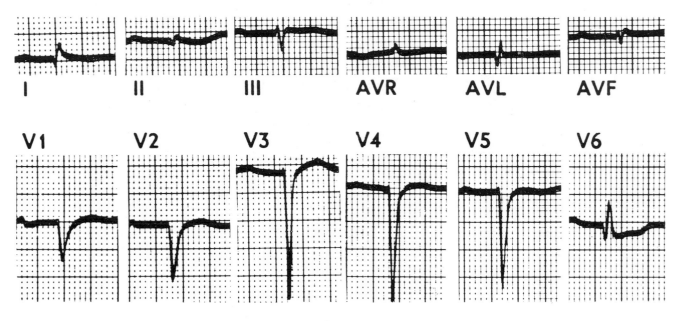

STUDY 39

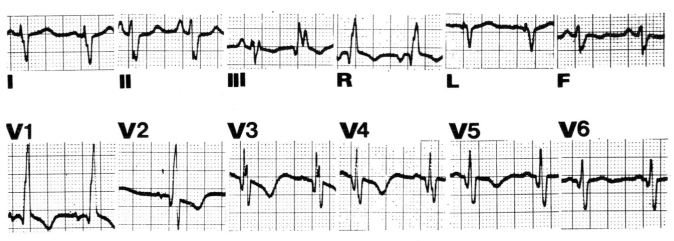

STUDY 40

41

Anterolateral Myocardial Infarction. Left Anterior Hemiblock Anterolateral Peri-Infarction Block

The left anterior hemiblock is evident from the following:

(a) The deep and wide S waves in Standard leads II and III, and lead AVF.

(b) The tall, wide R waves in Standard lead I, lead AVL and lead V6. These manifestations are an expression of a mean manifest frontal plane QRS axis of $-60°$.

(c) The rather prominent initial r waves in Standard leads II and III and leads AVF, and in leads V1–V3.

The acute, fully evolved phase of anterolateral myocardial infarction is revealed by the following:

(a) The deep and wide initial pathological Q waves in Standard lead I, lead AVL, and leads V5 and V6.

(b) The failure of increasing r wave progression from leads V1–V4.

(c) The elevated, coved S-T segments and the inverted T waves in Standard lead I, lead AVL, and leads V5 and V6.

There is a wide angle of 190° between the initial 0·04 sec QRS vector, directed at $+120°$, and the terminal 0·04 sec QRS vector, directed at $-70°$. This reflects the presence of anterolateral peri-infarction block.

COMMENT

The rather tall initial r waves in leads V1–V3 is an expression of the left anterior hemiblock associated with possible relatively low precordial electrode placement.

42

Old—Chronic—Anterolateral Myocardial Infarction with Left Anterior Hemiblock

The left anterior hemiblock is evident from:

(a) the deep and wide S waves and relatively prominent initial r waves in Standard leads II and III, and lead AVF, the mean manifest frontal plane QRS axis being directed at about $-60°$, and

(b) the rS complexes in the left lateral leads.

The precordial leads, leads V1–V6, reflect the following:

(a) Leads B were recorded with the electrodes in the correct position. They reflect the presence of an old anteroseptal myocardial infarction, as evidenced by the QS complexes in leads V2–V4.

(b) Precordial leads A were recorded with the electrodes in a minimally lower position. All the precordial leads now reflect rS complexes. The initial r waves in the right precordial leads are due to the left anterior hemiblock.

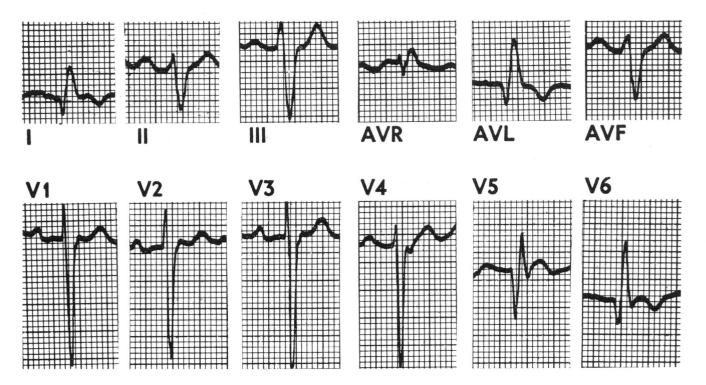

Study 41

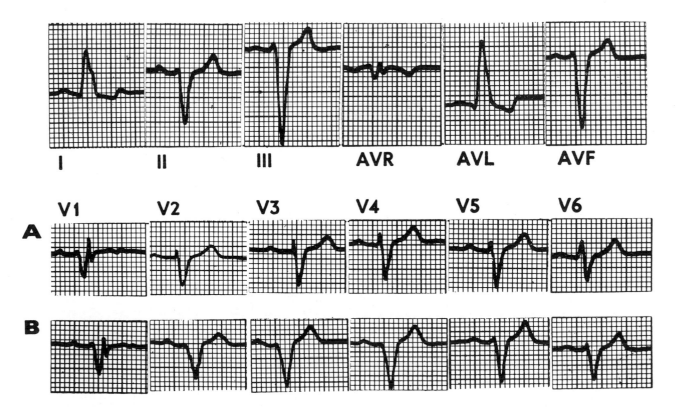

Study 42

43

Old High Lateral and Anteroseptal Myocardial Infarction with Left Anterior Hemiblock. Atrial Fibrillation

The left anterior hemiblock is reflected by the following:

(a) The deep *S* waves in Standard leads II and III, and lead AVF, the expression of a mean manifest frontal plane QRS axis of −60°.

(b) The prominent initial *r* waves in Standard leads II and III, and lead AVF.

(c) The rS complexes, the relative loss of positive deflections, in the left precordial leads.

The old high lateral myocardial infarction is revealed by the prominent initial *q* waves in Standard lead I, and lead AVL. These *q* waves could also be due to the left anterior hemiblock as such. However, they tend to be rather wide and therefore suggestive of high-lateral infarction.

The old anteroseptal myocardial infarction is revealed by the QS complexes in leads V1–V4. Note, this manifestation could also be due to a relatively high precordial electrode placement. See also Electrocardiographic Studies 42, 44, 45 and 60.

The *T* waves are low to inverted in Standard lead I, and leads AVL, V5 and V6. The mean *T* wave axis is deviated to the right in both the frontal and horizontal planes.

All the deflections are somewhat distorted by the 'f' waves of the atrial fibrillation. This is particularly so in the case of the *T* waves, and the initial *q* or QS deflection in Standard lead I, lead AVL, and leads V1 and V2.

44

Acute Anterior Wall Myocardial Infarction. Old—Chronic—Wall Myocardial Infarction with Left Anterior Hemiblock
(Courtesy of Dr V.Botoulas)

The electrocardiogram shows the fully evolved phase of acute anterior wall myocardial infarction. The necrosis is reflected by:

(a) the QS complexes in leads V1 to V5, and

(b) the diminished amplitude of the QRS complexes in lead V6, Standard lead I, and lead AVL.

The acute injury and ischaemia are reflected by the coved and elevated S-T segments and the low to inverted *T* waves in leads V1–V6, Standard leads I and II, and lead AVL.

COMMENT

The very small initial *r* waves in leads V3 and V4 (which therefore, in effect, reflect rS complexes rather than QS complexes) are probably due to the distorting effect of the initial vectors of the left anterior hemiblock.

There is left axis deviation of the mean manifest frontal plane QRS axis which is directed at −60°. Standard lead II reflects a prominent QS complex, whereas Standard lead III and lead AVF reflect small initial *r* waves. The *r* wave is taller in Standard lead III than in lead AVF.

This is the typical pattern of inferior wall myocardial infarction complicated by left anterior hemiblock. When this occurs, the initial *r* wave of the rS complex in Standard lead III is usually tallest, and Standard lead II usually shows a pure QS complex with no terminal *R* wave.

The initial *r* waves indicate that the posterior part of the inferior wall has been spared. The lack of associated S-T segment and *T* wave abnormalities indicates that the infarct is old or chronic.

The low to upright *T* waves in Standard leads II and III, and lead AVF may be due, in part, to the left anterior hemiblock.

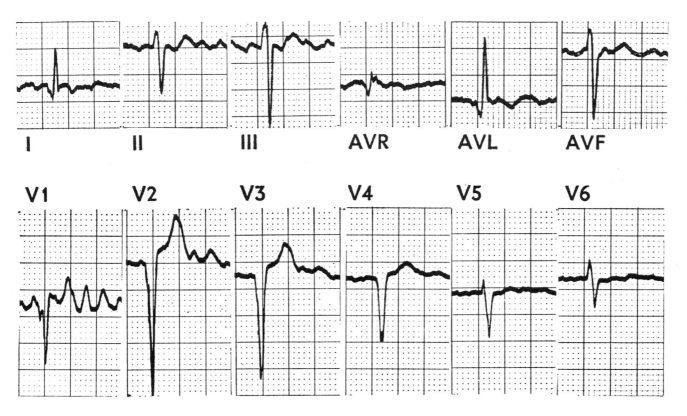

STUDY 43

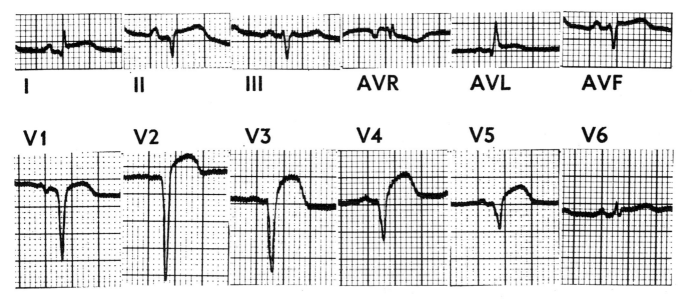

STUDY 44

45

Acute Inferolateral Myocardial Infarction with Left Anterior Hemiblock

The left anterior hemiblock is evident from the following manifestations:

(a) There are deep terminal S waves in Standard leads II and III, and lead AVF. The mean manifest frontal plane axis is directed at about −60°.

(b) There are prominent initial r waves in Standard leads II and III, and lead AVF.

(c) There is a prominent initial q wave in Standard lead I, and lead AVL.

The acute inferior wall myocardial infarction is reflected by the coved, elevated S-T segments and the inverted T waves in Standard leads II and III, and lead AVF.

The lateral, apical, extension of the infarction is reflected by the pathological Q wave, in effect a notched QS complex, the elevated, coved S-T segment and the inverted T wave in lead V6.

COMMENT

(a) The pathological Q waves or QS complexes of the inferior wall myocardial infarction is masked by the initial vectors of the left anterior hemiblock. These are directed inferiorly, and represent early activation of the posterior part of the inferior wall, which must, therefore, be spared by the infarction process.

(b) The rather tall R waves in the right precordial leads suggest the presence of a true posterior wall myocardial infarction. However, the absence of associated tall T waves makes this diagnosis questionable. Furthermore, as indicated above, the presence of initial r waves in Standard leads II and III, and lead AVF indicate that the postero-inferior wall is spared. The tall R waves in the right precordial leads are probably the expression of the inferior- and anterior-directed initial vectors resulting from the left anterior hemiblock associated with a rather low precordial electrode placement.

46

Old Lowseptal Myocardial Infarction. Left Posterior Hemiblock

The electrocardiogram was recorded from a 56-year-old man with a long history of coronary artery disease. It shows the manifestations of old lowseptal myocardial infarction as evidenced by the QS complex in lead V3 and the deep, wide, prominent pathological Q wave in lead V4. The coved, elevated S-T segments and inverted T waves of acute myocardial infarction are absent.

COMMENT

(a) Note that small initial r waves are present in leads V1 and V2, but these fail to progress and disappear in leads V3 and V4.

(b) Note that the Q wave in lead V4 is much deeper than the q wave in lead V6.

The left posterior hemiblock is reflected by the following:

(a) There is a right axis deviation of +100°.

(b) There is a small rs complex in Standard lead I.

(c) There are prominent q waves in Standard leads II and III, and lead AVF. The prominent q waves could conceivably reflect an old inferior wall infarction, but this is considered unlikely since the ensuing R waves are very tall. The right axis deviation indicates that these prominent q waves are more likely a manifestation of left posterior hemiblock.

There is a rightward deviation of the T wave vector in the horizontal plane, resulting in T waves which are tall and symmetrical in leads V1–V3, and low to inverted in leads V4–V6. This is the so-called TV1 greater than TV6 syndrome, and a manifestation of chronic coronary insufficiency.

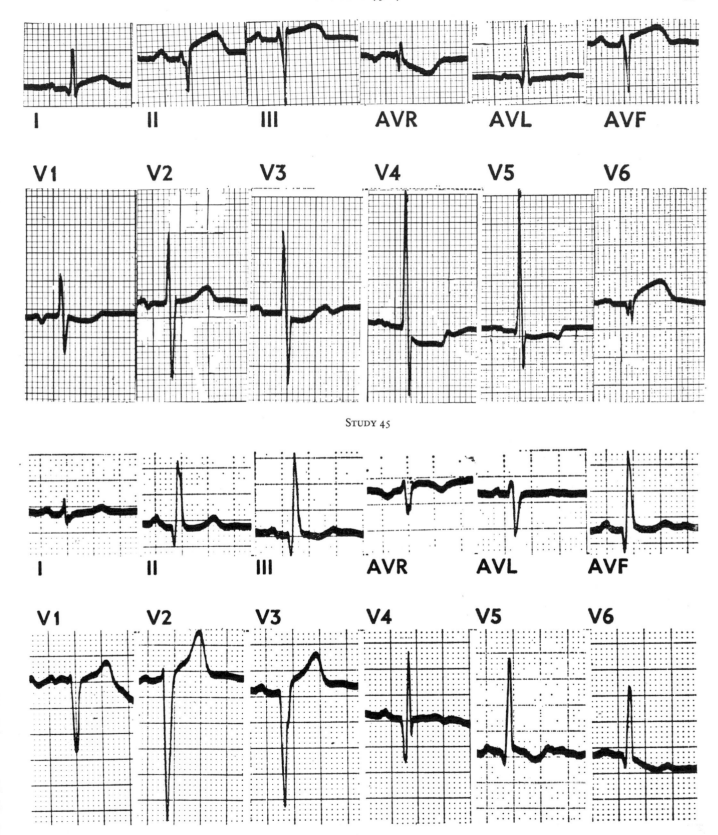

I II III AVR AVL AVF

V1 V2 V3 V4 V5 V6

Study 45

I II III AVR AVL AVF

V1 V2 V3 V4 V5 V6

Study 46

47

Left Posterior Hemiblock with Left Ventricular Hypertrophy and Strain

The electrocardiogram was recorded from a 60-year-old man with the Kimmelstiel-Wilson syndrome: diabetes, hypertension, and the nephrotic syndrome. The patient also had clinical stigmata of coronary artery disease.

The left posterior hemiblock is reflected by the following:

(a) The presence of right axis deviation. The mean manifest frontal plane QRS axis is directed at $+90°$.

(b) The presence of prominent initial q waves in Standard leads II and III, and lead AVF, and the initial prominent r waves in Standard lead I and lead AVL.

(c) The absence of clinical evidence of right ventricular dominance.

The inverted T waves in Standard leads II and III, and lead AVF are probably secondary changes, but could also be due to inferior wall myocardial ischaemia.

The presence of left ventricular hypertrophy and strain is reflected by the presence of deep S waves in the right precordial leads, the presence of tall R waves in the left precordial leads, and the deviation of the horizontal plane T wave axis to the right.

48

Acute Anteroseptal Myocardial Infarction Complicated by Right Bundle Branch Block and Transient Left Posterior Hemiblock[D11]

The electrocardiograms were recorded from a 56-year-old man who presented with the classic clinical features of acute myocardial infarction.

Electrocardiogram A was recorded on the day of admission to the coronary care unit, and shows the features of acute anteroseptal myocardial infarction complicated by right bundle branch block. The anteroseptal infarction is reflected by:

(a) the deep and wide pathological Q waves in leads V1–V4, and

(b) the coved and elevated S-T segments with the inverted T waves in leads V1–V5.

The anterolateral extension of the myocardial ischaemia is reflected by the low to inverted T waves in Standard lead I, and leads AVL and V6.

The right bundle branch block is reflected by:

(a) the slurred terminal S waves in Standard leads II and III, and leads AVF and V6, and

(b) the terminal R′ deflection in leads V1–V3.

Note that the right bundle branch block does not mask or distort the abnormal initial QRS forces of the myocardial infarction. These initial dominant QRS forces (excluding the forces of the right bundle branch block) are directed at $+50°$ on the frontal plane hexaxial reference system.

Electrocardiogram B recorded on the second day in hospital, and reflects the same features of the acute anteroseptal infarction as are depicted in Electrocardiogram A. The infarction pattern is now, however, associated with the following changes:

1. The mean manifest dominant frontal plane QRS axis (excluding the terminal force of the right bundle branch block) is now directed at $+110°$. This is reflected empirically by the tall R wave in Standard lead III, and lead AVF, and the deep terminal S wave in Standard lead I, and lead AVL. This right axis deviation represents the development of a left posterior hemiblock.

2. The QRS deflections in the horizontal plane leads (leads V1–V6) show a general diminution in amplitude and are now smaller than the QRS deflections of the frontal plane leads (Standard leads I, II and III, and leads AVR, AVL and AVF) which show a general increase in amplitude (compare with Electrocardiogram A).

3. The T waves are now upright in Standard lead I and lead AVL.

Electrocardiogram C was recorded on the third hospital day. The dominant QRS force (excluding the terminal QRS force of the right bundle branch block) is now directed at $-10°$ on the frontal plane hexaxial reference system. This consequently represents a regression from the right axis deviation shown in Electrocardiogram B. The regression has, however, so to speak overcompensated, since the dominant QRS force now reflects a slight left axis deviation. Furthermore, it is of interest to note that the QRS amplitude of the horizontal plane lead has deflections.

This direction of the dominant QRS force now remained stable throughout the evolution of the infarction, and no further episodes of left posterior hemiblock occurred. Furthermore, the patient did not develop any evidence of second or third degree A-V block.

He died suddenly 2 days later.

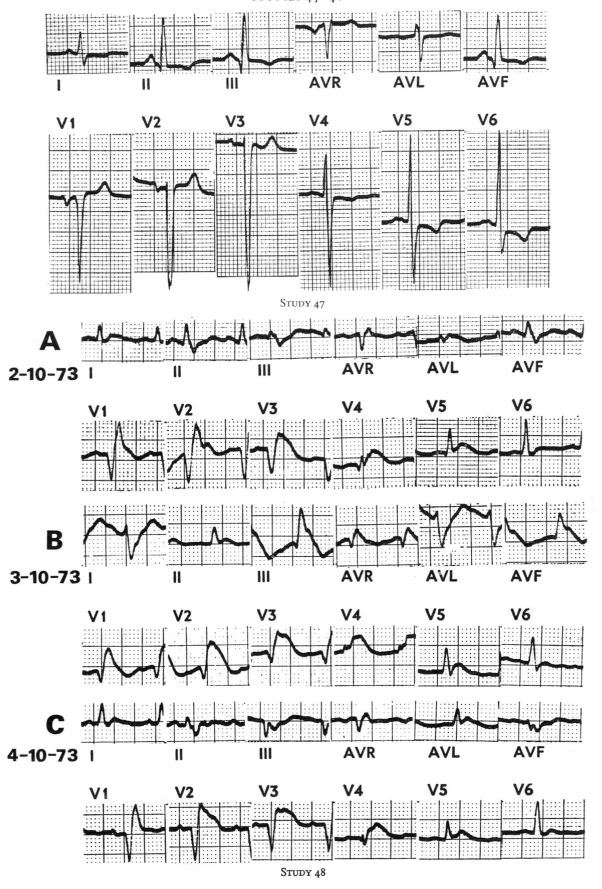

STUDY 47

A
2-10-73

B
3-10-73

C
4-10-73

STUDY 48

49

Acute Inferolateral Myocardial Infarction with Diaphragmatic Peri-infarction Block

The electrocardiogram shows the fully evolved phase of the inferolateral myocardial infarction which is evident from the following:

(a) The myocardial necrosis is reflected by the deep and wide pathological Q waves in Standard lead III and lead AVF, and the rather prominent q wave in Standard lead II.

(b) The myocardial injury and ischaemia is reflected by the elevated, coved S-T segments and the inverted T waves in Standard leads II and III, and lead AVF, the inferior wall myocardial infarction, and in lead V6, the lateral, apical, extension.

(c) The tall symmetrical T waves in leads V2–V5, Standard lead I and lead AVL are characteristic of the leads orientated to the uninjured surface during the phase of regression.

The diaphragmatic peri-infarction block is reflected by the terminal notched R waves of almost equal amplitude in Standard lead II and III, and lead AVF.

There is a wide frontal plane angle of 160° between the initial and terminal 0·04 sec QRS vectors: the initial 0·04 sec QRS vector is directed at −60°, and the terminal 0·04 sec QRS vector is directed at +100°.

50

Acute Inferior Wall Myocardial Infarction with Diaphragmatic Peri-infarction Block

The electrocardiogram shows the fully evolved phase of acute inferior wall myocardial infarction which is evident from the following:

(a) The myocardial necrosis is reflected by the deep and wide pathological Q waves in Standard lead III and lead AVF, and the rather prominent q wave in Standard lead II.

(b) The myocardial injury and ischaemia is reflected by the coved, elevated S-T segments, and the inverted T waves in Standard leads II and III, and lead AVF.

(c) There is reciprocal depression of the S-T segments in Standard lead I, lead AVL and leads V4–V6.

(d) The low to inverted T waves in leads V5 and V6 indicate lateral, apical, extension of the myocardial ischaemia.

The diaphragmatic peri-infarction block is reflected by the prominent terminal R waves in Standard leads II and III, and lead AVF. Note that these terminal R waves are of almost the same amplitude.

The angle between the initial and terminal 0·04 sec QRS vectors on the frontal plane is 150°.

The initial 0·04 sec QRS vector is directed at −60° on the frontal plane.

The terminal 0·04 sec QRS vector is directed at +90° on the frontal plane.

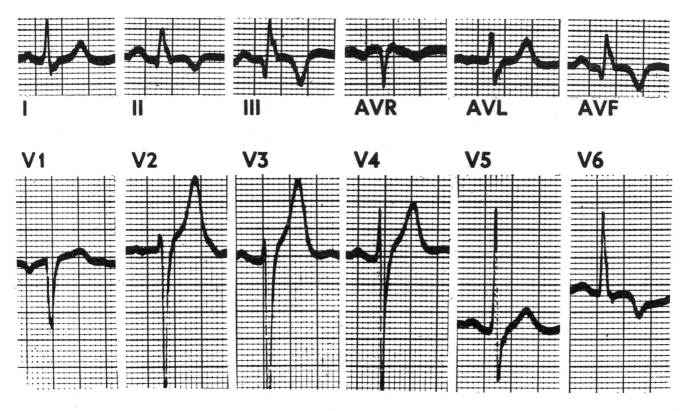

Study 49

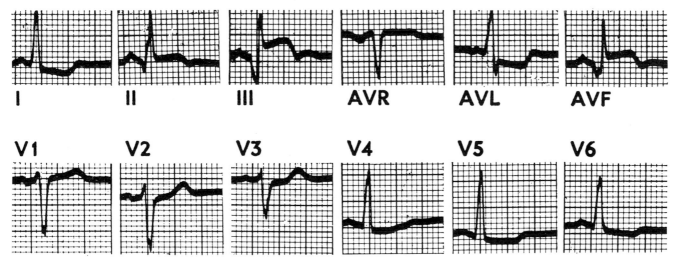

Study 50

51

Acute Anteroseptal Myocardial Infarction Associated with Right Bundle Branch Block, Possible Atrial Infarction

The right bundle branch block results in the inscription of a terminal QRS vector which is directed anteriorly and to the right. This is reflected by a prominent, wide and slurred S wave in Standard lead I, lead AVL and lead V6, and an R' deflection in the right precordial leads V1–V3.

The fully evolved phase of the acute anteroseptal myocardial infarction is revealed by the coved, elevated S-T segments, and the inverted T waves in leads V1–V6, lead AVL and Standard lead I. The region of necrosis is dominant over the mid- and lower-septal regions, as reflected by the absent initial r waves and deep wide Q waves in leads V1–V3. The left lateral leads (leads V4–V6, Standard lead I and lead AVL) reflect a loss of the initial q wave and a diminution in QRS amplitude.

COMMENT

(a) The effects of injury and ischaemia are extensive, being reflected in all the anterior and lateral orientated leads. The effects of necrosis are dominantly anteroseptal, although the loss of QRS amplitude in the left lateral leads would indicate a more extensive lesion.

(b) The complicating right bundle branch block does not disturb the basic patterns of the infarction, but merely results in the addition of a terminal QRS appendage.

(c) The rather horizontal P-R segment and sharp angled junction between the P wave and the P-R segment suggest the possible presence of an atrial infarction.

52

Anteroseptal Myocardial Infarction with Intermittent Right Bundle Branch Block

The electrocardiogram (lead V2) shows intermittent right bundle branch block: the first two beats reflect the right bundle branch block as evidenced by the terminal R wave; the last four beats do not.

The electrocardiogram shows the fully evolved phase of acute anteroseptal myocardial infarction. The myocardial necrosis is reflected by the deep and wide pathological Q waves in the first two beats, and the deep, wide and notched QS complexes in the last four beats. The myocardial injury and ischaemia is reflected by the elevated, coved S-T segments, and the inverted T waves.

COMMENT

(a) The right bundle branch block merely results in the addition of a terminal QRS appendage which does not obscure the essential features of the infarction.

(b) The notch in the QS complex of the last four beats represents intrainfarction block.

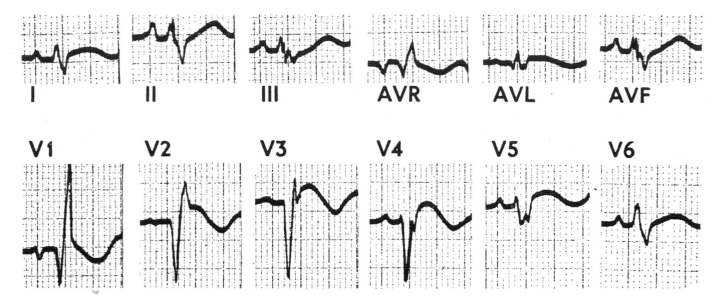

STUDY 51

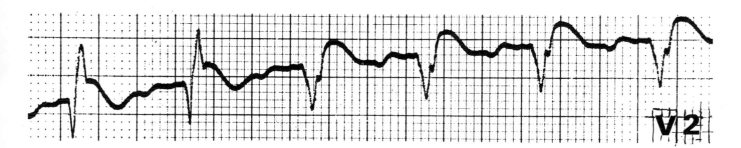

STUDY 52

53

Acute Inferior Wall Infarction Associated with Right Bundle Branch Block

The right bundle branch block is evident from the rightward and anteriorly directed terminal QRS vectors, as reflected by the deep, wide S waves in the left lateral leads, and the R' deflection in lead V1.

The acute inferior wall infarction is reflected by deep and wide pathological Q waves, coved and elevated S-T segments, and inverted T waves in Standard leads II and III, and lead AVF. Reciprocal S-T segment depression occurs in the left lateral leads, leads V4–V6, Standard lead I and lead AVL.

The initial, rather tall R waves in leads V1–V3 suggest possible true posterior extension.

COMMENT

The right bundle branch block does not obscure the diagnostic abnormal initial QRS vectors of the inferior wall infarction.

54

Acute Anterior Myocardial Infarction Complicated by Right Bundle Branch Block and Left Anterior Hemiblock

The acute, fully evolved, phase of anterior myocardial infarction is reflected by:

(a) pathological, widened, Q waves in leads V1–V5.
(b) the low amplitude QRS complex in lead V6.
(c) the coved and elevated S-T segments with inverted T waves in leads V1–V5, Standard lead I and lead AVL.

The right bundle branch block is reflected by the terminal R' wave in leads V1–V4 and the terminal slurred S waves in lead V6, Standard lead I and lead AVL. The right bundle branch block does not obscure the features of the infarction.

The initial vectors reflect a left anterior hemiblock. The axis is directed at −70 degrees.

Note that the initial r waves of the left anterior hemiblock in Standard leads II and III, and lead AVF are absent. Furthermore, the terminal S wave in Standard lead I and lead AVL is much diminished. The tracing therefore closely resembles the fully developed phase of masquerading bundle branch block, i.e. it tends to resemble left bundle branch block in the frontal plane leads.

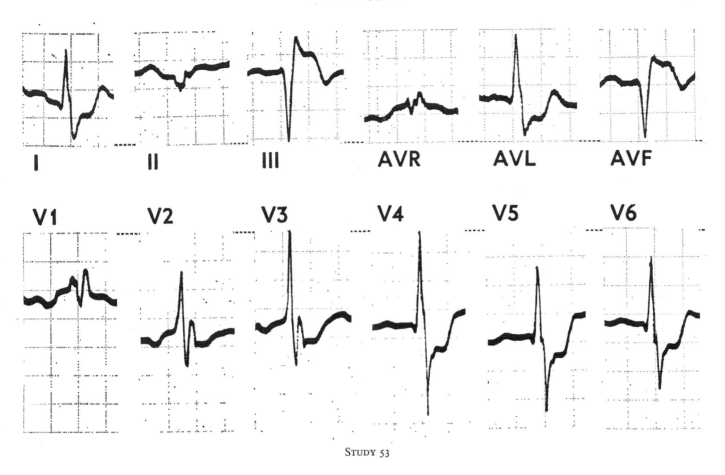

STUDY 53

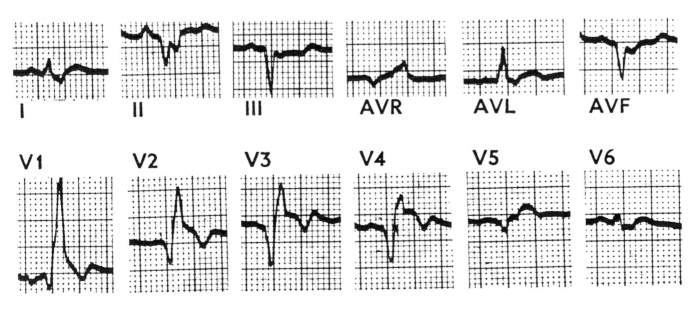

STUDY 54

55

Old Anteroseptal Myocardial Infarction. Right Bundle Branch Block with Left Anterior Hemiblock

The electrocardiogram shows right bundle branch block as evidenced by the terminal R wave in the right precordial leads V1 and V2, and the slurred terminal S wave in the left precordial leads, Standard lead I and lead AVL. This is an expression of a rightward and anteriorly directed terminal QRS vector.

There is, in addition, a left anterior hemiblock as evidenced by the following:

(a) There are deep S waves in Standard lead II and III and lead AVF, reflecting a mean manifest frontal plane QRS axis of $-50°$. The calculation of this axis excludes the terminal QRS deflection of the right bundle branch block.

(b) There are prominent initial r waves in Standard leads II and III and lead AVF.

There is an old, stabilized anteroseptal infarction. The necrotic scar of this infarction is evident from the absent initial r waves in leads V1–V3. These leads would consequently reflect QS complexes if it were not for the terminal R wave of the right bundle branch block. The coved and elevated S-T segments and the inverted T waves of acute myocardial infarction are absent.

The S-T segments reflect a primary change in that they are deviated in the same direction as the terminal QRS deflection. For example, they are depressed in leads V5 and V6 and Standard lead I, thus being deviated in the same direction as the terminal S wave.

The S-T segments in these leads also reflect a horizontality with a plane depression and a sharp angled ST-T junction. These S-T segment manifestations are an expression of chronic coronary insufficiency, chronic subendocardial myocardial injury.

COMMENT

The right bundle branch block does not affect the initial QRS deflections, which thus reflect the old anteroseptal infarction and the left anterior hemiblock.

56

Left Bundle Branch Block with Coronary Insufficiency

The electrocardiogram was recorded from a 57-year-old man who had frequent attacks of angina pectoris. It shows the features of complete left bundle branch block, as evidenced by the wide, bizarre and notched RR′ complexes in the left lateral leads, and the wide, bizarre and notched S waves of the rS complexes in the right precordial leads.

The S-T segment and T wave are opposite in direction to the terminal QRS vector, and hence reflect a basic secondary change to the abnormal intraventricular conduction. However, unlike uncomplicated left bundle branch block (see Electrocardiographic Study 59A), the T waves tend to be more pointed, symmetrical and increased in amplitude. Furthermore, the S-T segments tend to be more curved than in uncomplicated left bundle branch block. These features suggest the superimposition of the effects of epicardial ischaemia.

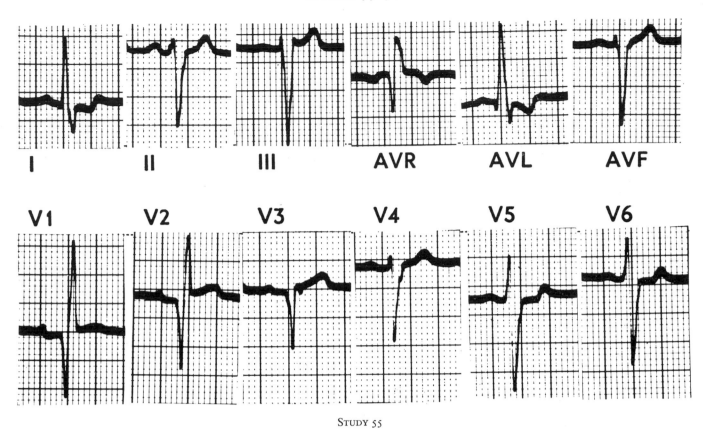

I II III AVR AVL AVF

V1 V2 V3 V4 V5 V6

STUDY 55

I II III AVR AVL AVF

V1 V2 V3 V4 V5 V6

STUDY 56

57

Left Bundle Branch Block Associated with Apical Subendocardial Ischaemia

The electrocardiogram shows left bundle branch as reflected by:

(a) the wide, bizarre, notched R-R′ complexes in leads V5 and V6, Standard lead I and lead AVL, and

(b) the deep wide rS complexes in leads V1–V3.

The apical subendocardial ischaemia is evidenced by:

(a) the upright, sharply pointed and symmetrical T waves in leads V5 and V6, Standard lead I and lead AVL, and

(b) the horizontal S-T segments with sharp-angled ST-T junction in leads V5 and V6, Standard leads I and II and lead AVL.

COMMENT

With left bundle branch block, the T wave is normally inverted in the left precordial leads, Standard lead I and lead AVL. This is a secondary change to the abnormal intraventricular conduction. An upright T wave thus reflects a primary change due to a primary myocardial disease. Since the T wave is upright in the left lateral leads, it is directed away from the apical subendocardium which, together with the T wave configuration, connotes subendocardial ischaemia.

58

Left Bundle Branch Block with Left Anterior Hemiblock Complicated by Acute Anteroseptal Myocardial Infarction

(Courtesy of Dr B.van Drimmelen)

Electrocardiogram A was recorded on the second day after the commencement of chest pain in a patient with acute myocardial infarction. It reflects left bundle branch block, as evidenced by the wide, bizarre and notched R waves in leads V5 and V6, Standard lead I and lead AVL.

There is left axis deviation of the initial 0·04 sec QRS vector ($-10°$) and the terminal 0·04 sec QRS vector ($-50°$). The presentation is thus one of left bundle branch block with left anterior hemiblock.

The S-T segments of the left lateral leads are within normal limits. The S-T segments of leads V1–V4 are abnormally elevated, more than is usual in uncomplicated left bundle branch block. In addition, these S-T segments tend to be *coved upward* instead of the usual initial concave-upward configuration. The presentation is compatible with an anterior wall subepicardial infarction.

Electrocardiogram B shows leads V1, V2, V3 of the tracing recorded on the first day (Tracing a), on the second day (Tracing b), and 2 weeks later (Tracing c).

The S-T segments of Tracing a are probably still within normal limits although they reflect a straightening of the normal upward concavity.

The S-T segments of Tracing b are elevated and coved, and show the fully evolved injury phase of the infarction as described under Electrocardiogram A.

The S-T segments of Tracing c have almost regressed to normal, but still reflect rather tall and symmetrical T waves of myocardial ischaemia.

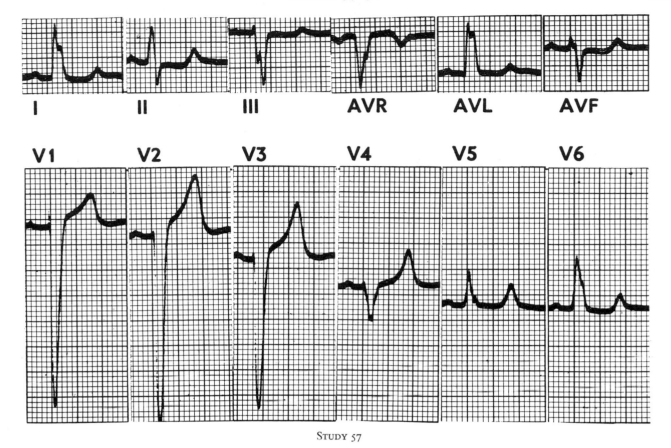

STUDY 57

STUDY 58A

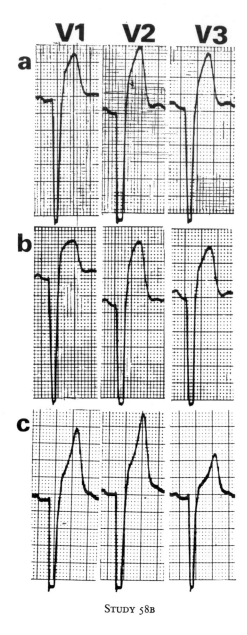

STUDY 58B

59

Left Bundle Branch Block Complicated by Anterior Wall Myocardial Infarction
(Courtesy of Dr D.Clark)

Electrocardiogram A shows uncomplicated left bundle branch block.

Note:

1. The small initial *r* waves in leads V1 and V2.
2. The relatively high QRS:S-T ratio of 3:1 in lead V2.
3. The slightly concave-upward S-T segment in leads V1–V3.

Electrocardiogram B was recorded 3 months later when the patient was seen with a classic clinical and biochemical presentation of myocardial infarction. It shows some of the typical features of left bundle branch block complicated by anterior wall infarction.

1. The initial *r* waves have become more prominent in leads V2 and V3.
2. The QRS:S-T ratio has diminished, and is now almost unity. This is due to some decrease in the depth of the QRS complex, and a marked elevation of the S-T segment.
3. The S-T segments in leads V2–V4 reflect prominent upward coving. The normal upward concavity of the S-T segment in leads V5 and V6 has become more pronounced.
4. Lead V4 has become markedly diminished in amplitude and shows a prominent initial *q* wave.
5. The proximal QRS deflection in leads V5 and V6 has become deformed. It is irregular and slurred, blending with the distal deflection.

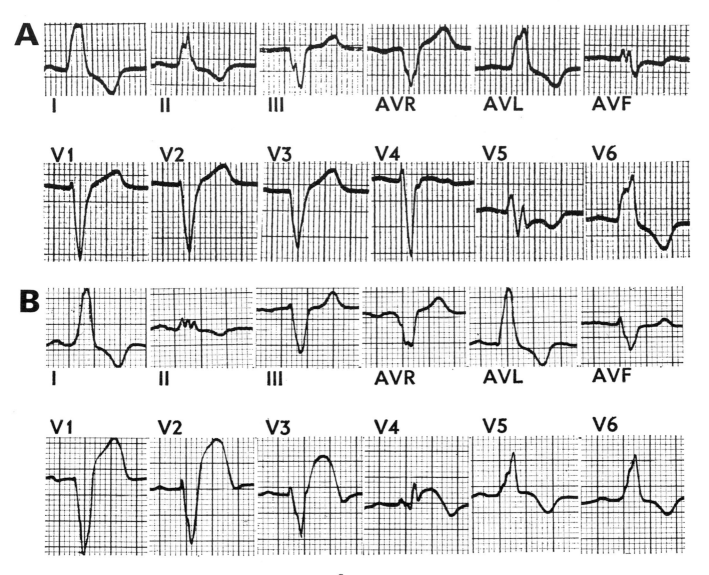

60

Acute Anterior Wall Myocardial Infarction Complicated by Left Anterior Hemiblock, Intermittent Right Bundle Branch Block and Left Bundle Branch Block

Electrocardiogram A was recorded (with twice normal sensitivity) on admission to the coronary care unit, and shows the features of acute anterior wall myocardial infarction complicated by left anterior hemiblock.

The left anterior hemiblock is reflected by the deep S waves and relatively prominent initial r waves in Standard leads II and III, and lead AVF. The mean manifest frontal plane QRS axis reflects a leftward shift, and is directed at about $-45°$. The left anterior hemiblock also results in initial r waves in leads V2–V4 (see below).

The acute anterior wall myocardial infarction is evident from the coved, elevated S-T segments and inverted T waves in leads V1–V6.

COMMENT

The pathological precordial Q waves or QS complexes of the anterior wall myocardial infarction are obscured by the initial inferior and anterior QRS vectors of the left anterior hemiblock. The effect may also, in part, be due to a relatively high precordial electrode placement. The infarction is, however, evident from the coved, elevated S-T segments and the failure of a progressive r wave increase from leads V2–V4. Electrocardiogram B was recorded on the following day and shows the anterior infarction complicated by left anterior hemiblock, and which is now further complicated by right bundle branch block.

The right bundle branch block does not change the initial QRS vectors which still reflect the features of the left anterior hemiblock as described above. However, the initial small r wave is now also absent in lead V2 and V3 and much less conspicuous in lead V4. This is probably due to a minimally higher precordial electrode placement of leads V1, V2 and V3. These leads thus reflect the initial deep, wide pathological Q waves—the equivalent of QS

complexes with uncomplicated intraventricular condution, and terminal R waves—the expression of right bundle branch block. The precordial S-T segments and T waves still reflect the acute myocardial injury and myocardial ischaemia pattern of the acute myocardial infarction.

Electrocardiogram C was recorded 2 days after Electrocardiogram B, and shows the acute myocardial infarction complicated by complete left bundle branch block with left anterior hemiblock. The acute anterior wall myocardial infarction is evident in the presence of the complicating left bundle branch block from the following features:

(a) There is marked diminution in the QRST amplitude of the precordial leads.

(b) The S-T segment amplitude is equal to the QRS magnitude in leads V2–V4, reflecting a QRS:S-T ratio of one.

(c) The S-T segments are elevated, coved and the T waves are low to inverted in leads V2–V4.

(d) Lead V4 reflects an initial small r wave followed by a bizarre, deep, wide and notched S wave.

(e) Lead V5 reflects a bizarre, deep and wide notched S wave.

(f) Standard lead I, lead AVL and lead V6 reflect the characteristic complex of infarction in the presence of complete left bundle branch block: an initial q wave followed by a dome and dart positive deflection. An enlargement of lead V6 is shown in Electrocardiogram D.

(g) Lead V6 also shows a terminal S wave.

(h) The left anterior hemiblock is evident from the deep terminal S waves in Standard leads II and III, and lead AVF.

COMMENT

(a) The bizarre, dominantly negative deflections in leads V4 and V5 as well as the initial q and ensuing slope of the complexes in leads V6, Standard lead I and lead AVL, reflect septal infarction.

(b) The terminal S wave in lead V6 reflects the infarction of the free wall of the left ventricle.

(c) The right bundle branch block does not mask the basic QRS manifestations of the myocardial infarction.

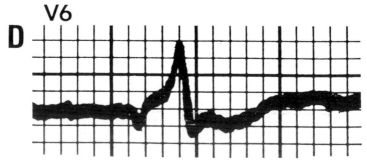

D V6

STUDY 60D

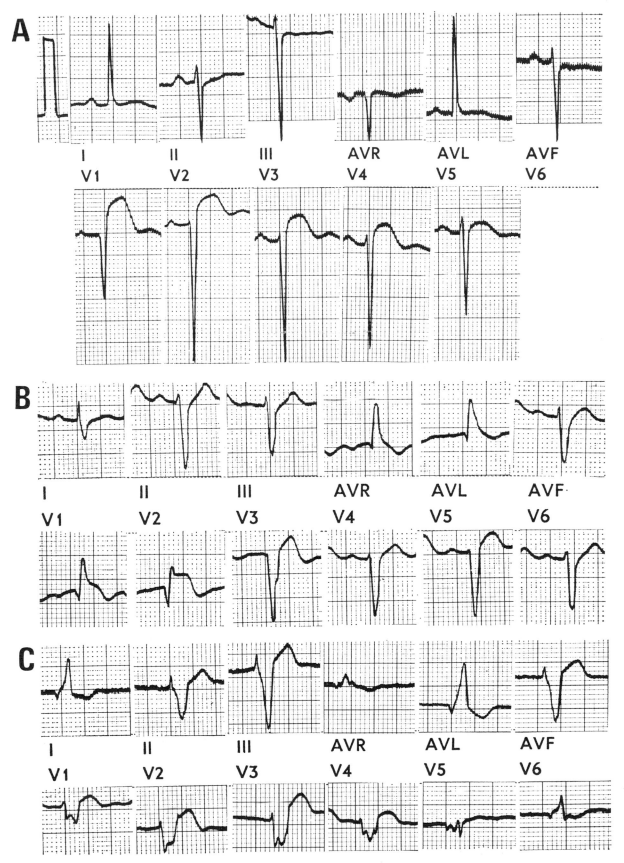

A

I   II   III   AVR   AVL   AVF
V1   V2   V3   V4   V5   V6

B

I   II   III   AVR   AVL   AVF
V1   V2   V3   V4   V5   V6

C

I   II   III   AVR   AVL   AVF
V1   V2   V3   V4   V5   V6

STUDY 60A, B, C

61

Acute Inferior Wall Myocardial Infarction Complicated by Complete Left Bundle Branch Block

Electrocardiogram A was recorded within a few hours of the onset of the myocardial infarction, and shows the early hyperacute phase of inferior wall myocardial infarction. This is reflected by the slope-elevation of the S-T segments and the increased amplitude and widening of the *T* waves in Standard leads II and III, and lead AVF.

The QRS complexes reveal the features of complete left bundle branch block.

Electrocardiogram B was recorded on the following day and shows the fully evolved phase of inferior wall myocardial infarction. This is reflected by the elevated, coved S-T segments and inverted *T* waves in Standard leads II and III, and lead AVF. A similar, though less marked, manifestation in leads V5 and V6 indicates lateral, apical, extension.

The following changes affect the QRS complexes:

(a) The frontal plane leads, Standard leads I, II and III and leads AVR, AVL and AVF, show a marked diminution in amplitude. None of these QRS complexes exceed 6 mm.

(b) There is also an appreciable diminution in the amplitude of the QRS complexes in leads V5 and V6.

(c) Standard lead II and lead AVF show very deep and prominent notches or *S* waves.

(d) Standard lead III shows a wide and deep pathological Q wave followed by a terminal *R* wave.

COMMENT

Note that the S-T segments in Standard leads II and III, and leads AVF, V5 and V6 reflect a *primary change* since they are displaced in the *same* direction as the terminal QRS deflection.

The S-T segments reflect the hyperacute phase (Electrocardiogram A) and the fully evolved phase (Electrocardiogram B) despite the presence of the left bundle branch block.

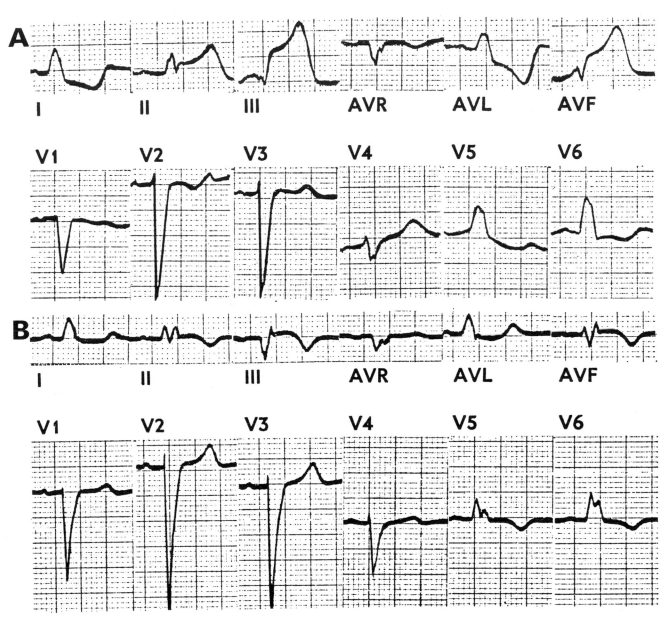

STUDY 61

62

Extensive Inferior and Anterior Wall Myocardial Infarction Complicated by Left Bundle Branch Block

The electrocardiogram shows the features of left bundle branch block which have been considerably modified by the advent of extensive myocardial infarction. The infarction is evident from the following:

1   *The QRS manifestations*

(a) There is a marked diminution in QRS amplitude in the frontal plane leads, Standard leads I, II and III, and leads AVR, AVL and AVF, and the left lateral precordial leads, leads V5 and V6. The amplitude of the QRS deflections does not exceed 4 mm in any of these leads.

(b) There are prominent initial *q* waves in leads V5 and V6 and Standard leads I and II. This reflects septal infarction.

(c) Leads V5 and V6 and Standard leads I and II also reflect terminal *S* waves. This indicates involvement of the free wall of the left ventricle.

(d) Lead V6 and Standard lead II show the characteristic initial *q* wave followed by a dome and dart deflection.

(e) The right precordial leads reflect very prominent, tall, initial *R* waves.

Note that all the precordial leads as well as Standard lead III, lead AVL and lead AVF also show ventricular extrasystoles (the second QRS complex in each of these leads).

2   *The S-T segment and* T *wave manifestations*

(a) The S-T segments are slightly coved and elevated, and the *T* waves are inverted in Standard leads II and III, and leads AVF, V5 and V6.

(b) The S-T segments are depressed in leads V2–V4.

COMMENT

Note that these S-T segments reflect a primary change, since they are displaced in the same direction as the terminal QRS deflections.

63

Left Bundle Branch Block Associated with Acute Anterolateral Myocardial Infarction
(Courtesy of Dr H.J.L.Marriott)

Electrocardiogram of 27 May 1966 shows left bundle branch block as reflected by the wide notched R-R' complexes in leads V5, V6, Standard lead I and lead AVL, and the deep wide *S* waves of the rS complexes in leads VI–V3.

There are primary S-T segment and *T* wave changes, i.e. changes which are not due to the abnormal intraventricular conduction of the left bundle branch block, but which connote primary myocardial disease. These are:

1. *T* waves which are upright in the left lateral leads: leads V5 and V6, Standard lead I and lead AVL.

2. S-T segments which are elevated in the left lateral leads.

These changes reflect the presence of the hyperacute injury phase of anterolateral myocardial infarction. There is reciprocal depression of the S-T segments in Standard leads II, III and lead AVF.

The electrocardiogram recorded on the next day shows the fully evolved phase of anterolateral myocardial infarction. This is evidenced by:

(a) the development of small initial *q* waves in Standard lead I and lead AVL, and

(b) the coved and elevated S-T segments with inverted *T* waves in Standard lead I and lead AVL.

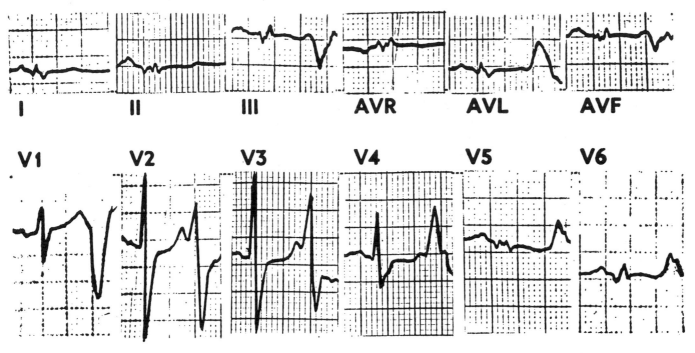

I   II   III   AVR   AVL   AVF

V1   V2   V3   V4   V5   V6

STUDY 62

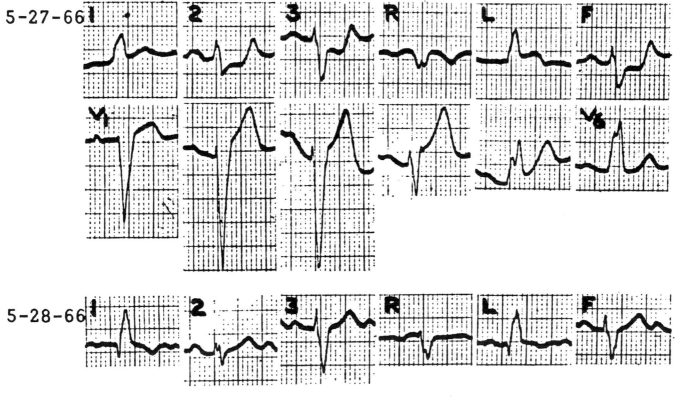

5-27-66

5-28-66

STUDY 63

64

Left Bundle Branch Block Associated with Acute Myocardial Infarction
(Courtesy of Dr H.J.L.Marriott)

The left bundle branch block is reflected by:

(a) the wide, bizarre, notched R-R′ deflection in leads V5 and V6, Standard lead I, and lead AVL, and

(b) the deep, wide, bizarre S waves of the rS deflection in leads V1–V4.

The acute extensive anterior wall infarction is reflected by:

(a) the prominent initial q waves in Standard lead I, and leads AVL and V5,

(b) the relatively low depth of the QRS complex in leads VI–V4,

(c) the markedly elevated S-T segments in leads V2–V4,

(d) the elevated S-T segments in Standard lead I and leads AVL and V5.

COMMENT

1. Note that the QRS:S-T ratio in leads V2–V4 is less than one; the normal usually being in the range of $1\frac{1}{2}:1$ to $2:1$ or even $3:1$.

2. Standard lead I, leads AVL and V6 reflect an S-T segment elevation, a deviation in the same direction as the terminal QRS vector, and thus connoting a primary change.

3. The relative normality of lead V6 indicates that the apex has probably been spared.

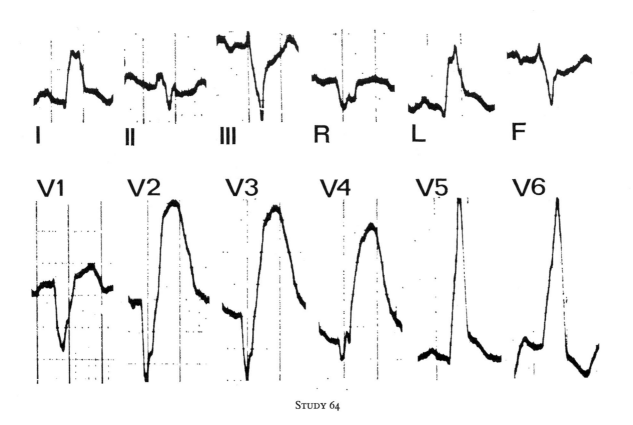

STUDY 64

65

Acute Extensive Anterior Wall Myocardial Infarction Complicated by Left Bundle Branch Block

The electrocardiograms were recorded from a 56-year-old man with a typical clinical and biochemical presentation of myocardial infarction.

Electrocardiogram A shows the fully evolved phase of an extensive anterior wall myocardial infarction. This is reflected by:

(a) QS complexes in leads V1–V5,

(b) Qr complexes in lead V6, Standard lead I and lead AVL, and

(c) elevated and coved S-T segments with inverted *T* waves in leads V1–V6, Standard lead I, and lead AVL.

Electrocardiogram B was recorded 2 days later, and shows the acute anterior wall myocardial infarction, which is now complicated by left bundle branch block. This is reflected by the following:

(a) There are rather prominent initial *r* waves of the rS complexes reflected by leads V1–V3.

(b) There is a diminution of the normal QRS:S-T segment ratio in leads V1–V3 (which is usually 2:1 or 3:1, see Electrocardiogram A) to unity, i.e. the magnitude of the QRS complex and the S-T segment being almost the same. This is due to a reduction in the depth of the QRS complex and an elevation, an increase in the amplitude, of the S-T segment.

(c) The S-T segments are coved in leads V1–V3.

(d) The left lateral leads, leads V5 and V6, Standard lead I, and lead AVL show:

(i) small initial *q* waves, and
(ii) initial slurring,

thereby giving a dome and dart appearance.

(e) The QRS complex is dominantly negative in lead V4.

(f) There is a generalized diminution in QRS voltage.

COMMENT

The frontal plane lead also reflects a dominant left axis deviation.

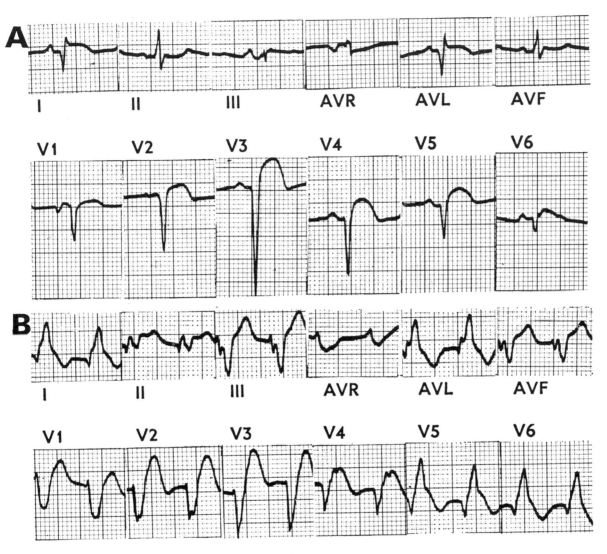

66

Acute Inferior Wall Myocardial Infarction Manifesting in Conducted Sinus Beats as well as in Interpolated Ventricular Extrasystoles

Standard leads II and III and lead AVF show marked S-T segment slope-elevation, reflecting the hyperacute phase of inferior wall myocardial infarction. Standard lead I shows reciprocal S-T segment depression. A prominent, though not pathological, Q wave is present in Standard lead II. The interpolated ventricular extrasystoles are dominantly positive in Standard leads II and III and lead AVF, and have prominent pathological Q waves with marked slope-elevation of the S-T segments.

COMMENT

(a) The S-T segments of the ventricular extrasystoles are deviated in the same direction as the terminal QRS deflection of the ventricular extrasystole, thereby indicating a primary abnormality of repolarization, in this case, the slope-elevation of the hyperacute injury phase.

(b) The infarction pattern is more manifest and more obvious in the ventricular extrasystoles than in the conducted sinus beats.

67

Hyperacute Phase of Anterior Wall Myocardial Infarction. Also Revealed in Complicating Ventricular Extrasystoles

The electrocardiogram shows the features of the hyperacute early injury phase of anterior wall myocardial infarction. This is evident from the slope-elevation of the S-T segments and the tall and widened T waves in leads V2–V5. Leads V4 and V5 also reflect QS complexes of myocardial necrosis.

Complicating ventricular extrasystoles are present in leads V1, V2, V3 and V6. The ventricular extrasystoles in leads V2 and V3 reflect the parameters of the acute myocardial infarction, as evidenced by the following:

(a) Initial q waves in the dominantly upright QRS complexes.

(b) Coved and elevated S-T segment, representing a primary repolarization change.

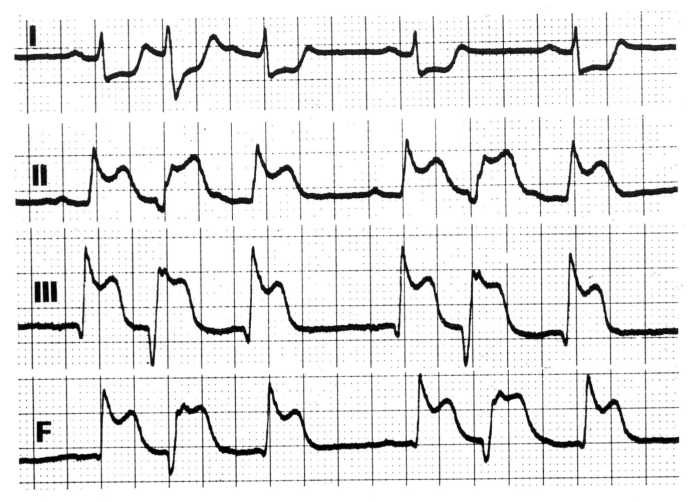

STUDY 66

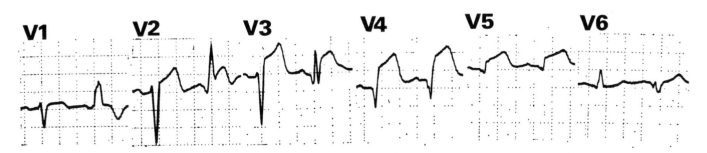

STUDY 67

68

Myocardial Infarction Evident in the Ectopic Beats of an Idioventricular Tachycardia[L37]

The electrocardiograms were recorded from a 54-year-old woman with acute myocardial infarction.

Electrocardiogram A shows an idioventricular tachycardia, as reflected by the bizarre QRS complexes which are dissociated from the P waves of the concomitant sinus rhythm. The rate of the ectopic rhythm is 94 beats/min, representing an enhanced idioventricular rhythm. The relatively slow rate of the tachycardia facilitates the occurrence of frequent ventricular capture beats, the momentary conduction to, and capture of, the ventricles by a sinus impulse. The capture beats are complete and incomplete. The complete capture reflects complete or total activation of the ventricles by the sinus impulse. The resulting QRS complex consequently represents the contour of the pure sinus beat. They are represented in the tracing by beats 5 and 11 of the top strip, beats 6 and 7 of the middle strip, and beats 6, 7, and 15 of the bottom strip.

The incomplete capture beats reflect partial activation of the ventricles by the sinus impulse synchronously with the ectopic impulse. The resulting QRS complex is a ventricular fusion beat, and has a configuration in between that of the pure sinus beat (the complete capture) and the pure ectopic beat. The configuration of these ventricular fusion beats will vary depending upon the relative contribution by the sinus and ectopic impulses to ventricular activation. Ventricular fusion beats (incomplete capture beats) are represented by beats 4, 6, 11, 13 and 14 of the top strip, beats 8, 9, 10, 11 and 12 of the middle strip, and beats 1, 6, 8 and 14 of the bottom strip. The presence of ventricular fusion complexes confirms the ventricular origin of the tachycardia.

Electrocardiogram B was recorded on the following day, and shows the idioventricular tachycardia which, on this occasion, is associated with retrograde conduction to the atria (the bottom strip Standard lead I). The 12 lead electrocardiogram shows complexes from each lead during the tachycardia. It is clearly evident that the complexes of leads V1–V6 are dominantly upright, and that they are all associated with wide and deep initial Q waves, reflecting the electrocardiographic parameter of necrosis. The S-T segments reflect the parameters of injury and ischaemia. The S-T segments are elevated in leads V2–V6, i.e. they are deviated in the same direction as the dominant QRS deflection, reflecting a primary change, a primary disease process. They also tend to be coved upward. The associated T waves are inverted, symmetrical, sharply pointed and of appreciable magnitude.

Electrocardiogram C is the 12 lead electrocardiogram recorded 2 days later during normal rhythm, and reflects the pattern of resolving extensive anterior infarction. This is represented by the QS complexes in leads V1–V5, the loss of positive deflection in lead V6 which only reflects a tiny initial r wave, and the rather prominent Q waves in Standard lead I and lead AVL. Standard lead I and lead AVL also reflect slightly elevated and coved S-T segments and inverted T waves.

COMMENT

The parameters of infarction are clearly evident in the complexes of the ectopic ventricular beats during the idioventricular tachycardia.

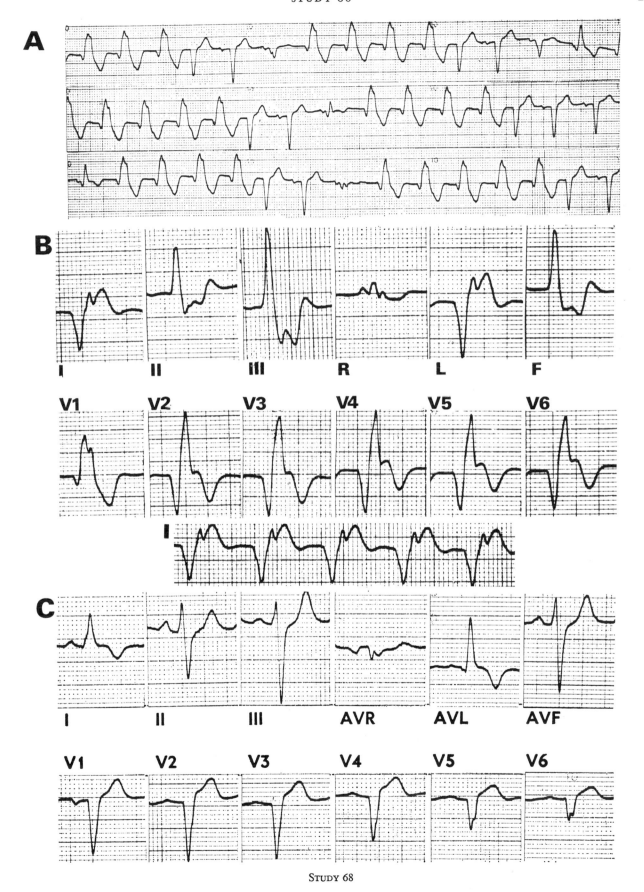

69

The Wolff-Parkinson-White Syndrome Simulating Chronic Inferior Wall Myocardial Infarction

The electrocardiogram shows the classic features of the Wolff-Parkinson-White syndrome: shortened P-R interval, delta wave, a slurred proximal limb of the QRS complex, and a minimally widened QRS complex.

The mean manifest frontal plane delta wave axis is directed at −50 degrees. The delta wave is consequently negative in Standard leads II and III, and lead AVF, simulating pathological Q waves in Standard lead III and lead AVF.

The correct diagnosis is evident from: (a) the parameters of the Wolff-Parkinson-White syndrome in all the complexes, and (b) the absence of any electrocardiographic manifestations of acute or chronic injury or ischaemia.

70

The Type A Wolff-Parkinson-White Syndrome Simulating Old Antero-lateral Myocardial Infarction and True Posterior Wall Myocardial Infarction

The electrocardiogram shows the Type A Wolff-Parkinson-White syndrome as evidenced by the following:

(a) There is a short P-R interval of 0·10 sec.

(b) There is a delta wave, a prominent, slurred deflection which deforms the proximal limb of the QRS complex. The mean manifest frontal plane delta wave axis is directed at +120°. It is consequently very tall in Standard lead III, also positive in Standard lead II, leads AVF and V1–V6, and negative in Standard lead I and lead AVL.

(c) The S-T segments are depressed with a tendency to a sharp-angled ST-T junction in Standard leads II and III, lead AVF and leads V1–V6. These represent secondary changes to the abnormal intraventricular conduction, the pre-excitation.

(d) The QRS complexes are dominantly upright in the right precordial leads, thereby reflecting the Type *A* Wolff-Parkinson-White syndrome.

COMMENTS

(a) The negative delta waves in Standard lead I and lead AVL simulate the pathological Q waves of old anterolateral myocardial infarction.

(b) The tall *R* waves in the right precordial leads simulate true posterior wall myocardial infarction.

(c) The secondary S-T segment and *T* wave changes may be mistaken for the primary changes of myocardial disease.

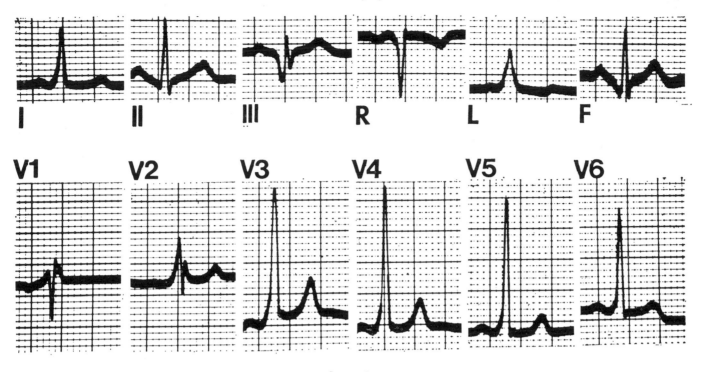

STUDY 69

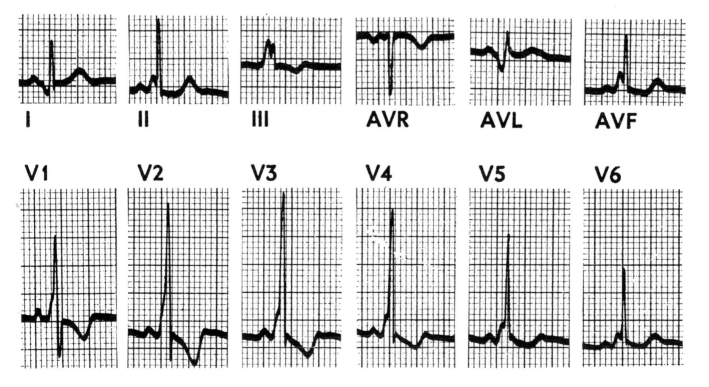

STUDY 70

71

Inferior, Anterior and True Posterior Myocardial Infarction Associated with the Type A Wolff-Parkinson-White Syndrome, Right Bundle Branch Block and Ventricular Extrasystoles[S36]

Electrocardiograms A–F were recorded from a 43-year-old man with coronary artery disease.

Electrocardiogram A shows the stable or chronic electrocardiographic pattern (recorded on 4 January 1966). It shows evidence of:

(a) an old inferior myocardial infarction, as reflected by deep, wide, pathological Q waves in Standard leads II and III, and lead AVF, and

(b) true posterior infarction, as reflected by tall R waves and tall symmetrical T waves in leads V1–V4.

Electrocardiogram B (recorded on 6 December 1969) shows the onset of the Wolff-Parkinson-White syndrome (WPW), Type A, as reflected by the dominantly positive QRS and delta waves in the right precordial leads. The delta wave vector is directed anteriorly and to the right at + 120°. The delta waves are clearly seen in Standard leads II and III, lead AVF, and leads V1–V6. This results in:

(a) obliteration of the pathological Q waves in Standard leads II and III, and lead AVF,

(b) prominent negative delta deflections in Standard lead I and lead AVL, which simulate the pathological Q waves of anterolateral myocardial infarction, and

(c) taller R waves in leads V1–V4, an augmentation of the tall R waves of the true posterior infarction.

Electrocardiogram C shows the electrocardiogram of 29 January 1971, during an attack of clinical myocardial infarction with extreme shock. The electrocardiogram shows the WPW syndrome pattern which is now complicated by an anterior wall subepicardial injury pattern; depressed and horizontal S-T segments in Standard leads I and II, lead AVF, and leads V5 and V6, with elevated S-T segments and tall T waves in leads V1–V4.

Electrocardiogram D shows the electrocardiogram recorded 8 hours later. The WPW syndrome pattern is again evident. There is, in addition, a right bundle branch block pattern, and this is associated with primary S-T segment and T wave changes; convex-upward S-T segments in leads V1–V4.

Electrocardiogram E was recorded 2 months later, during a further admission with the patient in shock. The WPW syndrome pattern is now absent, revealing once again the deep wide Q waves in Standard leads II and III, and lead AVF of the old inferior myocardial infarction. The right bundle branch block pattern is also absent. The tall R waves in the precordial leads, the manifestation of the true poster-

ior infarction and/or the Type A WPW syndrome, have also disappeared, revealing deep, wide, pathological Q waves associated with raised and coved S-T segments of acute anteroseptal myocardial infarction.

Electrocardiogram F (recorded 7 months later, on 10 September (1971), shows sinus rhythm complicated by ventricular ectopic beats. The conducted sinus beats again show the WPW syndrome which masks both the old inferior and anterior myocardial infarctions. The ventricular ectopic beats, however, show evidence of the old anterior and inferior myocardial infarctions (deep, wide Q waves, followed by tall R waves, in Standard leads II and III, lead AVF, and in leads V1–V4). There are also primary S-T segment changes associated with the ventricular ectopic beats, best seen in leads V2 and V3.

The electrocardiographic manifestation of the old inferior myocardial infarction is obliterated by the advent of the WPW syndrome (compare Electrocardiograms A and E, which show the infarction pattern, with Electrocardiograms B, C, D and F which do not). The tall precordial R waves of the old posterior infarction are augmented by the advent of the WPW syndrome, i.e. the tall precordial R waves become taller (compare Electrocardiogram A with Electrocardiogram B). The anterior infarction is nullified by the advent of the WPW syndrome (compare Electrocardiogram E with Electrocardiogram F). The infarction pattern, is, however, still evident in the complicating ventricular ectopic beats which are not influenced by pre-excitation. Since ventricular ectopic beats arise ectopically in the ventricles, they are not affected by pre-excitation, as is evident in Electrocardiogram F.

When the WPW syndrome Type B complicates right bundle branch block, it frequently normalizes the right bundle branch block pattern. This is because the pre-excitation wave may gain access to a region of the right bundle branch that is below the block, and hence completes the activation of the right ventricle in a normal manner. It is consequently rare for the WPW syndrome Type B to be seen in association with right bundle branch block. The Type A WPW syndrome, however, activates the left ventricle and thus cannot normalize a right bundle branch block form of conduction. The two may, therefore, be seen in association, as is evident in this case.

Thus, pre-excitation which is in this case situated in the posterosuperior region of the left ventricle (illustrated in Fig. 43 of the text) and which results in a delta wave vector directed anteriorly and inferiorly, has the following effects on the pattern of infarction:

1. It masks the pattern of inferior infarction.
2. It masks the pattern of anterior infarction.
3. It augments the pattern of true posterior infarction.
4. It obviously has no effect on the infarction pattern in a ventricular extrasystole which arises in the ventricle and, therefore, cannot be affected by pre-excitation.

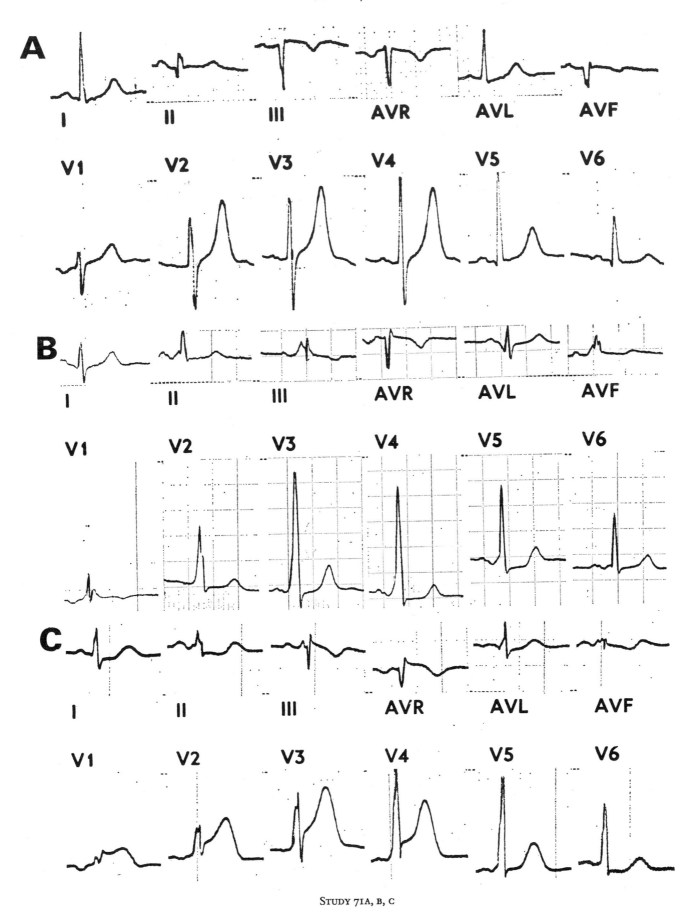

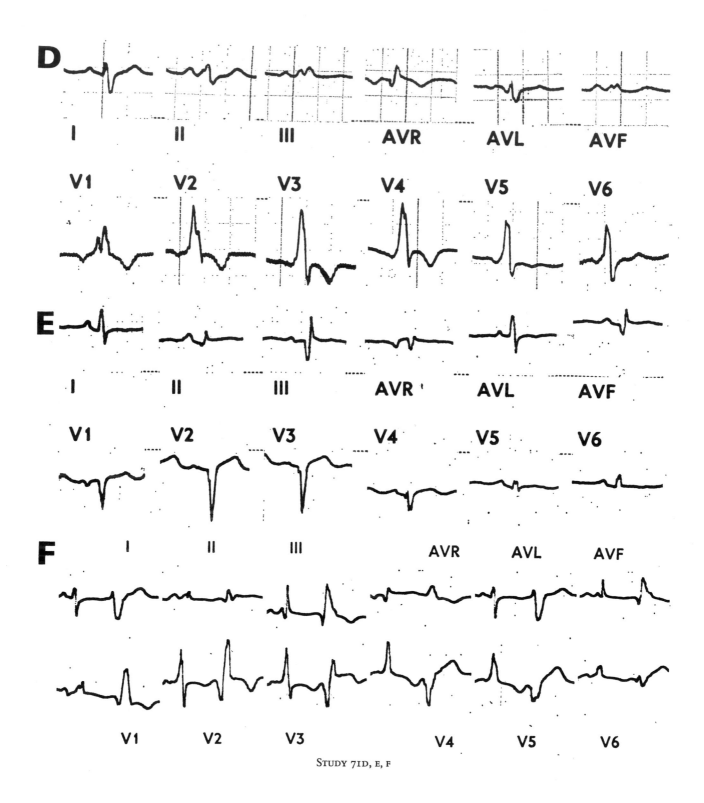

STUDY 7ID, E, F

72

**The Wolff-Parkinson-White Syndrome Compli-
cated by Acute Anterior Wall Myocardial Infarction**
(Courtesy of Dr D.Pittaway)

The electrocardiogram was recorded from a man with the
typical clinical presentation of acute myocardial infarction.
It shows the Wolff-Parkinson-Syndrome, as reflected by
the shortened P-R interval and the prominent delta wave,
which is well seen in all the leads (except lead AVF, where

it is equiphasic) as a slurred, initial deformity. The mean
manifest frontal plane delta wave axis is directed at 0°.

The infarction is evident from the T waves and S-T
segments only. The T waves are deeply inverted,
symmetrical and arrow-head in appearance in leads V2 and
V6, Standard leads I and II and lead AVL. The S-T segments also tend to be coved upward in these leads.

COMMENT

The delta wave masks the initial pathological Q wave of
the infarction. Compare Electrocardiographic Study 71.

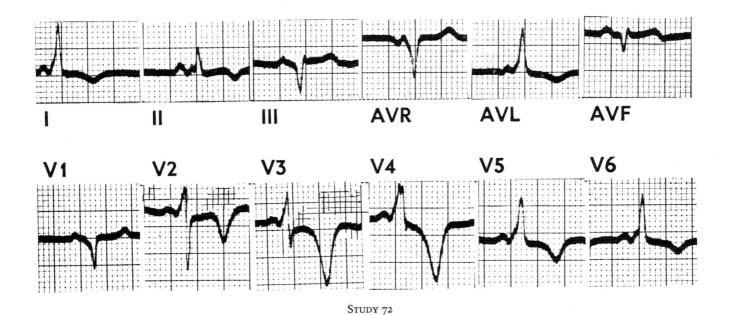

I   II   III   AVR   AVL   AVF

V1   V2   V3   V4   V5   V6

Study 72

73

Acute Subendocardial Infarction

Electrocardiogram A was recorded from a 49-year-old man with a typical clinical and biochemical (enzyme) presentation of acute myocardial infarction.

The acute subendocardial infarction is reflected by:

(a) the depressed S-T segments, and

(b) the inverted *T* waves which are widened and of increased magnitude, in Standard leads II and III, lead AVF and leads V1–V6.

The S-T segment vector is directed posteriorly and at −140°. The *T* wave vector is directed posteriorly and at −100°. The small initial *q* waves are absent from the left precordial leads, but the QRS complexes are otherwise unaffected.

The manifestation is analogous to (a) the hyperacute early injury phase of transmural or dominant epicardial infarction, and (b) the variant form of angina pectoris. In this case, however, the endocardium rather than the epicardium is dominantly affected. Hence the presentation is the mirror-image of the S-T segment slope-elevation and the increased and widened *T* wave which is typical of the early hyperacute injury phase of epicardial infarction (Electrocardiogram B).

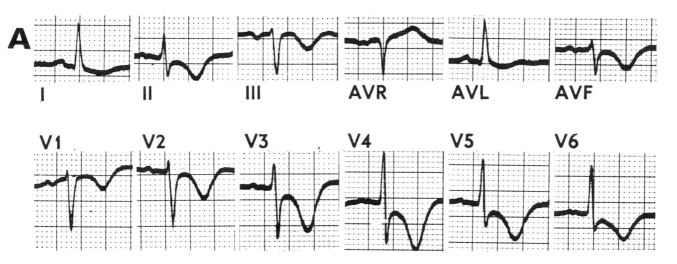

STUDY 73A

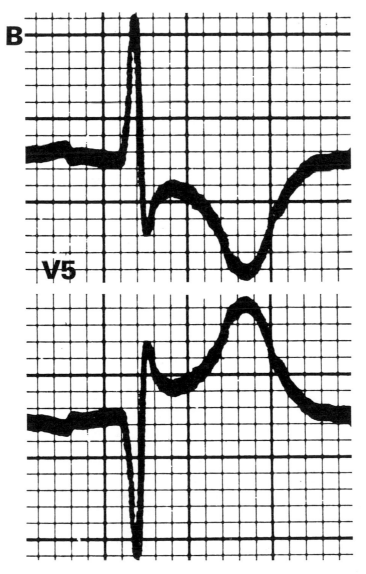

V5

STUDY 73B

74

Acute Subendocardial Infarction

The electrocardiogram was recorded from a 51-year-old man with a typical clinical and biochemical (enzyme) presentation of myocardial infarction. The tracing shows the features usually associated with acute subendocardial infarction.

1. The S-T segment is depressed with a downward, slightly convex-upward slope in Standard leads I and II, and leads AVL, V5 and V6. The S-T segment vector is directed at ±180 degrees and flush with the frontal plane.

2. The T waves are widened and inverted in Standard lead I and leads AVL, V5 and V6. The T wave axis is directed at ±150 degrees on the frontal plane and slightly anteriorly.

COMMENT

1. The S-T segment depression with inverted T wave is the mirror-image of the hyperacute early injury phase of dominant subepicardial infarction or the variant angina pectoris. See also Electrocardiographic Study 73.

2. These features regressed within a week.

75

Acute Extensive Subendocardial Infarction

The electrocardiogram was recorded from a 49-year-old man with a typical clinical and biochemical (enzyme) presentation of myocardial infarction. The tracing shows the features commonly associated with acute subendocardial infarction:

1. The S-T segment is depressed with a downward convex-upward slope in Standard leads I, II and III, and leads AVF and V2-V6. The S-T segment vector is directed posteriorly and at −100 degrees on the frontal plane hexaxial reference system.

2. The T waves are widened and inverted in Standard leads I, II and III, and leads AVF, and V2-V6. The T wave axis is directed posteriorly and at −110 degrees on the frontal plane hexaxial reference system.

COMMENT

1. The S-T segment depression with inverted T wave, best seen in Standard leads II and III, leads AVF and V2-V5, is the mirror-image of classic electrocardiographic presentation of the hyperacute early injury phase of dominant subepicardial infarction of the variant angina pectoris. See also Electrocardiographic Studies 73 and 74.

2. These features regressed within 10 days.

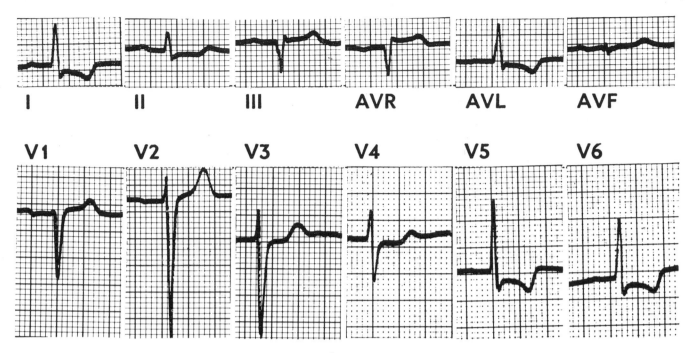

I   II   III   AVR   AVL   AVF

V1   V2   V3   V4   V5   V6

STUDY 74

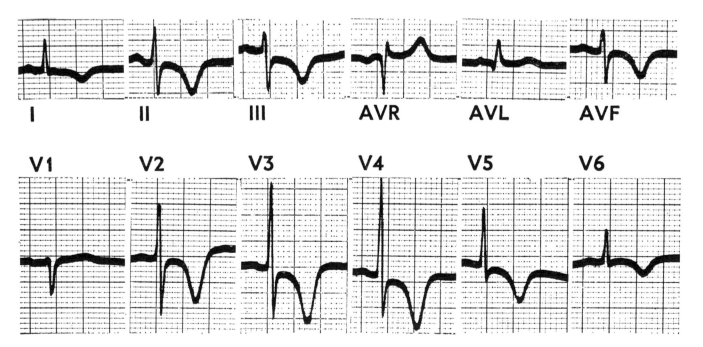

I   II   III   AVR   AVL   AVF

V1   V2   V3   V4   V5   V6

STUDY 75

76

Extensive Regressing Subendocardial Infarction

The electrocardiogram was recorded from a 49-year-old woman with severe diabetes mellitus on the fifth day following a classic clinical and biochemical presentation of acute myocardial infarction. It shows the electrocardiographic features commonly associated with regressing subendocardial infarction.

1. The S-T segments are depressed and concave-upward in Standard leads I and II, and in leads AVL, AVF, V4–V6. The S-T segments are reciprocally elevated in leads AVR and V1. The S-T segments vector is directed at −140° on the frontal plane hexaxial reference system, and is almost flush with the frontal plane.

2. The T waves are isoelectric in most leads, thereby indicating the regression from the acute phase (compare Electrocardiographic Studies 73 and 74). The abnormal features resolved completely 1 week later.

3. The S-T segments are, in effect, the mirror-image of acute anterior wall epicardial infarction.

77

Normal Electrocardiogram Simulating Pathological S-T Segment Horizontality

The electrocardiogram is normal. The mean manifest frontal plane QRS axis is directed at +50°. The mean manifest T wave axis is directed at 0°. The T wave is consequently negative in Standard lead III and positive in Standard lead I. Standard lead II reflects a transition T wave which effects the appearance of S-T segment horizontality. This horizontality, unlike pathological S-T segment horizontality, was only present in this one transition lead.

78

Coronary Insufficiency. Inferior Wall Subendocardial Injury and Ischaemia

The electrocardiogram (Standard lead II) was recorded from a 57-year-old man with angina pectoris. The presence of coronary insufficiency is evident from the following:

1. The T wave is tall, sharply pointed, and symmetrical.

2. The U wave is isoelectric, and consequently invisible.

3. There is junctional S-T segment depression. This S-T segment is, however, significant since the parabola (dotted line), joining the P-R segment, the S-T segment, and the proximal limb of the T wave, is broken.

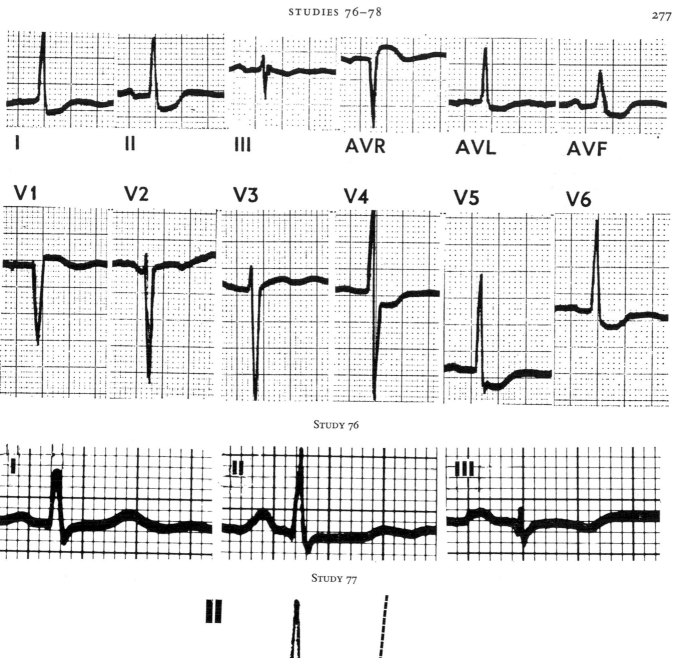

I   II   III   AVR   AVL   AVF

V1   V2   V3   V4   V5   V6

STUDY 76

STUDY 77

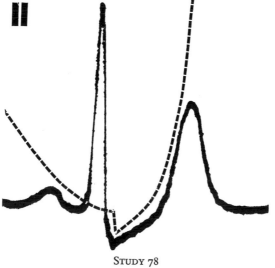

II

STUDY 78

79

Chronic Coronary Insufficiency

The electrocardiogram reflects the presence of chronic coronary insufficiency as evidenced by 1 mm plane S-T segment depression with sharp angled ST-T junction, and an inverted *U* wave.

80

Acute Coronary Insufficiency. Acute Apical Subendocardial Myocardial Injury

The electrocardiogram was recorded during an attack of angina pectoris and shows the following:

(a) *Sinus tachycardia.* The rate is 125 beats/min.

(b) *Acute subendocardial injury.* This is reflected by the marked plane depression of the S-T segments with sharp angled ST-T junction in leads V4–V6, Standard leads I and II, and lead AVL. Lead AVR shows reciprocal elevation of the S-T segment. The mean manifest frontal plane S-T segment vector is directed at $-150°$.

COMMENT

The subendocardial injury is dominantly apical, as evidenced by the S-T segment depression in the left lateral leads, and the typical S-T segment vector deviation to $-150°$. This reflects the classic localization usually associated with angina pectoris.

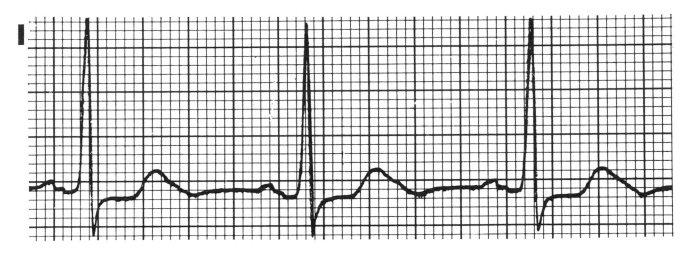

STUDY 79

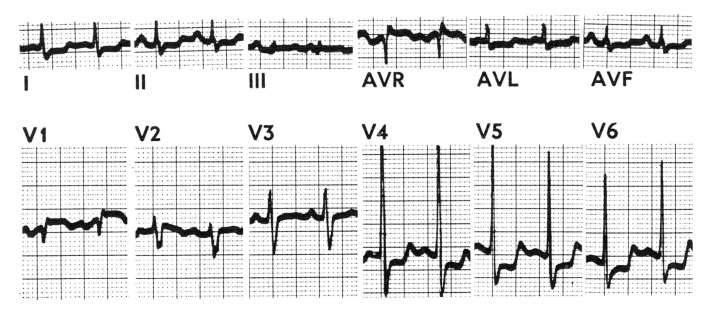

STUDY 80

81

Chronic Coronary Insufficiency

The electrocardiogram shows the signs of chronic coronary insufficiency as evidenced by the following:

(a) Rather tall and symmetrical *T* waves in Standard leads II and III, lead AVF and leads V2–V6. This indicates anterior and inferior wall subendocardial myocardial ischaemia.

(b) The tendency to horizontality of the S-T segment with a sharp angled ST-T junction in Standard leads II and III, and lead AVF. Note that the S-T segment in Standard lead III and lead AVF tends to hug the baseline for the relatively long period of about 0·12 sec. (3 mm.).

82

Chronic Coronary Insufficiency. Chronic Subendocardial Injury

The electrocardiogram was recorded from a 54-year-old diabetic patient with extensive xanthomatosis. The presence of chronic coronary insufficiency is reflected by plane or sagging S-T segment depression, and sharp angled ST-T junction in Standard leads II and III, and lead AVF, and leads V2–V6. The *U* wave is rather flat or absent in these leads.

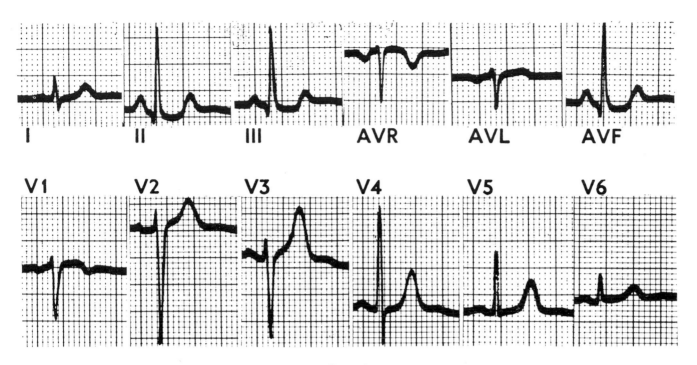

STUDY 81

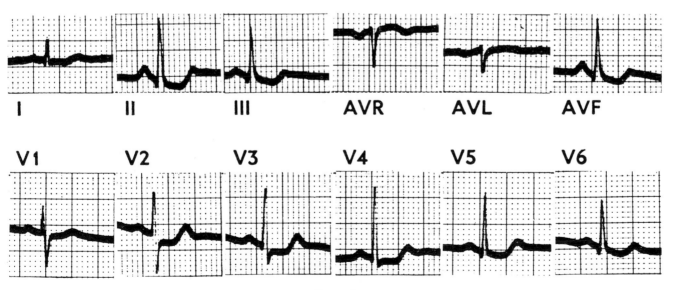

STUDY 82

83

Chronic Coronary Insufficiency

The electrocardiogram shows the manifestations of chronic coronary insufficiency, which is evident from the following manifestations:

(a) The *T* waves are symmetrical and pointed in Standard leads II and III, lead AVF, and leads V3–V6.

(b) There is horizontality of the S-T segment with a tendency to a sharp angled ST-T junction in Standard lead II and leads AVL, V5 and V6.

(c) The *U* wave is inverted in Standard leads II and III and leads AVF, V4, V5 and V6.

(d) There is a tendency to a wide mean manifest frontal plane QRS-T angle; an angle of 70°. The mean manifest frontal plane QRS axis is directed at about −10°, whereas the mean manifest frontal plane *T* wave axis is directed at +60°.

COMMENT

These features indicate the presence of subendocardial apical and inferior wall myocardial injury and ischaemia.

84

Chronic Coronary Insufficiency

Electrocardiogram A shows some manifestations of chronic coronary insufficiency, which is evident from the following:

(a) The *T* waves are rather tall in leads V2–V5.

· (b) The *T* waves tend to be symmetrical and sharply pointed in Standard leads I and II, and leads AVF, V2–V6.

(c) The *U* waves are low to inverted throughout. The inversion is well seen in lead V5, an enlargement of which is shown in Electrocardiogram B.

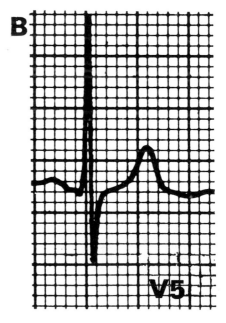

STUDY 84B

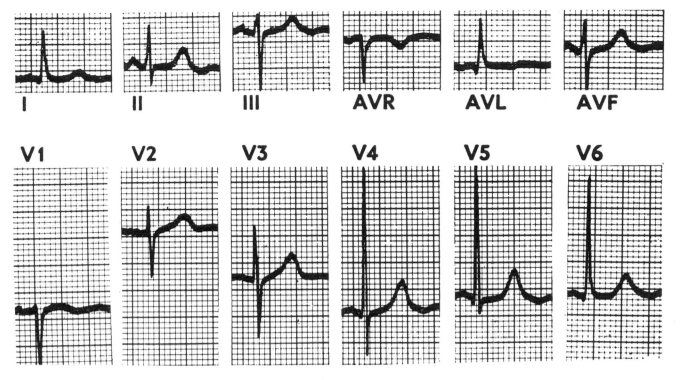

STUDY 83

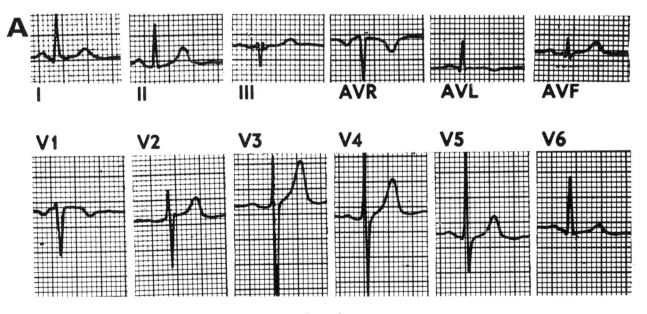

STUDY 84A

85

Extensive Subendocardial Ischaemia

The electrocardiogram was recorded from a 58-year-old man with frequent attacks of angina pectoris, and reflects the features of extensive subendocardial ischaemia. This is evident from the tall, peaked and symmetrical *T* waves in Standard leads I and II, and leads AVL, AVF and V2–V6. The subendocardial ischaemia involves the anterior wall and extends into the lateral (superior) and inferior walls.

COMMENT

The patient developed a typical extensive anterior wall infarction 3 weeks later.

87

A Comparative Study of the S-T Segment and T Wave Abnormalities of Coronary Insufficiency, Left Ventricular Strain, and Digitalis Effect

Electrocardiogram A reflects the pattern of coronary insufficiency. The *T* wave is symmetrical, sharply pointed and deep. The S-T segment hugs the baseline for the relatively long period of 0·24 sec.

Electrocardiogram B reflects the pattern of left ventricular hypertrophy and strain. The strain is manifested by the depressed minimally concave-upward S-T segment which leaves the QRS complex immediately, i.e. it is not isoelectric for any period. The inverted *T* wave is blunt, not particularly deep, and *a*symmetrical.

Electrocardiogram C reflects the pattern of digitalis effect. The depressed S-T segment is not isoelectric for any period. It shows a straight downward slope with a sharp terminal rise, the mirror-image of a check or correction mark. The inverted *T* wave is very blunt.

86

Extensive Subendocardial Ischaemia

The electrocardiogram was recorded from a 66-year-old man with chronic angina pectoris, and reflects the features of extensive subendocardial ischaemia. This is evident from the tall, peaked and symmetrical *T* waves in Standard leads II and III, and leads AVF, V2–V6. The presence of these *T* waves in the inferior as well as the anterior orientated leads connotes an extensive subendocardial 'rind' of ischaemia.

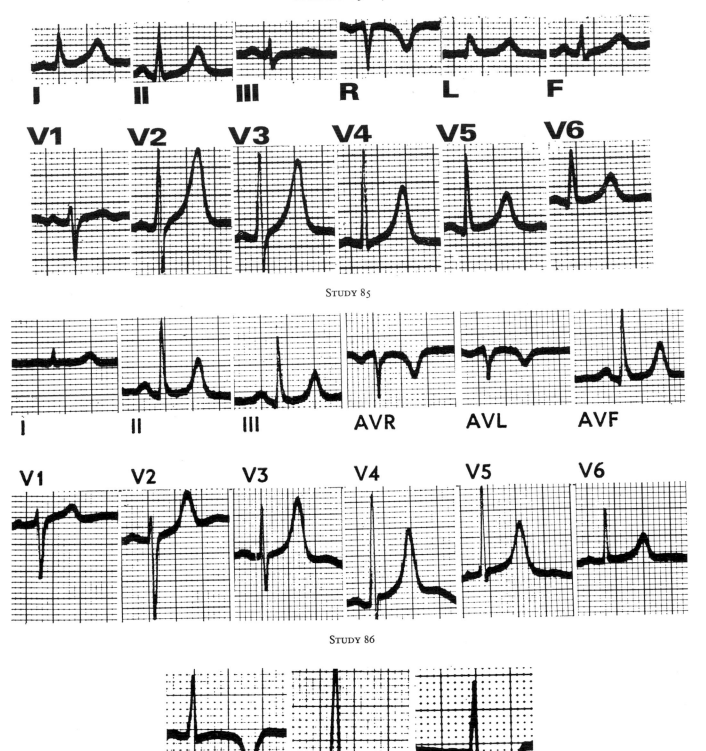

STUDY 85

STUDY 86

STUDY 87

88

Anterolateral Epicardial Ischaemia. Wide Frontal and Horizontal Plane QRS-T Angles

The electrocardiogram reflects anterolateral myocardial ischaemia as evidenced by the inverted and symmetrical T waves in Standard lead I, and leads AVL, V5 and V6. The T waves are upright and symmetrical in the right precordial leads, V1–V3.

These features represent wide frontal and horizontal plane QRS-T angles. The mean manifest frontal plane QRS axis is directed at +30° and the mean manifest frontal plane T wave is directed at +150°, thereby resulting in the very wide frontal plane QRS-T angle of 120°. In the horizontal plane, the dominant T wave axis is directed to the right, whereas the dominant QRS axis is directed to the left.

89

Coronary Insufficiency. Wide Frontal and Horizontal Plane QRS-T Angles. T V1 Taller than T V6 Syndrome

The electrocardiogram was recorded from a 56-year-old man, a heavy smoker, with frequent attacks of angina pectoris.

The electrocardiogram shows the stigmata of coronary insufficiency as reflected by the following:

1. There is a wide frontal plane QRS-T angle of 100°. The mean manifest frontal plane T wave axis is directed at +40°. The mean manifest frontal plane T wave axis is directed at −60°. This results in negative T waves in Standard leads II and III, and lead AVF.

2. The T waves tend to be rather symmetrical and pointed in Standard leads II and III, and lead AVF.

3. The S-T segments tend to be isoelectric, i.e. they tend to hug the baseline for a relatively long period, in Standard leads II and III, and lead AVF.

4. There is a tendency to a wide frontal plane QRS-T angle. The T wave axis is directed towards the right, resulting in T waves which are taller in the right precordial leads than in the left precordial leads; the T V1 taller than T V6 syndrome.

5. The T waves tend to be tall and symmetrical and sharply pointed in the precordial leads.

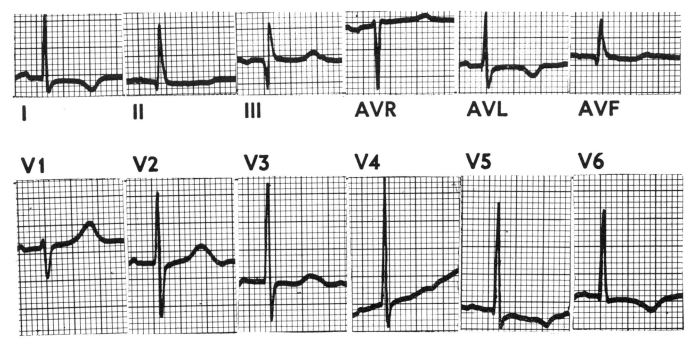

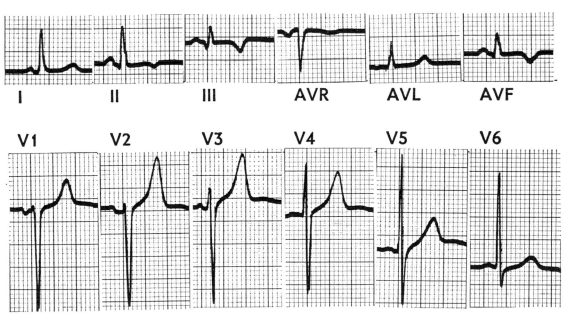

STUDY 89

90

The Variant Form of Angina Pectoris (Prinzmetal's, Atypical, Angina Pectoris) Manifesting in Complicating Ventricular Extrasystoles

The electrocardiograms were recorded from a 59-year-old woman who presented with a history of recurrent attacks of severe angina pectoris.

Electrocardiogram A was recorded at rest, and when the patient was asymptomatic. The tracing is equivocal. The T waves tend to be a little symmetrical in Standard lead I and II, and leads V2–V6. There is also a tendency to horizontality of the S-T segment in Standard lead I and lead V6. The normal initial small q waves are absent in the left lateral leads, leads V4–V6, and Standard lead I, suggesting the possible presence of early incomplete left bundle branch block.

Electrocardiogram B (a continuous strip of lead V6) was recorded a few seconds later and concomitant with the development of severe spontaneous substernal chest pain. The pain had, in fact, begun when lead V6 of Electrocardiogram A was being recorded. The sinus rhythm is now complicated by ventricular extrasystoles. The conducted sinus beats now clearly reflect a 1½ mm. S-T segment elevation. The associated T waves have maintained their symmetry, which is perhaps a little more marked than in Electrocardiogram A. The ventricular extrasystoles reflect these changes, as primary S-T segment and T wave changes (see below) more clearly. The S-T segments are markedly elevated to about 3 mm. The S-T segment configuration is clearly horizontal with a very sharp angled ST-T junction. The associated T waves are tall and very symmetrical. No ensuing U wave is visible, thereby indicating a flattening of the U wave. In fact, there may be an ensuing depression, indicating some U wave inversion.

The fourth ventricular extrasystole is slightly different. It has a shorter coupling interval (0·42 sec as compared with the coupling interval of 0·49 sec of the other ventricular extrasystoles). The S-T segment reflects a greater elevation, 4 mm. The ensuing T wave is less marked. The ensuing U wave reflects a clear inversion. The most striking feature, however, is the development of a small initial q wave, followed by a tall R wave, taller than those of the other ventricular extrasystoles. These abnormal changes regressed within a few seconds to that of the pattern shown in Electrocardiogram A.

Electrocardiogram C was recorded the next day, and reflects coved and elevated S-T segments with inverted symmetrical T waves in leads V2–V6. The QRS complexes reflect a slightly lower R wave in lead V6 than in either electrocardiogram A or Electrocardiogram B, but otherwise reflect no change from that of tracing A. The tracing represents an anterolateral subepicardial infarction.

COMMENT

The electrocardiographic manifestations of the variant form of angina pectoris are, in this case, more obvious and more definitive in the ectopic beat than in the conducted sinus beat.

91

The Electrocardiographic Features of the Variant Form of Angina Pectoris: Atypical, Prinzmetal's, Angina, Precipitated by the Exercise Test[S34]
(Courtesy of Dr M.M.Suzman)

The electrocardiograms were recorded from a 47-year-old man with angina pectoris.

Leads V4 and V5 of Electrocardiogram A were recorded at rest. The T wave is possibly a little symmetrical in lead V5, and there is a tendency to a T-U dip in both leads; but the tracings are essentially within normal limits.

Leads V4 and V5 of Electrocardiogram B were recorded immediately after exercise and show the following abnormal features:

(a) The S-T segments are markedly elevated in lead V4.

(b) The T waves are increased in magnitude in lead V4.

(c) The T waves are more symmetrical in both leads V4 and V5.

(d) The U waves are inverted in leads V4 and V5.

(e) There are 3 consecutive extrasystoles in lead V4, and four consecutive extrasystoles in lead V5. The first of these ventricular extrasystoles tends to resemble the conducted sinus impulse, whereas the ensuing ones are more bizarre. These extrasystoles are probably A-V nodal in origin with the bizarre complexes showing aberration of right bundle branch block with left anterior hemiblock. They, therefore, probably constitute paroxysms of extrasystolic A-V nodal tachycardia. The alternative diagnosis of extrasystolic ventricular tachycardia cannot be excluded with certainty.

COMMENT

These manifestations of the variant form of angina pectoris may occur spontaneously, and may also be precipitated by the exercise test.

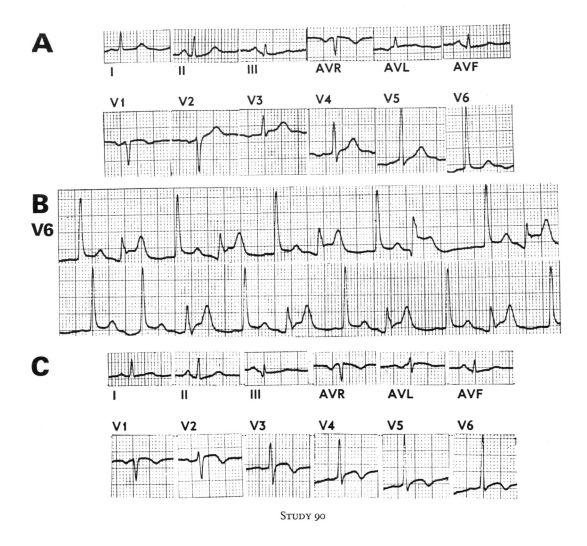

A

I   II   III   AVR   AVL   AVF

V1   V2   V3   V4   V5   V6

B

V6

C

I   II   III   AVR   AVL   AVF

V1   V2   V3   V4   V5   V6

STUDY 90

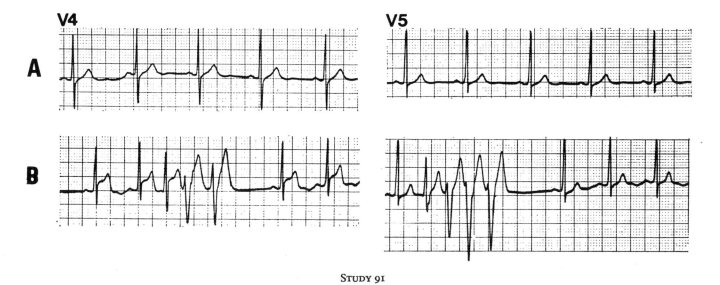

V4   V5

A

B

STUDY 91

92

Acute Subendocardial Injury and Ischaemia Precipitated by Exercise

The electrocardiograms (all complexes of Standard lead II) were recorded with the patient at rest, and at ½ minute, 2 minutes, and 4 minutes after effort. They reflect the following:

1. *The control tracing recorded at rest.* This shows a prolonged P-R interval of 0·26 sec. The *T* wave tends to be somewhat symmetrical and there is also a slight tendency towards the formation of a sharp-angled ST-T junction. The *U* wave is rather flattened. These features are equivocal.

2. *The tracing recorded ½ minute after effort.* This shows a shortening of the P-R interval to 0·20 sec with an increase in the height of the *P* wave and a downward-sloping P-R segment. The S-T segment reflects a plane depression of 1·25 mm with a sharp angled ST-T junction. The *T* wave is more symmetrical and sharply pointed. The ensuing *P* wave is superimposed upon, and thus obscures, the *U* wave, due to the sinus tachycardia.

3. *The tracing recorded 2 minutes after effort.* This shows essentially the same features as the ½ minute tracing. However, the sinus rate has slowed and the *P* wave is no longer superimposed upon the *U* wave which is clearly inverted.

4. *The tracing recorded 4 minutes after effort.* This tracing is essentially the same as the control tracing.

COMMENT

The plane depression, sharp angled ST-T junction, symmetrical *T* waves and inverted *U* wave are clear manifestations of acute subendocardial injury and ischaemia and constitute an abnormal response to exercise.

93

Coronary Insufficiency. Acute Subendocardial Injury. Abnormal Exercise Test

Electrocardiogram a (Standard lead II) was recorded at rest. The *P* wave, QRS complex, S-T segment and *T* wave are all within normal limits. Note how the S-T segment leaves the baseline immediately after the QRS complex and blends smoothly and imperceptibly with the proximal limb of the *T* wave. The *U* wave is not visible and is probably isoelectric.

Electrocardiogram b (Standard lead II) was recorded immediately after effort, and reflects an abnormal response. It shows 0·75 mm *plane depression* with a sharp angled ST-T junction. The S-T segment is horizontal for over 3 mm. The *P* wave is minimally taller and the P-Ta segment has a downward slope.

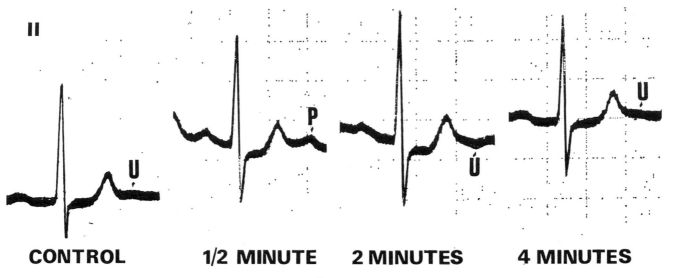

CONTROL   1/2 MINUTE   2 MINUTES   4 MINUTES

Study 92

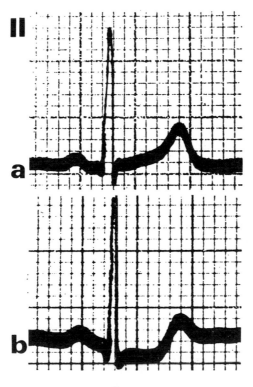

Study 93

94

Acute Coronary Insufficiency. An Abnormal Exercise Test

The electrocardiograms were recorded from a 52-year-old man with a history of angina pectoris.

Electrocardiogram A was recorded at rest and is equivocal but nevertheless suggestive of coronary insufficiency.

1. The *T* waves in leads V2 to V6, and Standard leads II and III, and lead AVF are rather tall and symmetrical.

2. The *U* waves are rather flat in the left precordial leads. Lead V4 reflects a T-U dip or possibly frank *U* wave inversion.

Electrocardiogram B was recorded after the exercise test which precipitated an attack of angina pectoris, and reflects a markedly abnormal response. This is evidenced by the plane depression with sharp angled ST-T junction in leads V3–V6, Standard leads I and II, and lead AVF. The S-T segment depression is most marked in lead V4, measuring 3 mm.

95

Acute Coronary Insufficiency. Acute Subendocardial Injury Associated with Right Bundle Branch Block
(Courtesy of Dr M.M.Suzman)

Leads V5 and V6 of Electrocardiogram A were recorded at rest, and show the features of uncomplicated right bundle branch block. This is reflected by the wide, notched and slurred terminal *S* waves. The S-T segments are slightly elevated, i.e. they are opposite in direction to the terminal QRS deflection and thus represent a secondary change to the abnormal intraventricular conduction. Note the smooth upward slope of the S-T segment resulting in a blunt, obtuse ST-T junction. The S-T segment leaves the baseline almost immediately, and there is virtually no part of it that is isoelectric.

Leads V5 and V6 of Electrocardiogram B were recorded after the performance of the electrocardiographic exercise test. They reflect the parameter of acute subendocardial injury, as evidenced by the plane depression of the S-T segments and the sharp angled ST-T junction.

COMMENT

Note that the S-T segment is deviated in the *same direction* as the terminal QRS deflection, and hence connotes a primary change.

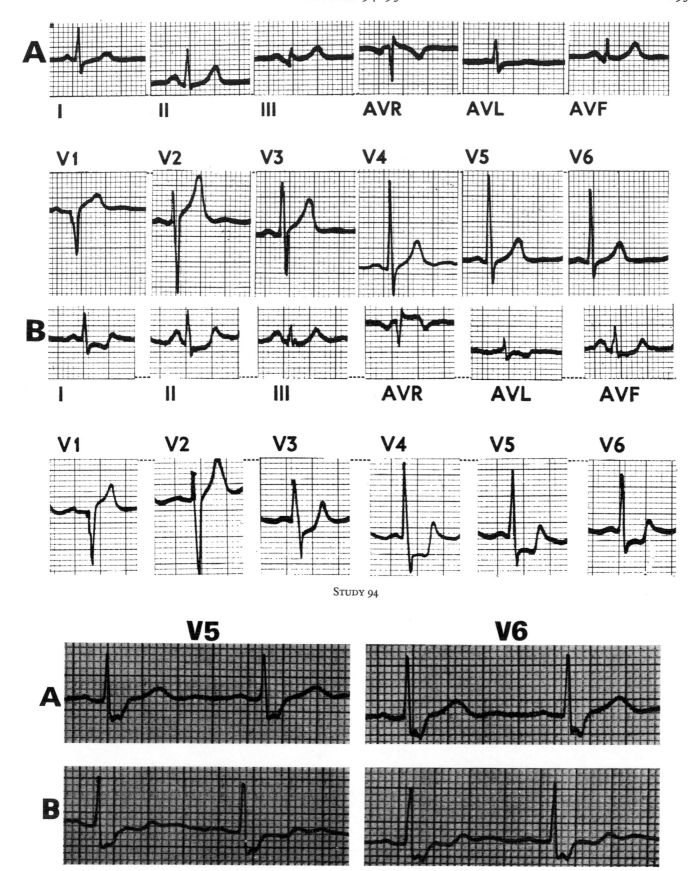

STUDY 94

STUDY 95

96

Coronary Insufficiency. Post-Extrasystolic T Wave Change

The electrocardiogram (continuous strip of lead V1) was recorded from a 60-year-old man with chronic coronary insufficiency, which is evident from the following:

1. There is post-extrasystolic T wave inversion. The third beat in the top strip and the fifth beat in the bottom strip are conducted atrial extrasystoles. The fifth beat in the top strip, the bizarre QRS complex, is a ventricular extrasystole. The conducted sinus beat *following* the long compensatory pause of each of these extrasystoles shows a T wave change. This change consists of marked T wave inversion. The T wave is moreover symmetrical, sharply pointed and arrow-head in appearance, the typical configuration of the coronary T wave.

2. The T wave is dominantly upright in the other conducted sinus beats. Since lead V1 normally reflects a low to inverted T wave, this would indicate a deviation of the T wave axis to the right in the horizontal plane. This reflects a wide QRS-T angle in the horizontal plane and constitutes further corroborative evidence of the coronary insufficiency.

97

Chronic Coronary Insufficiency. Post-extrasystolic U Wave Inversion

The electrocardiogram was recorded from a 47-year-old man with a history suggestive of angina pectoris. The tracing (Standard lead II) was recorded at rest with the patient asymptomatic, and reflects the following changes of myocardial ischaemia:

1. The T waves are tall, symmetrical and sharply pointed.

2. There is first degree A-V block. The P-R interval measures 0·24 sec.

3. There is post-extrasystolic U wave change. The third QRS complex is preceded by a premature and abnormal P' wave, and reflects a conducted atrial extrasystole which is probably interpolated. The two ensuing sinus beats reflect clear evidence of U wave inversion. The first and last beats of the tracing are associated with normal U waves. The distorted baseline between the first and second beats is due to artifact.

98

Acute Pulmonary Embolism[P14]
(Courtesy of Dr M.M.Perlman)

The electrocardiogram was recorded from a 63-year-old man on the eighth postoperative day following cholecystectomy, when he suddenly experienced severe retrosternal pain and dyspnoea, accompanied by cyanosis and collapse. He failed to respond to emergency measures and died 3 hours later. Post-mortem examination revealed a large embolus lodged in the right main pulmonary artery without evidence of coronary artery or myocardial disease.

The Standard leads reveal the classical S1 Q3 T3 pattern; there is a deep S wave in Standard lead I with a Q wave and inverted T wave in Standard lead III. The main QRS frontal plane axis is $+80°$. Right precordial leads V1–V4 show T wave inversion. S-T segment depression of acute pulmonary embolism is evident in Standard leads II and II, and leads V2–V4.

There is slight slurring of the S wave in lead V2. Note the marked diminution in the amplitude as well as flattening of the bottom of the S wave in lead V1.

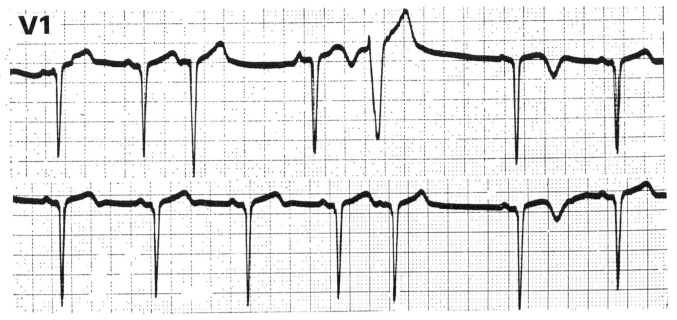

STUDY 96

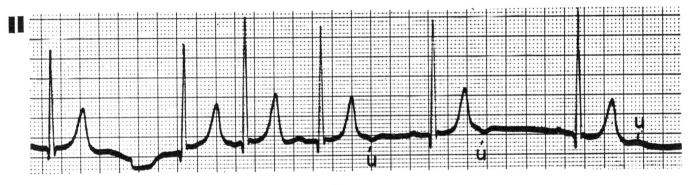

STUDY 97

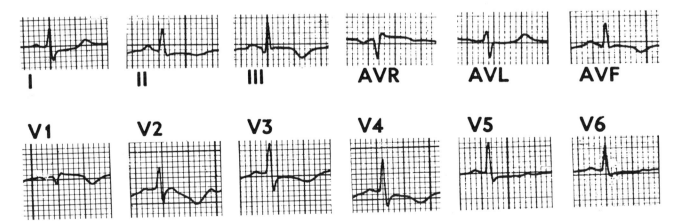

STUDY 98

99

Acute Pericarditis

The electrocardiogram shows the features of acute pericarditis. This is reflected by the following:

(a) The S-T segments are elevated and concave-upward in Standard leads I and II, and leads AVL, AVF, and V2–V6. The S-T segment is isoelectric in Standard lead III and depressed in lead AVR. The mean manifest frontal plane S-T segment vector is directed at +30°.
cavity and base of the biventricular chamber.

(b) The *T* waves are pointed and increased in amplitude in Standard leads I and II, leads AVR, AVL, AVF and V2–V6.

(c) There is sinus tachycardia.

100

Normal Variant: Vagotonia
(Courtesy of Dr D. Wilton)

The electrocardiogram is a normal variant, and shows the features usually associated with vagotonia.

(a) The S-T segments are concave-upward and minimally elevated in Standard leads I, II and III, leads AVL and AVF, and leads V2–V6. The proximal part of the S-T segment is well-marked and hook-like in Standard lead II, lead AVF, and leads V4–V6. Note that the S-T segment elevation is most marked in those leads with the tallest *T* waves, viz. leads V2–V4.

(b) The associated *T* waves are tall and symmetrical.

(c) The associated QRS complexes are of increased amplitude, and show prominent, deep but narrow, initial *q* waves in Standard leads II and III, and lead AVF.

(d) The mean manifest plane QRS and *T* wave axes are similarly directed. The QRS is at +50°, and the *T* wave axis is at +45°, i.e. the QRS-T angle is narrow.

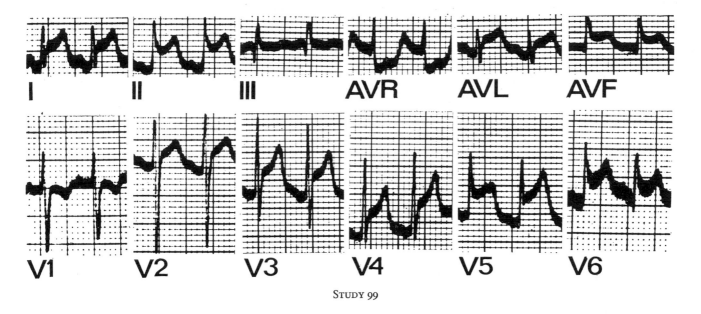

STUDY 99

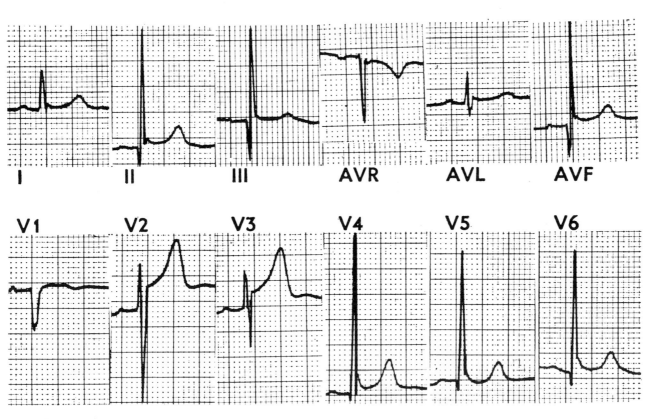

STUDY 100

101

Normal Variant: Vagotonia

The electrocardiogram was recorded from a normal 22-year-old athletic man. It shows the following features:

(a) There is sinus bradycardia with respiratory sinus arrhythmia. The rate varies from 50–55 beats/min.

(b) The S-T segments are slightly elevated in Standard leads I and II, and leads AVF and V1–V6.

(c) There is a proximal hook or positivity to the S-T segments in leads V4–V6.

(d) The *T* waves are relatively tall and tend to be pointed. They are nevertheless still asymmetrical.

(e) There are deep, narrow though prominent, *q* waves, in leads V4–V6.

Note. There is a narrow frontal plane QRS-T angle of 10°. The mean manifest frontal plane QRS axis is directed at +50°, and the mean manifest frontal plane *T* wave axis is directed at +40°.

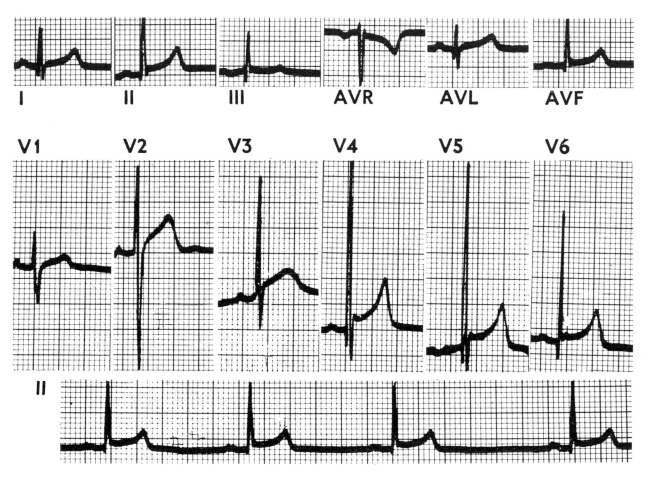

102

Normal Variant. S1 S2 S3 Syndrome
(Courtesy of Dr B.Gentin)

The electrocardiogram was recorded from a thin, anxious young adult man with no evidence of organic disease.

Tracing A recorded at rest, reflects a wide frontal plane QRS-T angle of 110°. The mean manifest frontal plane QRS axis is directed at +80°, and the mean manifest frontal plane T wave axis at −30°. This particular location of the QRS and T wave axes may, in the absence of heart disease, reflect a normal variant, the so-called 'half-past-two' pattern, the T wave axis representing the short arm of the clock and the QRS axis the long arm. The T waves are also inverted in leads V1 and V2, probably representing the persistent 'juvenile' pattern.

Tracing B was recorded after effort, and reflects a normalization of the variant depicted in Tracing A. The QRS axis is still directed at +80°, but the T wave axis is now directed at +30°, thus normalizing the previously inverted T waves in Standard leads II and III, and lead AVF.

Both tracings reflect the S1 S2 S3 syndrome, terminal s waves in all three Standard leads which, in this case, is also a normal variant.

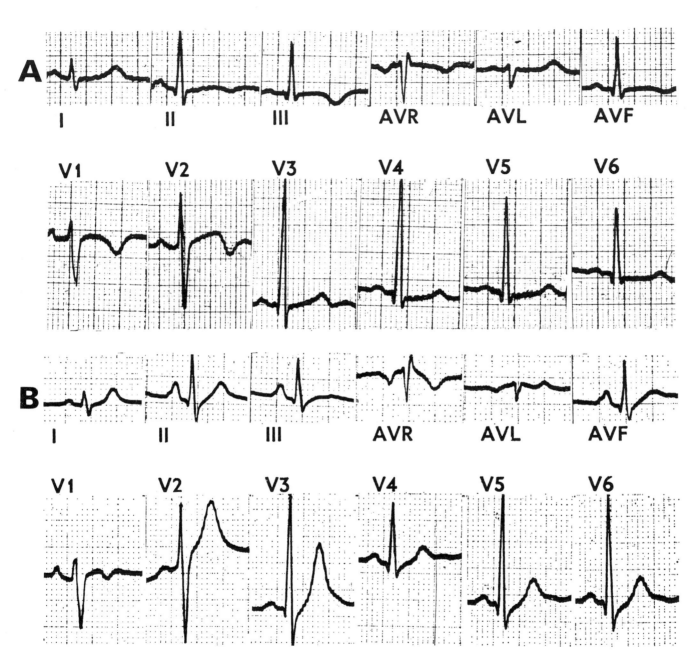

103

Hyperkalaemia

The electrocardiogram was recorded from a patient in chronic renal failure. The serum potassium level was greater than 8 mEq/100 ml.

The hyperkalaemia is evidenced by the following:

(a) Absent *P* waves.

(b) Tall widened *T* waves in Standard leads II and III, and leads AVF, V2–V6, which blend with the widened and bizarre QRS complexes. No clear-cut S-T segment can be defined.

(c) The QRS complexes are bizarre, and widened, resembling the pattern of right bundle branch block with left anterior hemiblock.

104

Hypocalcaemia
(Courtesy of Dr A.Dubb)

The electrocardiogram was recorded from a woman with hypoparathyroidism and a low serum calcium. It shows the following features:

(a) There is a prolonged Q-T interval. The Q-Tc was calculated to be 145 per cent.

(b) The prolongation of the Q-T interval is due to a prolongation of the S-T segment. Note that the *T* wave is not particularly widened. Note, too, that the S-T segment reflects marked horizontality and is isoelectric, hugging the baseline for 6 mm, a relatively long period of 0·24 sec. There is also a tendency to a sharp angled ST-T junction.

COMMENT

Although coronary insufficiency can also manifest with horizontality, the S-T segment does not remain isoelectric for as long a period as in hypocalcaemia.

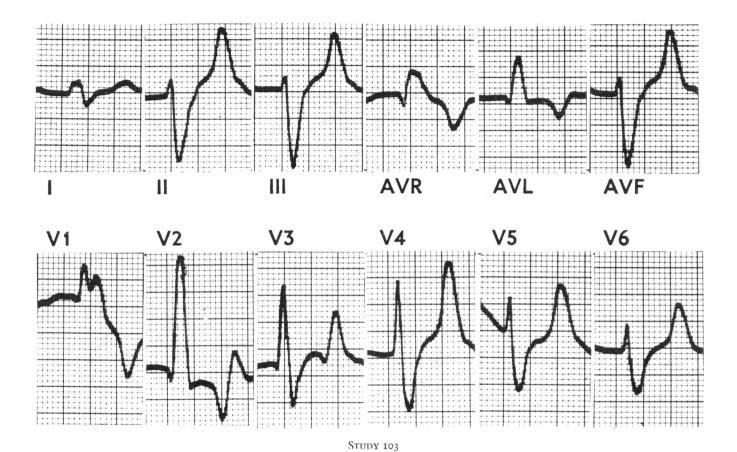

I   II   III   AVR   AVL   AVF

V1   V2   V3   V4   V5   V6

STUDY 103

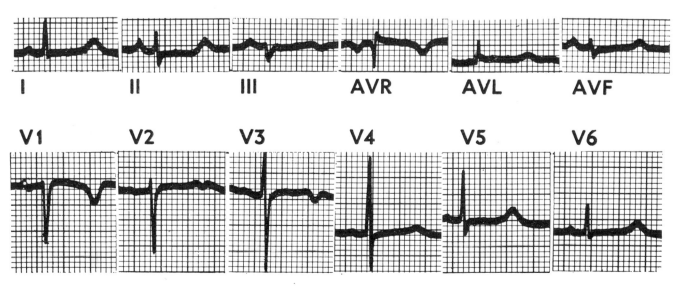

I   II   III   AVR   AVL   AVF

V1   V2   V3   V4   V5   V6

STUDY 104

105

The CVA Pattern

The electrocardiogram was recorded from a 40-year-old man with a subarachnoid haemorrhage. It reflects the electrocardiographic features frequently associated with an intracranial haemorrhage, and is known as the CVA pattern. These are: a prolonged Q-Tc which measured 130 per cent, and tall wide symmetrical *T* waves in Standard leads I, II and III, leads AVL, AVF and V3–V6.

The pattern occurs particularly with haemorrhage of the anterior cranial fossa.

106

Right Bundle Branch Block. Right Ventricular Dominance. Tricuspid Incompetence

The electrocardiogram was recorded from a 26-year-old woman with chronic rheumatic heart disease. She was in cardiac failure with tricuspid incompetence.

The tracing shows right bundle branch block as evidenced by the deep terminal *S* waves in Standard lead I, lead AVL and lead V6, and the *R'* waves in leads V1–V5. The right ventricular dominance is reflected by:

(a) the right axis deviation of the initial 0·04 sec vector which is directed at $+100°$, resulting in tall *R* waves in Standard lead III and lead AVF, and
(b) the initial tall *R* waves in leads V1–V4.

The qR pattern in leads V1 and V2 reflects a positional change as a result of marked right atrial enlargement, and is most commonly due to tricuspid incompetence.

COMMENT

A qR pattern in leads V1 and V2 could also be due to midseptal infarction, but there is no other electrocardiographic or clinical evidence of this.

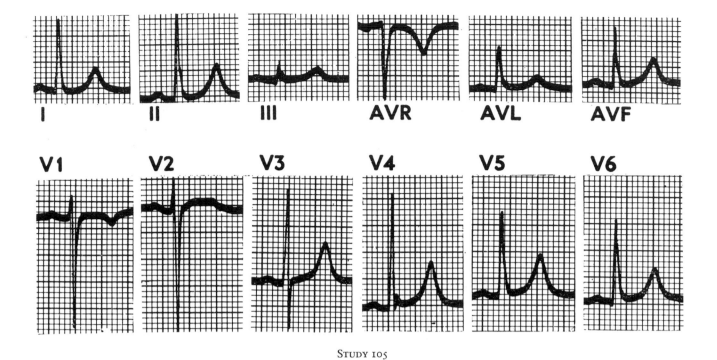

I   II   III   AVR   AVL   AVF

V1   V2   V3   V4   V5   V6

STUDY 105

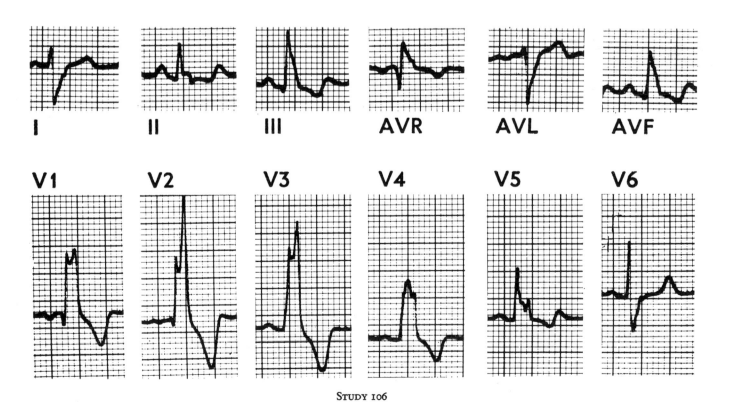

I   II   III   AVR   AVL   AVF

V1   V2   V3   V4   V5   V6

STUDY 106

107

Annular Subvalvular Mitral Aneurysm[C24]

The electrocardiogram was recorded from an 18-year-old man with a congenital annular, subvalvular, mitral aneurysm which was surgically corrected.

The electrocardiogram shows the features of high-lateral infarction and true posterior wall infarction.

The high-lateral infarction is reflected by the pathological Q waves of the QR complexes in Standard lead I and lead AVL, and the coved and elevated S-T segments and symmetrically inverted T waves in Standard lead I and lead AVL.

The true posterior wall myocardial infarction is reflected by the tall R waves and the very tall and widened T waves in the right precordial leads V1–V4. The manifestation was due to pressure of the aneurysm on the left circumflex coronary artery.

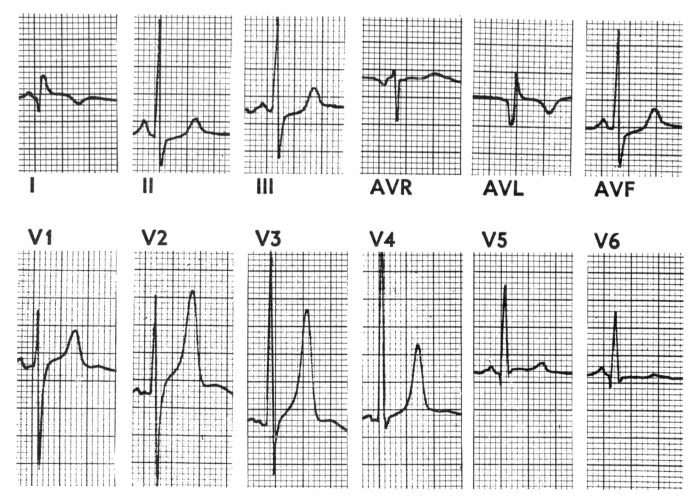

STUDY 107

108

The Erb-Duchenne Type Muscular Dystrophy

The electrocardiogram was recorded from a 12-year-old boy with the Erb-Duchenne type of muscular dystrophy. It reflects the electrocardiographic features usually associated with this disorder.

1. The right precordial leads V1-V3 show tall R waves. This is associated with rather tall and widened T waves in leads V2 and V3.

2. The left lateral leads, leads V5, V6, Standard leads I and II, leads AVL and AVF, reflect prominent initial q waves.

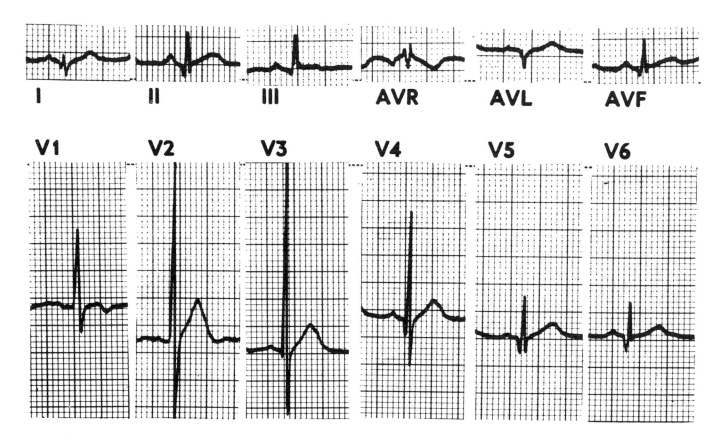

STUDY 108

109

Ventricular Septal Defect

The electrocardiogram reflects the classic features of a ventricular septal defect, a combination of right ventricular systolic overload and left ventricular diastolic overload.

1. The right ventricular systolic overload is reflected by:
(a) the tall *R* waves in leads V1–V3, and
(b) the inverted *T* wave in lead V1.

Note the initial slurring of the R wave in lead V1, a feature commonly seen in right ventricular dominance.

2. The left ventricular diastolic overload is reflected by:
(a) the tall *R* waves in leads V4–V6,
(b) the tall, upright and symmetrical *T* waves, and
(c) the deep but narrow initial *q* waves in leads V4–V6.

3. Note the presence of the Katz-Wachtel phenomenon, large amplitude equiphasic QRS complexes in the midprecordial leads V2–V4. This is characteristically seen in cases of ventricular septal defect.

110

Ventricular Parasystole

The electrocardiogram (continuous strip of lead V1) shows:

1. Normal conducted sinus rhythm. This is represented, for example, by the first and second P-QRS complexes in the second strip. The *P* waves are normal. The P-P intervals measure 0·80 sec, reflecting a rate of 68–75 beats/min. The P-R interval measures 0·16 sec.

2. Ventricular parasystole. This is represented by the premature and bizarre QRS complexes. The independent, parasystolic, character of the ectopic rhythm is evident from the following:

(a) The QRS complexes are unrelated to the *P* waves.

(b) The coupling intervals vary markedly. For example, the coupling interval of the first abnormal QRS complex in the second strip measures 0·87 sec, whereas the coupling interval of the last abnormal QRS complex in the second strip measures 0·50 sec.

(c) Ventricular fusion complexes. These are represented by QRS complexes which have a configuration in between that of the pure ectopic ventricular complex and the pure QRS complex of the conducted sinus beat. These fusion complexes are indicated by the half-shaded circles. The configurations of the fusion complexes vary, depending upon the relative contribution of each pacemaker. For example, the seventh QRS complex is but little changed from the pure conducted sinus complex, and reflects a dominant contribution by the sinus impulse. The other fusion complexes are more bizarre, and reflect a greater contribution by the ectopic pacemaker.

(d) Mathematically related interectopic intervals. The interectopic intervals are all in multiples of 1·33 sec (±0·02 sec), reflecting a close relationship between the ectopic beats. The positions of the ectopic discharges, measured at the calculated ectopic cycle length of 1·33 sec, are indicated by the circles and dots. The black dots indicate the manifest ectopic beats. The open circles indicate the non-manifest ectopic discharges. Note that these non-manifest ectopic discharges occur during the refractory period of the ventricular myocardium consequent to the activation by the sinus impulses, i.e. they occur during the periods represented by the S-T segments and *T* waves of the conducted sinus impulses.

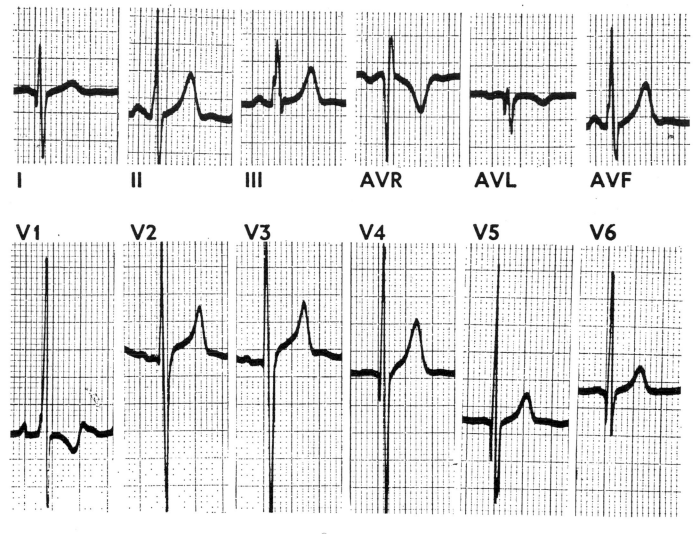

STUDY 109

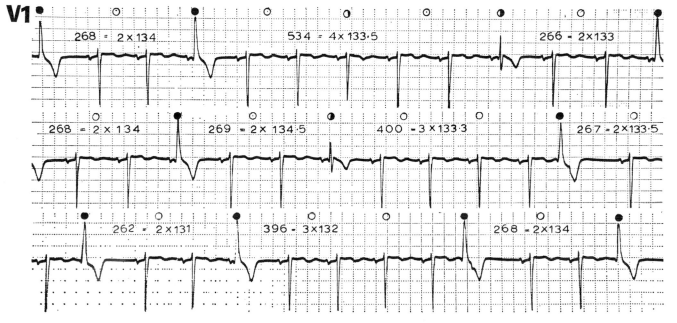

STUDY 110

111

Ventricular Flutter Associated with High-grade A-V Block. Giant T Wave Inversion. The R on T Phenomenon

The electrocardiograms were recorded from a 56-year-old woman with atherosclerotic heart disease and frequent syncopal attacks.

The electrocardiograms show the following:

Features in Standard lead II (continuous strip):

(a) Sinus rhythm. The R-P intervals measure about 0·70 sec, representing a rate of approximately 86 beats/min.

(b) High-grade A-V block. The second, fourth and seventh QRS complexes in the upper strip are preceded by P-R intervals of 0·14 sec, and represent conducted sinus beats. The fifth QRS complex may also represent a conducted sinus beat (with aberration). The third and fourth sinus P waves are not conducted, and are followed by an A-V nodal escape beat.

(c) Ventricular flutter. This is represented by the bizarre QRS complexes. The R-R intervals measure 0·28 sec., reflecting a rate of 214 beats/min. The syncopal attacks in this patient were due to the attacks of ventricular flutter.

(d) Giant inverted *T* waves: see below.

Features in lead V3:
This was also recorded during this period, and shows:

(a) Sinus rhythm with 2:1 A-V block. The P-R intervals of the conducted beats measure 0·14 sec. The *P* waves representing the blocked sinus impulses are superimposed upon the proximal limbs of the large, bizarre 'Giant' *T* waves. The second, fifth and eighth QRS complexes are bizarre, and represent either ventricular extrasystoles or aberrant ventricular conduction of the preceding sinus impulses (thereby reflecting momentary 3:2 A-V conduction).

(b) Giant inverted *T* waves. The *T* waves in lead V3 and Standard lead II are widened and prolonged.

(c) Prolonged Q-T interval. The Q-Tc is markedly prolonged, and measures 200 per cent.

COMMENT

1. The Giant *T* waves with prolonged Q-Tc are the result of syncopal attacks and are virtually pathegnemonic of preceding episodes of unconsciousness.

2. The prolongation of the Q-T interval results in the R on T phenomenon. The coupling intervals of the ventricular extrasystoles are relatively long (0·60 sec). Thus, the prolongation of the Q-T interval to 0·84 sec results in the ventricular extrasystole falling on or near the apex of the *T* wave. This R on T phenomenon precipitates the period of ventricular flutter.

112

Extrasystolic Ventricular Tachycardia

The *P* waves and the P:QRS relationship cannot be accurately identified. The electrocardiogram nevertheless reflects the following features which indicate a diagnosis of extrasystolic ventricular tachycardia.

1. The mean manifest frontal plane axis is directed at −150°. This is a bizarre and unusual axis. In the case of phasic aberrant ventricular conduction the axis would tend to be normally directed.

2. The QRS complexes do not resemble the typical forms of either left or right bundle branch block.

3. The horizontal plane leads reflect the *concordant pattern*; the QRS complexes are upright in *all* the precordial leads.

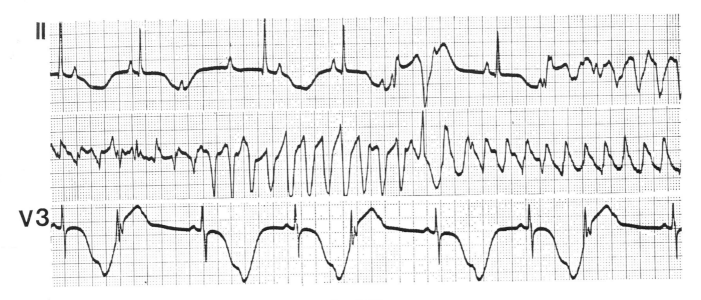

STUDY 111

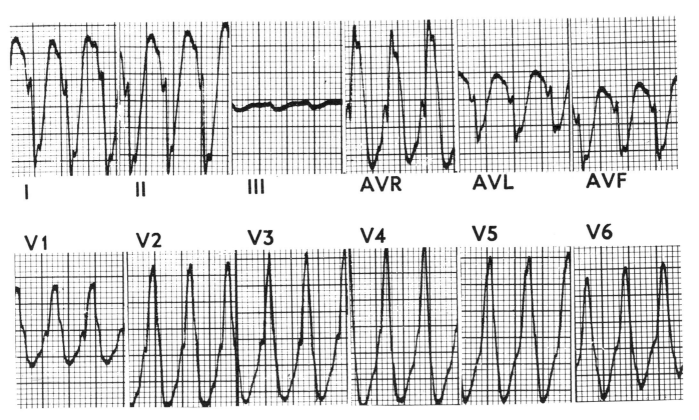

STUDY 112

References

A

A1 ABARQUEZ R.F., FREIMAN A.H., REICHEL F. & LaDUE J.S. (1960) The precordial electrocardiogram during exercise. *Circulation* **22**, 1060.

A2 ABILDSKOV J.A., MILLAR K., BURGESS M.J. & VINCENT, W. (1970) The electrocardiogram and the central nervous system. *Progr. Cardiovasc. Dis.* **13**, 210.

A3 ABRAMSON D.I., FENICHEL N.M. & SHOOKHOFF C. (1938) Study of electrical activity in auricles. *Am. Heart J.* **15**, 471.

A4 ACHESON E.D. (1957) The electrocardiogram after exercise in the detection of latent coronary disease in R.A.F. personnel. *Lancet* **272**, 26.

A5 ADGEY A.A.J., GEDDES J.S., MULHOLLAND H.C., KEEGAN D.A.J. & PANTRIDGE J.F. (1968) Incidence, significance and management of early bradyarrhythmia complicating acute myocardial infarction. *Lancet* **2**, 1097.

A6 ADGEY A.A.J. & PANTRIDGE J.F. (1970) Acute phase of myocardial infarction. *Circulation Suppl.* **3**, 41 and **42**, 96 (Abstr.).

A7 ALESSI R., NUSYNOWITZ M., ABILDSKOV J.A. & MOE G.K. (1958) Non-uniform distribution of vagal effects on the atrial refractory period. *Am. J. Physiol.* **194**, 406.

A8 ALTIERI P. & SCHAAL S.F. (1973) Inferior and anteroseptal myocardial infarction concealed by transient left anterior hemiblock. *J. Electrocardiol.* **6**, 257.

A9 ALZAMORA-CASTRO V., ABUGATTAS R., RUBIO C., BOURONCLE J., ZAPATA C., SANTA-MARIA BATTILANA G., BINDER T., SUBIRIA R. & PAREDAS D. (1953) Parietal focal block: an experimental and electrocardiographic study. *Circulation* **7**, 108.

A10 AMER N.S., STUCKEY J.H., HOFFMAN B.F., CAPPELLETTI R.R. & DOMINGO R.T. (1960) Activation of the interventricular septal myocardium studied during cardiopulmonary bypass. *Am. Heart J.* **59**, 224.

A11 ANGLE W.D. (1958) Myocardial infarction in the W.P.W. syndrome. A method of vector analysis of E.C.G. changes. *Am. Heart J.* **56**, 36.

A12 ANTTONEN V.M., LESKINEN E., MEURMAN L., OKA M. & RAUNIO H. (1962) The diagnostic value of unipolar precordial patterns of ventricular premature beats in myocardial infarction. *Acta Med. Scand. Suppl.* **387**, 1.

A13 ARESKOG, N.H., BJÖRK, L., BJÖRK, V.O., HALLEN, A. & STRÖM, G. (1967) Physical work capacity, ECG reaction to work tests and coronary angiograms in coronary artery disease. *Acta Med. Scand. Suppl.* **472**, 9.

A14 ATTERHÖG J.H., EKELUND L.G. & KAIJSER J. (1971) Electrocardiographic abnormalities during exercise three weeks to eighteen months after anterior myocardial infarction. *Brit. Heart J.* **33**, 871.

A15 AVERBUCK S.H. (1942) Acute generalized postoperative peritonitis simulating coronary artery disease. *J. Mt. Sinai Hosp.* **8**, 335.

B

B1 BAER C.G. (1956) Die maskierung elektrokardiographischer infarktzeichen durch ein W.P.W. syndrom. *Ztschr. Kreislfschg.* **45**, 301.

B2 BAHL O.P., WALSH T.J. & MASSIE E. (1970) Electrocardiography and vectorcardiography in idiopathic hypertrophic subaortic stenosis. *Am. J. Med. Sci.* **259**, 262.

B3 BANTA H.D., GREENFIELD J.C. JR. & ESTES E.H. (1964): Left axis deviation. *Am. J. Cardiol.* **14**, 330.

B4 BARBATO E., DELES A.C., FRUIJOKA T., PILEGGI F., ZERBINI DE J.E. & DECOURT L.V. (1959) Direct epicardial and thoracic leads: their relationship in man. *Am. Heart J.* **58**, 238.

B5 BARGER A.C., HERD J.A. & LIEBOWITZ M.R. (1961) Chronic catheterization of coronary artery: induction of ECG pattern of myocardial ischaemia by intracoronary epinephrine. *Proc. Soc. Exp. Biol. Med.* **107**, 474.

B6 BARKER J.M. & VALENCIA F. (1949) The precordial electrocardiogram in incomplete right bundle branch block. *Am. Heart J.* **38**, 376.

B7 BARKER J.P. & WALLACE J.J. (1952) *The Unipolar Electrocardiogram*, p. 233. New York: Appleton-Century-Crofts.

B8 BARKER P.S., SCHRADER E.L. & RONZONI E. (1939) The effects of alkalosis and of acidosis upon the human electrocardiogram. *Am. Heart J.* **17**, 169.

B9 BARLOW J.B., BOSMAN C.K., POCOCK W.A. & MARCHAND P. (1968) Late systolic murmurs and non-ejection ('mid late') systolic clicks. *Brit. Heart J.* **30**, 203.

B10 BARNES A.R. (1939) *Electrocardiographic Patterns*, p. 43. Springfield, Illinois: Charles C.Thomas.

B11 BARNES A.R. & WHITTEN M.B. (1929) Study of the R-T interval in myocardial infarction. *Am. Heart J.* **5**, 142.

B12 BARROW W.H. & OUER R. (1943) Electrocardiographic changes with exercise. *Arch. Int. Med.* **71**, 547.

B13 BASHOUR F.A., JONES E. & EDMONSON R. (1967) Cardiac arrhythmias in acute myocardial infarction. II. Incidence of the common arrhythmias with special reference to ventricular tachycardia. *Dis. Chest* **5**, 520.

B14 BAUER G.E. (1964) Transient bundle branch block. *Circulation* **29,** 730.

B15 BAUER G.E., JULIAN D.G. & VALENTINE P.A. (1965) Bundle branch block in acute myocardial infarction. *Brit. Heart J.* **27,** 724.

B16 BAUERLEIN T.C. & STOBBE L.H.O. (1954) Acute pancreatitis simulating myocardial infarction with characteristic electrocardiographic changes. *Gastroenterology* **27,** 861.

B17 BAYLEY R.H. (1942) An interpretation of the injury and the ischemic effects of myocardial infarction in accordance with laws which determine the flow of electric currents in homogeneous volume conductors and in accordance with relative pathologic change. *Am. Heart J.* **24,** 514.

B18 BAYLEY R.H. (1958) *Biophysical Principles of Electrocardiography*, Vol. I. New York: Hoeber.

B19 BAYLEY R.H. & LaDUE J.S. (1944) Electrocardiographic changes of impending infarction, and the ischemia-injury pattern produced in the dog by total and subtotal occlusion of a coronary artery. *Am. Heart J.* **28,** 54.

B20 BAYLEY R.H., LaDUE J.S. & YORK D.J. (1944) Electrocardiographic changes (local ventricular ischemia and injury) produced in the dog by temporary occlusion of a coronary artery, showing a new stage in the evolution of myocardial infarction. *Am. Heart J.* **27,** 164.

B21 BEAN W.B. (1938) Infarction of Heart: Clinical course and morphological findings. *Ann. Int. Med.* **12,** 71.

B22 BECK R.N. & MONTGOMERY D.A.D. (1957) Treatment of hypopituitrism. *Brit. Med. J.* **1,** 441.

B23 BECKNER G.L. & WINSOR T. (1954) Cardiovascular adaptations to prolonged physical effort. *Circulation* **9,** 835.

B24 BEDFORD D.E. & THOMAS G. (1954) The sickle-shaped R-T plateau. A common RS-T pattern in health. *Brit. Heart J.* **16,** 469.

B25 BEFELER B., GOMEZ J., AGHA A.S. & CASTELLANOS A. JR. (1971) Changes in the inferior wall myocardial infarction pattern produced by acute fascicular block. *Circulation* **44** (*Suppl. II*), 11–63 (Abstr.).

B26 BELLET S., DELIYIANNIS S. & ELIAKIM M. (1961) The electrocardiogram during exercise as recorded by radio-electrocardiography: Comparison with the post-exercise electrocardiogram (Master two-step test). *Am. J. Cardiol.* **8,** 385.

B27 BELLET S., ELIAKIM M., DELIYIANNIS S. & FIGALLO E.M. (1962) Radioelectrocardiographic changes during strenuous exercise in normal subjects. *Circulation* **25,** 686.

B28 BELLET S., ELIAKIM M., DELIYIANNIS S. & LA VAN D. (1962) Radioelectrocardiography during exercise in patients with angina pectoris. Comparison with the postexercise electrocardiogram. *Circulation* **25,** 5.

B29 BELLET S., MULLER O.F., HERRING A.B. & LA VAN, D. (1963) Effect of erythrotil tetranitrate on the electrocardiogram as recorded during exercise by radioelectrocardiography. *Am. J. Cardiol.* **11,** 600.

B30 BELLET S., ROMAN L.R., NICHOLS G.J. & MULLER O.F. (1967) Detection of coronary-prone subjects in a normal population by radioelectrocardiographic exercise tests. *Am. J. Cardiol.* **19,** 783.

B31 BENCHIMOL A. & BARRETO E.C. (1969) Serial vectorcardiograms with the Frank system in patients with acute inferior wall myocardial infarction. *J. Electrocardiol.* **2,** 159.

B32 BENCHIMOL A., BARRETO E.C. & PEDRAZA A. (1971) The Frank vectorcardiogram in left anterior hemiblock. *J. Electrocardiol.* **4,** 116.

B33 BENCHIMOL A. & DESSER K.B. (1972) Co-existing left anterior hemiblock and inferior wall myocardial infarction. *Am. J. Cardiol.* **29,** 7.

B34 BENCHIMOL A., LEGLER J.F. & DIMOND E.G. (1963) The carotid tracing and apex cardiogram in subaortic stenosis and idiopathic myocardial hypertrophy. *Am. J. Cardiol.* **11,** 427.

B35 BENGTSSON E. (1956) The exercise electrocardiogram in healthy children and in comparison with adults. *Acta med. Scand.* **154,** 225.

B36 BENGTSSON E. (1956) Working capacity and exercise electrocardiogram in convalescence after acute infectious diseases without cardiac complications. *Acta med. Scand.* **154,** 359.

B37 BEREGOVICH J., FENIG S. & LASSERS J. (1969) Management of acute myocardial infarction complicated by advanced atrioventricular block: role of artificial pacing. *Am. J. Cardiol.* **23,** 54.

B38 BERKMAN F. & ROY O.Z. (1969) Estimation of internal cancellation effects during ventricular depolarisation. In *Electrical Activity of the Heart*, ed. Manning G.W. & Ahuja S.P. p. 106. Springfield, Illinois: Charles C.Thomas.

B39 BERMAN R., SIMONSON E. & HERON W. (1954) Electrocardiographic effects associated with hypnotic suggestion in normal and coronary sclerotic individuals. *J. Appl. Physiol.* **7,** 89.

B40 BERNART W.F. & DE ANDINO A.M. (1958) Electrocardiographic changes in hypopituitarism of pregnancy. *Am. Heart J.* **55,** 231.

B41 BERNREITER M. (1958) Cardiac amyloidosis. *Am. J. Cardiol.* **1,** 644.

B42 BERSANO E., DICOSKY C. & ZIMMERMAN H.A. (1968) Left atrial infarction. *Dis. Chest* **54,** 249.

B43 BEYER E., TOTH L.A. & ASHMAN R. (1947) Electrocardiographic changes induced by cooling or warming the inner surface of the dog's ventricle. *Am. J. Physiol.* **149,** 264.

B44 BIBERMAN L., SARMA R.N. & SURAWICZ B. (1971) T wave abnormalities during hyperventilation and isoproterenol infusion. *Am. Heart J.* **81,** 166.

B45 BIERRING E., LARSEN K. & NIELSEN E. (1936) Some cases of slow pulse associated with electrocardiographic changes in cardiac patients after maximal work on the Krogh ergometer. *Am. Heart J.* **11,** 416.

B46 BIÖRCK G.S. (1946) Anoxemia and exercise tests in diagnosis of coronary disease. *Am. Heart J.* **32,** 689.

B47 BISTENI A., MEDRANO G.A. & SODI-PALLARES D. (1961) Ventricular premature beats in the diagnosis of myocardial infarction. *Brit. Heart J.* **23,** 521.

B48 BISTENI A., SODI-PALLARES D., MEDRANO G.A. & PILEGGI, F. (1960) A new approach for the recognition of ventricular premature beats. *Am. J. Cardiol.* **5,** 358.

B49 BISTENI A., TESTELLI M.R., DE MICHELI A. & MEDRANO G.A. (1961) La activation ventricular y las morfologias unipolares en condiciones normales y en los bloqueos de rama. *Cardiologia, Homenaje al Dr. Demetrio Sodi-Pallares*. Mexico: Ed. Interamericana S.A.

B50 BITTAR N. & SOSA J.O. (1968) The billowing mitral valve leaflet: report on fourteen patients. *Circulation* **38,** 763.

B51 BLACKBURN H., KEYS A., SIMONSON E., RAUTAHARJU P. & PUNSAR S. (1960) The electrocardiogram in population studies. *Circulation* **21,** 1160.

B52 BLACKBURN H., TAYLOR H.L. & KEYS A. (1970) The electrocardiogram in prediction of five-year coronary heart disease incidence among men aged forty through fifty-nine. In

Coronary Heart Disease in Seven Countries, ed. Keys A. *Circulation* **41** (*Suppl. I*), 1–154.

B53 BLACKMAN N.S. & KUSKIN L. (1964) Inverted *T* waves in the precordial electrocardiogram of normal adolescents. *Am. Heart J.* **67**, 204.

B54 BLOMQUIST C.G. (1971) Use of exercise testing for diagnosis and functional evaluation of patients with arteriosclerotic heart disease. *Circulation* **44**, 1120.

B55 BLONDEAU M., MAURICE P., REVERDY V. & LENEGRE J. (1967) Troubles du rhythme et de la conduction auriculoventriculaire dans l'infarctus du myocarde recent. Consideration anatomiques. *Arch. Mal. Coeur* **60**, 1733.

B56 BLONDEAU M., RIZZON P. & LENEGRE J. (1961) Les troubles de la conduction auriculo-ventriculaire dans l'infarctus myocardique recent. II Etude anatomique. *Arch. Mal Coeur* **54**, 1104.

B57 BLOOM N.B. (1942) The auricular complex in coronary thrombosis. *Am. Heart J.* **24**, 602.

B58 BLOUNT S.G. JR., MUNYAN E.A. JR. & HOFFMAN M. (1957) Hypertrophy of the right ventricular outflow tract. *Am. J. Med.* **22**, 784.

B59 BLUMENSCHEIN S.D., BOINEAU J.P., SPACH M.S., BARR R.C., GALLIE T.M. & EBERT P.A. (1969) Correlation of epicardial excitation with body surface potentials in ostium primum atrial defect In, *Electrical Activity of the Heart*, ed. Manning G.W. & Ahuja S.P. p. 69. Springfield, Illinois: Charles C. Thomas.

B60 BLUMGART H.L., GILLIGAN D.R. & SCHLESINGER M.J. (1941) Experimental studies of the effect of temporary occlusion of coronary arteries. *Am. Heart J.* **22**, 374.

B61 BOBBA O., CASARI A., PELLEGRINO L. & SALERNO J.A. (1970) Emiblocco anteriore sinistro reversibile od a carattere evolutivo mell'infarto acuto del miocardio. *Atti. Soc. Ital. Cardiol.* **3**, 25.

B62 BOBBA P., CASARI A., SALERNO J.A. & PELLEGRINO L. (1971) Sulle sindromi elletrocardiografiche indicative di bloco intraventricolare di tipo 'trifascicolare'. *Giorn. It. Cardiol.* **1**, 138.

B63 BOBBA P., DI GUGLIELMO L., VECCHIO C. & MONTEMARTINI C. (1971) Coronarographic patterns in Prinzmetal's variant angina. *Acta Cardiol.* **26**, 568.

B64 BOBBA P., SALERNO J.A. & CASARI A. (1972) Transient left posterior hemiblock. Report of four cases induced by the exercise test. *Circulation* **46**, 931.

B65 BOBBA P., VECCHIO C., DI GUGLIELMO L., SALERNO J., CASARI A. & MONTEMARTINI C. (1972) Exercise-induced RS-T elevation. Electrographic and angiographic observations. *Cardiology* **57**, 162.

B66 BOHNING A. & KATZ L.N. (1935) The four-lead electrocardiogram in coronary sclerosis. A study of a series of consecutive patients. *Am. J. Med. Sci.* **189**, 833.

B67 BOINEAU J.P., BLUMENSCHEIN S.D., SPACH M.S. & SABISTON D.C. (1968) Relationship between ventricular depolarisation and electrocardiogram in myocardial infarction. *J. Electrocardiol.* **1**, 233.

B68 BOINEAU J.P., SPACH M.S. & AYERS C.R. (1967) Time-normalized correlation of ventricular excitation with the vectorcardiogram. *Am. Heart J.* **73**, 64.

B69 BOTTI R.E. (1966) A variant form of angina pectoris with recurrent transient complete heart block. *Am. J. Cardiol.* **17**, 443.

B70 BOURNE G. (1957) Paradoxical electrocardiogram in coronary exercise test. *Lancet* **2**, 1320.

B71 BOUSFIELD G. (1918) Angina pectoris: changes in electrocardiogram during paroxysm. *Lancet* **2**, 457.

B72 BOWERS D. (1961) An electrocardiographic pattern associated with mitral valve deformity in Marfan's syndrome. *Circulation* **23**, 30.

B73 BRAUDO M., WIGLE E.D. & KEITH J.D. (1964) A distinctive electrocardiogram in muscular subaortic stenosis due to ventricular septal hypertrophy. *Am. J. Cardiol.* **14**, 599.

B74 BRAUNWALD E., MORROW A.G., CORNELL W.P., AYGEN M.M. & HILBISH T.F. (1960) Idiopathic hypertrophic subaortic stenosis. *Am. J. Med.* **29**, 924.

B75 BREITWIESER R. (1947) Electrocardiographic observations in chronic cholecystitis before and after surgery. *Am. J. Med. Sci.* **213**, 598.

B76 BRENES P.C., MEDRANO G.A. & SODI-PALLARES D. (1970) El bloqueo de la subdivision posterior de la rama izquierda de haz de His. *Arch. Inst. Cardiol. Mexico* **40**, 621.

B77 BRIQUEMONT F. (1961) Le syndrome d'hyperventilation. *Acta Cardiol. (Brux).* **16**, 539.

B78 BRODY A.J. (1959) Master two-step exercise test in clinically unselected patients. *JAMA* **171**, 1195.

B79 BRODY D.A. (1956) A theoretical analysis of intracavitary blood mass influence on the heart-lead relationship. *Circulation Res.* **4**, 731.

B80 BROUSTET P. (1948) Grande onde coronarienne transitoire au cours d'une crise angineuse. *Arch Mal. Coeur* **41**, 767.

B81 BROWN K.W.G., MACMILLAN R.L., FORBATH N., MEL'-GRANO F. & SCOTT J.W. (1963) Coronary unit—an intensive care centre for acute myocardial infarction. *Lancet* **2**, 349.

B82 BRUCE R.A., MAZARELLA J.A. & JORDAN J.W. (1966) Quantitation of QRS and ST segment responses to exercise. *Am. Heart J.* **71**, 455.

B83 BRYANT J.M. (1958) Intraventricular conduction. In *Recent Advances in Electrocardiography*, ed. Kossmann C.E. New York: Grune and Stratton.

B84 BRYANT J.M., SAID S.I. & YOUN H.B. (1956) 'Incomplete left bundle branch block' a frequent normal electrocardiographic variant. *J. Lab. and Clin. Med.* **48**, 793.

B85 BUNN W.H. JR. & CHREMOS A.N. (1963) Clinical evaluation of sublingial nitrates. *Angiology* **14**, 48.

B86 BURCH G.E. (1956) An electrocardiographic syndrome characterized by absence of Q in leads I, V5 and V6. *Am. Heart J.* **51**, 487.

B87 BURCH G.E. & DE PASQUALE N.P. (1961) Electrocardiographic and vectorcardiographic detection of heart disease in the presence of pre-excitation syndrome (W.P.W. syndrome). *Ann. Int. Med.* **54**, 387.

B88 BURCH G.E., HORAN L.G., ZESKIND J. & CRONVICH J.A. (1958) Correlative study of post-mortem, electrocardiographic and spatial vectorcardiographic data in myocardial infarction. *Circulation* **18**, 3.

B89 BURCH G.E., MEYERS R. & ABILDSKOV J.A. (1954) A new electrocardiographic pattern observed in cerebrovascular accidents. *Circulation* **9**, 719.

B90 BURCHELL H.B. (1968) The value of exercise tests in the diagnosis of coronary disease. *Symposium on Coronary Heart Disease*, 2nd Edn., Monograph No. 2, American Heart Association, p. 49.

B91 BURCHELL H.B. & PRUITT R.D. (1951) The value of the esophageal electrocardiogram in the elucidation of post-infarction intraventricular block. *Am. Heart J.* **42**, 81.

B92 BURDA C.D. (1966) Electrocardiographic changes in lightning stroke. *Am. Heart J.* **72,** 521.

B93 BURSTEIN J. & ELLENBOGEN L. (1938) Electrocardiograms in which the main ventricular deflections are directed downward in the standard leads. *Am. Heart J.* **16,** 165.

C

C1 CABRERA E. & FRIEDLAND C. (1953) La onda de activacion ventricular en el bloqueo de rama izquierda con infarto (un nuevo signo electrocardiografico). *Arch. Inst. cardiol. Mexico* **23,** 441.

C2 CABRERA E., ROCHA J.C. & FLORES C. (1959) El vectrocardiograma de los infartos iocardicos contrastornos en la conduccion intraventricular. *Arch. Inst. Cardiol. Mexico* **29,** 625.

C3 CALLEJA H.B. & GUERRERO H.B. (1973) Prolonged P-R interval and coronary artery disease. *Brit. Heart J.* **35,** 372.

C4 CALZAVARA G., LUSIANI G.B. & SARACENI G. (1966) Contributo clinico alla conoscenza della 'variant form' di angina pectoris. Descrizione de 4 casi. *Folia cardiol.* **25,** 283.

C5 CAMERINI F. & DAVIES L.G. (1955) Secondary *R* waves in right chest leads. *Brit. Heart J.* **17,** 28.

C6 CASKEY T.D. & HARVEY ESTES JR. E. (1964) Deviation of the S-T segment. *Am. J. Med.* **36,** 424.

C7 CASTELLANOS A. JR., CHAHINE R.A., CHAPUNOFF E., GOMEZ J. & PORTILLO B. (1971) Diagnosis of left anterior hemiblock in the presence of inferior wall myocardial infarction. *Chest* **60,** 543.

C8 CASTELLANOS A. JR. & CHAPUNOFF E. (1970) The vectorcardiogram in left posterior hemiblock. Presented at the XI International Symposium on Vectorcardiography. Long Island Jewish Medical Center. New York.

C9 CASTELLANOS A. JR. & LEMBERG L. (1969) Vectorcardiography. A programmed introduction. New York: Meredith Corporation.

C10 CASTELLANOS A. JR., LEMBERG L. & ARCEBAL A.G. (1969) Mechanisms of slow ventricular tachycardias in acute myocardial infarction. *Dis. Chest* **56,** 470.

C11 CASTELLANOS A. JR., LEMBERG L. & IOANNIDES G. (1966) The vectorcardiogram in right bundle branch block co-existing with left ventricular focal block. *Am. J. Cardiol.* **18,** 705.

C12 CASTELLANOS A. JR., MAYTIN O. & ARCEBAL A.G. (1970) Significance of complete right bundle branch block with right axis deviation in absence of right ventricular hypertrophy. *Brit. Heart J.* **32,** 85.

C13 CASTELLANOS A. JR., MAYTIN O., ARCEBAL A.G. & LEMBERG L. (1969) Alternating and co-existing block in the divisions of the left bundle branch. *Dis. Chest* **56,** 103.

C14 CASTLEMAN B. (ed.) (1957) Clinico-pathological conference. *New England J. Med.* **257,** 1185.

C15 CERQUEIRA-GOMES M. (1970) Novas ideias sobre a activacao septal. *O Medico* **975,** 492.

C16 CERQUEIRA-GOMES M., DE ABEU E LIMA C. & RAMALHAO C. (1972) Estudo vectorcardiografico sistematico do chamado hemibloqueio anterior. *Separata do Boletim da Soc. Portug. de Cardiologia* **10,** 361.

C17 CERQUEIRA-GOMES M., TEIXEIRA LOPES A.M., SOUSA MAGALHAES L., FREITAS S. & BRAGANCA-TENDER (1970) Estudo retrospectivo das perturbacoes da conducao intraventricular na populacao de um Hospital *Geral. J. Medico* **1445,** 392.

C18 CHADHA J.S., ASHBY D.W. & BROWN J.O. (1968) Abnormal electrocardiogram after adder bite. *Brit. Heart J.* **30,** 138.

C19 CHAPMAN M.G. & PEARCE M.L. (1957) Electrocardiographic diagnosis of myocardial infarction in the presence of left bundle branch block. *Circulation* **16,** 558.

C20 CHATTERJEE K., HARRIS A., DAVIES G. & LEATHAM, A. (1969): Electrocardiographic changes subsequent to artificial ventricular depolarisation. *Brit. Heart J.* **31,** 770.

C21 CHATTERJEE K., HARRIS A. & LEATHAM A. (1969) The risk of pacing after infarction and current recommendations. *Lancet* **2,** 1061.

C22 CHELTON H.G. & BURCHELL H.B. (1955) Unusual RS-T segment deviations in electrocardiograms of normal persons. *Am. J. M. Sci.* **230,** 54.

C23 CHENG I.O. (1971) Incidence of ventricular aneurysm in Coronary artery disease. An angiographic appraisal. *Am. J. Med.* **50,** 340.

C24 CHESLER E., JOFFE N., SCHAMROTH L. & MEYERS A. (1965) Annular subvalvular left ventricular aneurysms in the South African Bantu. *Circulation* **32,** 43.

C25 CHEVALIER H. & LENEGRE J. (1949) Angine de Poitrine et Epreuve d'effort. *Arch. Mal. Coeur* **42,** 613.

C26 CHICHE P., BAILLET J. & SAUVAN R. (1956) Epreuve d'effort et hypertrophie ventricular gauche. *Arch. Mal. Coeur* **49,** 894.

C27 CHICHE P., BERKMAN M. & HAIAT R. (1971) Ondes Q transitoires et 'a eclipse' au cours de l'insuffisance coronarienne aiguë. *Arch. Mal. Coeur* **5,** 657.

C28 CHRISTENSEN B.C. (1946) Variations of the carbon dioxide tension in the arterial blood and the electrocardiogram in man. *Acta Physiol. Scand.* **12,** 389.

C29 CHRISTENSEN B.C. (1946) Studies in hyperventilation. II. Electrocardiographic changes in normal man during voluntary hyperventilation. *J. Clin. Invest.* **25,** 880.

C30 CHRISTIAN N. & BOTTI R.E. (1972) Prinzmetal's variant angina pectoris with prolonged electrocardiographic changes in the absence of obstructive coronary disease. *Am. J. Med. Sci.* **263,** 225.

C31 CHOU TE-CHUON & SUSILAVORN B. (1969) Electrocardiographic changes in intracranial haemorrhage. *J. Electrocardiol.* **2,** 193.

C32 CLARKE N.E. (1945) Electrocardiographic changes in active duodenal and gall-bladder disease. *Am. Heart J.* **29,** 628.

C33 CLOWE G.M., KELLERT E. & GORHAM L.W. (1934): Rupture of the right auricle of the heart: case report with electrocardiographic and postmortem findings. *Am. Heart J.* **9,** 324.

C34 COHEN J. (1961) Acute myocardial infarction early and objectively diagnosed through ventricular extrasystoles. *Am. J. Cardiol.* **7,** 882.

C35 COHEN S.I., LAU S.H. & STEIN E. (1968): Variations of aberrant conduction in man: evidence of isolated block within the specialised conduction system. An electrocardiographic and vectorcardiographic study. *Circulation* **38,** 899.

C36 COHN P.F., VOKONOS P.S. & MOST A.S. (1972) Diagnostic accuracy of two-step post-exercise ECG. Results in 305 subjects studied by coronary arteriography. *JAMA* **220,** 501.

C37 COL J.J. & WEINBERG S.L. (1972) The incidence and mortality of intraventricular conduction defects in acute myocardial infarction. *Am. J. Cardiol.* **29,** 344.

C38 COLUCCI C.F. (1957) Le syndrome decalage superior concave en haut du segment S-T avec T positif, ample et asymetrique recherches d'electrocardiographie clinique. *Arch. Mal. Coeur* **50**, 758.

C39 CONNOR R.C.R. (1969) Myocardial damage secondary to brain lesions. *Am. Heart J.* **78**, 145.

C40 CONRAD L.L., CUDDY T.E. & BAYLEY R.H. (1959) Activation of the ischemic ventricle and acute peri-infarction block in experimental coronary occlusion. *Circulation Res.* **7**, 555.

C41 COOCH J.W. & SCHOENFELD H.H. (1949) Electrocardiographic changes in acute appendicitis. *M. Ann. District of Columbia* **18**, 569.

C42 COOK R.W., EDWARDS J.E. & PRUITT R.D. (1958) Electrocardiographic changes in acute subendocardial infarction: I. Large subendocardial and large nontransmural infarcts. *Circulation* **18**, 603.

C43 COOK R.W., EDWARDS J.E. & PRUITT, R.D. (1958) Electrocardiographic changes in acute subendocardial infarction: II. Small subendocardial infarcts. *Circulation* **18**, 613.

C44 COOPER E.L., O'SULLIVAN J. & HUGHES E. (1937) Athletics and the heart: an electrocardiographic and radiological study of the response of healthy and diseased heart to exercise. *M. J. Australia* **1**, 569.

C45 COOPER T., WILLAM V.L. & HANLON C.R. (1964) Drug responses of the transplanted heart. *Dis. Chest* **45**, 284.

C46 CORDAY E., WILLIAMS J.H., DE VERA L.B. & GOLD H. (1959) Effect of systemic blood pressure and vasopressor drugs on coronary blood flow and the electrocardiogram. *Am. J. Cardiol.* **3**, 626.

C47 CORNE R.A., PARKIN T.W., BRANDENBURG R.O. & BROWN A.L. (1965) Significance of marked left axis deviation. Electrocardiographic–pathologic correlative study. *Am. J. Cardiol.* **15**, 605.

C48 COSBY R.C. & BERGERON M. (1963) Electrocardiographic changes in carbon monoxide poisoning. *Am. J. Cardiol.* **11**, 93.

C49 COSBY R.S. & MAYO M. (1959) The value of the Master two-step exercise test in coronary artery disease. *Am. J. Cardiol.* **3**, 444.

C50 COWAN J. & RITCHIE W.T. (1922) *Diseases of the Heart.* London: Edward Arnold.

C51 CRAIB W.H. (1927–29): A study in the electrical field surrounding active heart muscle. *Heart* **14**, 71.

C52 CREDE R.H., CHIVERS N.S. & SHAPIRO A.P. (1951) Electrocardiographic abnormalities associated with emotional disturbances. *Psychosom. Med.* **13**, 277.

C53 CROMPTON M.R. (1963) Hypothalamic lesions following the rupture of cerebral (berry) aneurysms. *Brain* **86**, 301.

C54 CROPP G.J. & MANNING G.W. (1960) Electrocardiographic changes simulating myocardial ischaemia and infarction associated with spontaneous intracranial haemorrhage. *Circulation* **22**, 25.

C55 CUMMING G.R., BORYSYK L. & DUFRESNE C. (1972) The maximal exercise ECG in asymptomatic men. *Canad. med. Ass. J.* **106**, 649.

C56 CUSHING E.H., FEIL H., STANTON E.J. & WARTMAN W.B. (1942): Infarction of cardiac auricles (atria): clinical pathological and experimental studies. *Brit. Heart J.* **4**, 17.

C57 CUTFORTH R.H. & ORAM S. (1958) The electrocardiogram in pulmonary embolism. *Brit. Heart J.* **20**, 41.

D

D1 DANZIG R., ALPERN H. & SWAN J.H.C. (1969) The significance of atrial rate in patients with atrioventricular conduction abnormalities complicating acute myocardial infarction. *Am. J. Cardiol.* **24**, 707.

D2 DAOUD F.S. & SURAWICZ B. (1967) The effect of isoproterenol (ISP) on the electrocardiogram in patients with intracranial lesions. *Am. J. Cardiol.* **19**, 148 (Abstr.).

D3 DAUCHOT P. & GRAVENSTEIN J.S. (1971) Effects of atropine on the electrocardiogram in different age groups. *Clin. Pharmacol. Ther.* **12**, 274.

D4 DAVIES H. & EVANS W. (1960) The significance of deep S waves in leads II and III. *Brit. Heart J.* **22**, 551.

D5 DAVIES C.T.M., KITCHIN A.H., KNIBBS A.V. & NEILSON J.M. (1971) Computer quantitation of S-T segment response to graded exercise in untrained and trained normal subjects. *Cardiovasc. Res.* **5**, 201.

D6 DAVIS M.J. (1971) *Pathology of Conducting Tissue of the Heart.* London: Butterworths.

D7 DAVIS F.W. JR., SCARBOROUGH W.R., MASON R.E., SINGERWALD M.L. & BAKER B.M. JR. (1953) Effects of exercise and smoking on electrocardiograms and ballistocardiograms of normal subjects and patients with coronary artery disease. *Am. Heart J.* **46**, 529.

D8 DAY H.W. (1967) Effectiveness of an intensive coronary care area. *Am. J. Cardiol.* **15**, 51.

D9 DAY W. (1968) Acute coronary care—a five year report. *Am. J. Cardiol.* **21**, 252.

D10 DEGLAUDE L. & LAURENS P. (1954) Diagnostic vectorgraphique de l'infarctus du myocarde associe a un bloc de branche. *Arch. mal. Coeur* **47**, 579.

D11 DE KOCK J. & SCHAMROTH L. (1974) Right bundle branch block associated with transient left posterior hemiblock in a case of acute anteroseptal myocardial infarction. *S. Afr. med. J.* **48**, 1237.

D12 DEL CASTILLO E.B., SCHARER R.F., GUARDO A.H., LARATONDA A. & ZUCAL C.A. (1963) Considerations à propos de quelques troubles cardioaques au cours du syndrome de Simmonds-Sheehan. *Presse méd.* **71**, 806.

D13 DEMOULIN J.C. & KULBERTUS H.E. (1972) Histopathological examination of concept of left hemiblock. *Brit. Heart J.* **34**, 807.

D14 DHURANDHAR R.W., MacMILLAN R.L. & BROWN K.W.G. (1971) Primary ventricular fibrillation complicating acute myocardial infarction. *Am. J. Cardiol.* **27**, 347.

D15 DICOSKY C. & ZIMMERMAN H.A. (1969) Atrial injury. *J. Electrocardiol.* **2**, 51.

D16 DI IELSI A.J., PINSKY H.A. & EYNON H.K. (1952) Auricular infarction; report of two cases. *Ann. Int. Med.* **36**, 640.

D17 DIMOND E.G. (1961) The exercise test and prognosis of coronary heart disease. *Circulation* **24**, 736.

D18 DODGE H.T., GRANT R.P. & SEAVEY P.W. (1953) The effect of induced hyperkalemia on the normal and abnormal electrocardiogram. *Am. Heart J.* **45**, 725.

D19 DOLARA A. (1967) Early premature ventricular beats with repetitive ventricular fibrillation. *Am. Heart J.* **74**, 332.

D20 DOLARA A., MORANDO P. & PAMPALONI M. (1967) Electrocardiographic findings in 98 consecutive non-penetrating chest injuries. *Dis. Chest* **52**, 50.

D21 DOLARA A. & POZZI L. (1971) Electrical alternation of T

wave without change in QRS complex. *Brit. Heart J.* **33**, 161.

D22   DONOSO E., WACHTEL F. & GRISHMAN A. (1957) Polarity of the S-T vector. *Am. J. Physiol.* **189**, 219.

D23   DORRA M., WAYNBERGER M., NEZRY R. & SLAMA R. (1968) A propos d'une observation d'angor dit de Prinzmetal à forme syncopale. Etude coronarographique. *Arch. Mal Coeur* **61**, 1043.

D24   DOYLE J.T. & KINCH S.H. (1970) Prognosis of an abnormal electrocardiographic stress test. *Circulation* **41**, 545.

D25   DREIFUS L. (1967) In *Cardiac Pacing and Cardioversion*, ed. Meltzer E.L. & Kitchell J.R. p. 93. Philadelphia: The Charles Press Publishers, Inc. U.S.A.

D26   DREIFUS L.S., BAROLUCCI G. & LIKOFF W. (1960) Nodal tachycardia: etiology and therapy. *Circulation* **22**, 741 (Abstr.).

D27   DRESSLER W.A. (1943) A case of myocardial infarction masked by bundle branch block but revealed by occasional premature ventricular beats. *Am. J. Med. Sc.* **206**, 361.

D28   DRESSLER W. (1943) Myocardial infarction indicated by an electrocardiographic pattern in which T1 is lower than T3. *Am. Heart J.* **71**, 642.

D29   DRESSLER W. (1944) Myocardial infarction indicated by angina pectoris of effort or by brief attacks of angina of rest. *Am. Heart J.* **28**, 81.

D30   DRESSLER W. & ROESLER J. (1947) High *T* waves in the earliest stage of myocardial infarction. *Am. Heart J.* **34**, 627.

D31   DRESSLER W. & ROESLER J. (1948) The diagnostic value of the pattern T1 lower than T3 compared with the information yielded by multiple chest leads in myocardial infarction. *Am. Heart J.* **36**, 115.

D32   DRESSLER W. & ROESLER H. (1949) *An Atlas of Electrocardiography*. Springfield, Illinois: Charles C.Thomas.

D33   DRESSLER W., ROESLER H. & SCHWAGER A. (1950) The electrocardiographic signs of myocardial infarction in the presence of bundle branch block. I. Myocardial infarction with left bundle branch block. *Am. Heart J.* **39**, 217.

D34   DUBNOW M.H., BURCHELL H.B. & TITUS J.L. (1965) Postinfarction ventricular aneurysm—a clinico-morphologic and electrocardiographic study of 80 cases. *Am. Heart J.* **70**, 753.

D35   DUCHOSAL P.W. & GROSGURIN J.R. (1959) *Atlas d'Electorcardiographie et de Vectorcardiographie*. Basel: S. Karger.

D36   DUNN F.L. & BEENKEN H.G. (1959) Short distance radio telemetering of physiological information. *JAMA* **169**, 1618.

D37   DUNN F.L. & RAHM W.E. JR. (1950) Electrocardiography: modern trends in instrumentation and visual and direct recording electrocardiography. *Ann. Int. Med.* **32**, 611.

D38   DUNN W.J., EDWARDS J.E. & PRUITT R.D. (1956) The electrocardiogram in infarction of the lateral wall of the left ventricle. *Circulation* **14**, 540.

D39   DURANT T.M., GINSBURG I.W. & ROESLER H. (1939) Transient bundle branch block and other electrocardiographic changes in pulmonary embolism. *Am. Heart J.* **17**, 423.

D40   DURANT T.M., LONG J. & OPPENHEIMER M.J. (1947) Pulmonary (venous) air embolism. *Am. Heart J.* **33**, 269.

D41   DURANT T.M., OPPENHEIMER M.J., WEBSTER M. & LONG J. (1949) Arterial air embolism. *Am. Heart J.* **38**, 481.

D42   DURRER D., FORMIJNE P., VAN DAM R.T.H., BÜLLER J., VAN LIER A.A.W. & MEIJLER F.L. (1961) The electrocardiogram in normal and in some abnormal conditions. *Am. Heart J.* **61**, 303.

D43   DURRER D., ROOS J.P. & BÜLLER J. (1965) The spread of

excitation in canine and human heart. *Electrophysiology of the Heart*, ed. Taccardi B. & Marchetti G. p. 203. London: Pergamon Press.

D44   DURRER D., ROOS J.P. & VAN DAM R.T.H. (1966) The genesis of the electrocardiogram of patients with ostium primum defects (ventral atrial septal defects). *Am. Heart J.* **71**, 642.

D45   DURRER D. & VAN DER TWEEL L.H. (1957) Excitation of the left ventricular wall of the dog and goat. *Ann. N.Y. Acad. Sci.* **65**, 779.

D46   DURRER D., VAN DER TWEEL L.H., BERREKLOUW S. & VAN DER WEY L.P. (1955) Spread of activation in the left ventricular wall of the dog: 2 and 3 dimensional analysis. IV. *Am. Heart J.* **50**, 860.

D47   DURRER D., VAN DER TWEEL L.H., BLICKMAN J.R., BERREKLOUW S. & VAN DER WEY L.P. (1953) I. Spread of activation in the left ventricular wall of the dog. *Am. Heart J.* **46**, 683.

D48   DURRER D., VAN DER TWEEL L.H., BLICKMAN J.R., BERREKLOUW S. & VAN DER WEY L.P. (1954) II. Activation conditions at the epicardial surface. *Am. Heart J.* **47**, 192.

D49   DURRER D., VAN DER TWEEL L.H., BLICKMAN J.R., BERREKLOUW S. & VAN DER WEY L.P. (1954) III. Transmural and intramural analysis. *Am. Heart J.* **48**, 13.

D50   DURRER D., VAN DER TWEEL L.H., BLICKMAN J.R., BERREKLOUW S. & VAN DER WEY L.P. (1955) IV. Two and three dimensional analysis. *Am. Heart J.* **50**, 860.

D51   DURRER D., VAN LIER A.A.W. & BÜLLER J. (1964) Epicardial and intramural excitation in chronic myocardial infarction. *Am. Heart J.* **68**, 765.

E

E1   EAST T. & ORAM S. (1952) The cardiogram in ventricular aneurysm following cardiac infarction. *Brit. Heart J.* **14**, 125.

E2   EDEIKEN J. (1954) Elevation of the RS-T segment, apparent or real, in the right precordial leads as a probable normal variant. *Am. Heart J.* **48**, 331.

E3   Editorial (1971) Atypical angina. *Brit. Med. J.* **1**, 62.

E4   EHLERS K.H., ENGLE M.A., LEVIN A.R., GROSSMAN H. & FLEMING R.J. (1970) Left ventricular abnormality with late mitral insufficiency and abnormal electrocardiogram. *Am. J. Cardiol.* **26**, 333.

E5   EICHERT H. (1944) Wolff-Parkinson-White syndrome simulating myocardial infarction. *Ann. Int. Med.* **21**, 907.

E6   EINTHOVEN W. (1908) Weiteres ueber das Elektrokardiogram. *Arch. ges. Physiol.* **122**, 517.

E7   EKELUND L.-G. & STRANDELL T. (1960) EKG-reaktionen under och efter arbete hos män med tidigare genomgangen jhärtinfarkt. Report given at the meeting of the Swedish Society for Clinical Physiology.

E8   EKMEKCI A., TOYOSHIMA H., KWOCZYNSKI J.K., NAGAYA T. & PRINZMETAL M. (1961) Angina pectoris. IV. Clinical and experimental difference between ischemia with ST-T elevation and ischemia with ST depression. *Am. J. Cardiol.* **7**, 412.

E9   ELISBERG E.J. (1958) Electrocardiographic changes associated with pectus excavatum. *Ann. Int. Med.* **49**, 130.

E10   ELLESTAD M.H., ALLEN W. & WAN M.C.K. (1969) Maximal treadmill stress testing for cardiovascular evaluation. *Circulation* **39**, 517.

E11   EMSLIE-SMITH D. (1956) The late intracardiac *R* wave and the precordial pattern of right ventricular hypertrophy. *Brit. Heart J.* **18**, 78.

E12   EPSTEIN E.J., COULSHED N. MCKENDRICKS C.S., CLARKE J. & KEARNS W.E. (1966) Artificial pacing by electrode catheter for heart block or asystole: complicating acute myocardial infarction. *Brit. Heart J.* **28**, 546.

E13   ERICKSON R.V., SCHER A.M. & BECKER R.A. (1957) Ventricular excitation in experimental bundle branch block. *Circulation Res.* **5**, 5.

E14   ESTES E.H. JR., WHALEN R.E., ROBERTS S.R. JR. & MCINTOSH H.D. (1963) The electrocardiographic and vectorcardiographic findings in idiopathic hypertrophic subaortic stenosis. *Am. Heart J.* **65**, 155.

E15   EVANS R.W., MERSHON J.C., EDGETT J. & NELSON W.P. (1971) Diagnostic changes of acute myocardial infarction in the electrocardiogram and vectorcardiogram with co-existing complete left bundle branch block. *J. Electrocardiol.* **4**, 267.

E16   EVANS W. & WRIGHT G. (1942) The electrocardiogram in Friedreich disease. *Brit. Heart J.* **4**, 91.

E17   EYSTER J.A.E. & MEEK W.J. (1913–14) Experiments on the origin and propagation of the impulse of the heart. I. The point of primary negativity in the mammalian heart and the spread of negativity of other regions. *Heart* **5**, 119.

F

F1   FAZZINI P.F. & MARCHI F. (1970) Atrioventricular block in acute myocardial infarction. *Acta Cardiologica* **25**, 517.

F2   FEIL H. (1958) The problems of acute coronary attacks without classic electrocardiographic signs of acute myocardial infarction. *Prog. Cardiovasc. Dis.* **1**, 165.

F3   FEIL H. & BROFMAN B.L. (1953) The effect of exercise in the electrocardiogram of bundle branch block. *Am. Heart J.* **45**, 665.

F4   FEIL H., CUSHING E.H. & HARDESTY J.T. (1938) Accuracy in diagnosis and localization of myocardial infarction. *Am. Heart J.* **15**, 721.

F5   FEIL H. & SIEGEL M.L. (1928) Electrocardiographic changes during attacks of angina pectoris. *Am. J. Med. Sci.* **175**, 255.

F6   FEINCHEL N.N. (1962) A long-term study of concave RS-T elevation—A normal variant of the electrocardiogram. *Angiology* **13**, 360.

F7   FENICHEL N.M., SHOOKHOFF C. & ABRAMSON D.I. (1936) Theoretical considerations regarding the variations of the RS-T segment and subsequent *T* wave following local ventricular trauma. *Am. Heart J.* **12**, 406.

F8   FENTZ V. & GORMSEN J. (1962) Electrocardiographic patterns in patients with cardiovascular accidents. *Circulation* **25**, 22.

F9   FERNANDEZ F., HELLER J., TREVI G.-P., RABENOU S., SCEBAT L. & LENEGRE J. (1972) The QRS loop in left anterior and posterior hemiblocks. Vectorcardiographic study during selective coronary arteriography. *Am. J. Cardiol.* **29**, 337.

F10   FERNANDEZ F., SCEBAT L. & LENEGRE J. (1970) Electrocardiographic study of left intraventricular hemiblock in man during selective coronary arteriography. *Am. J. Cardiol.* **26**, 1.

F11   FERNANDEZ F., SCEBAT L. & LENEGRE J. (1971) Caracteristiques electrocardiographiques et criteres diagnostiques des 'hemiblocs gauches'. *Arch. Mal. Coeur* **2**, 153.

F12   FERNANDEZ F., TREVI G.P. & RABENAU S. (1970) Contribution de l'arteriographie coronaire a la connaissance electrocardiographique des troubles de la conduction intraventriculaire: à propos du 'peri-infarction block' et de bloc droit avec forte deviation axiale de QRS. *Arch. Mal Coeur* **10**, 1353.

F13   FINKELSTEIN D. & NIGAGLIONI A. (1961) Electrocardiographic alterations after neurosurgical procedures. *Am. Heart J.* **62**, 772.

F14   FIRST S.R., BAYLEY R.H. & BEDFORD D.R. (1950) Peri-infarction block; electrocardiographic abnormality occasionally resembling bundle branch block and local ventricular block of other types. *Circulation* **2**, 31.

F15   FISCH C. (1961) Giant negative *T* wave. *J. Indiana State Med. Ass.* **54**, 1664.

F16   FISCHER R. (1938) Influence d'une thrombose coronarienne aïgue sur l'electrocardiogramme d'un block de branche. *Arch. Mal. Coeur* **31**, 397.

F17   FORD A.B. & HELLERSTEIN H.K. (1957) Energy cost of the Master two-step test. *JAMA* **164**, 1868.

F18   FORTUIN N.J. & FRIESINGER G.C. (1970) Exercise-induced S-T segment elevation. Clinical, electrocardiographic and arteriographic studies in twelve patients. *Am. J. Med.* **49**, 459.

F19   FREEDBERG A.S., RISEMAN J.E.F. & SPIEGL E.D. (1941) Objective evidence of the efficacy of medicinal therapy in angina pectoris. *Am. Heart J.* **22**, 494.

F20   FREEDBERG A.S., SPIEGL E.D. & RISEMAN J.E.F. (1944) Effect of external heat and cold on patients with angina pectoris. Evidence for the existence of a reflex factor. *Am. Heart J.* **27**, 611.

F21   FREIMAN A.H., TOLLES W., CARBERY W.J., RUEGSEGGER P., ABARQUEZ R.F. & LADUE J.S. (1960) The electrocardiogram during exercise. *Am. J. Cardiol.* **5**, 506.

F22   FREMONT R.E., KLOPSTOCK R. & GLASS P. (1959) Controlled studies on the efficiency of bilateral internal mammary artery ligation in patients with angina pectoris. *Angiology* **10**, 20.

F23   FRENCH A.J. & DOCK W. (1944) Fatal coronary arteriosclerosis in young soldiers. *JAMA* **124**, 1233.

F24   FREUNDLICH J. & SERENO L.R. (1959) Auricular infarction. *Am. Heart J.* **57**, 654.

F25   FRIEDBERG C.K. (1967) *Disease of the Heart*. Philadelphia: Saunders.

F26   FRIEDBERG C.K., COHEN H. & DONOSO E. (1968) Advanced heart block as a complication of acute myocardial infarction: role of pacemaker therapy. *Prog. Cardiovasc. Dis.* **10**, 466.

F27   FRIEDBERG C.K., COHEN H. & DONOSO E. (1968) L'impiego degli stimolatori artificiali nella terapia del blocco di cuore avanzato complicante l'infarto miocardico acuto. *Progr. Patol. Cardiovasc.* **11**, 345.

F28   FRIEDBERG C.K., DONOSO E. & STEIN W.G. (1964) Non-surgical acquired heart block. *Ann. N.Y. Acad. Sci.* **3**, 835.

F29   FRIEDBERG C.K., JAFFE H.L., PORDY L. & CHESKY K. (1962) The two-step exercise electrocardiogram. *Circulation* **26**, 1254.

F30   FRIEDBERG C.K. & ZAGER A. (1961) 'Nonspecific' ST- and *T*-wave changes. *Circulation* **23**, 655.

F31   FRITZLAR G. (1940) Das verhalten der nachschwankung im belastungselektrokardiogramm bei schweren myokardschäden und kammerextrasystolen. *Z. Kreislaufforschg.* **32**, 409.

F32 FRUSCELLA R. & BOCCARDELLI V. (1954) Difficolta diagnostiche in caso di infarto associato a blocco di branca sinistro. Osservazioni su un nuovo segno elettrocardiografico. *Folia Cardiol.* **13,** 371.

F33 FULTON M.C. & MARRIOTT H.J.L. (1963) Acute pancreatitis simulating myocardial infarction in the electrocardiogram. *Ann. Intern Med.* **59,** 730.

F34 FURBERG C. (1967) Adrenergic beta-blockade and electrocardiographical ST-T changes. *Acta Med. Scand.* **181,** 21.

F35 FURBERG C. & TENGBLAD C.F. (1966) Adrenergic beta receptor blockade and the effect of hyperventilation on the electrocardiogram. *Scand. J. Clin. Lab. Invest.* **18,** 467.

F36 FURBETTA D., BUFALARI A., SANTUCCI F. & SOLINAS P. (1956) Abnormality of the *U* wave and the T-U segment of the electrocardiogram. The syndrome of the papillary muscles. *Circulation* **14,** 1129.

G

G1 GALLIVAN G.J., LEVINE H. & CANZONETTI A.J. (1970) Ischaemic electrocardiographic changes after truncal vagotomy. *JAMA* **211,** 798.

G2 GAMBETTA M. & CHILDERS R.W. (1973) Rate-dependent right precordial Q waves: 'Septal Focal Block'. *Am. J. Cardiol.* **32,** 196.

G3 GAMBOA R., PENALOZA D., SIME F. & BANCHERO N. (1962) The role of the right and left ventricles in the ventricular pre-excitation (WPW) syndrome. An experimental study in man. *Am. J. Cardiol.* **10,** 650.

G4 GARB S. (1953) Effects of epinephrine, arterenol and isuprel on the electrical potentials of mammalian heart muscle: Inability of nitrites to block effects. *Am. J. Physiol.* **172,** 399.

G5 GARDBERG M. & ASHMAN R. (1943) The QRS complex of the electrocardiogram. *Arch. Int. Med.* **72,** 210.

G6 GASPAR H., BASHOUR F.A. & TAYLOR W.P. (1968) Cardiac arrhythmias in acute myocardial infarction. IV. Further observations in complete heart block. *Dis. Chest* **53,** 775.

G7 GAZES R. (1966) In *The Current Status of Intensive Coronary Care*, p. 71. New York: The Charles Press.

G8 GAZES P.C., CULLER M.R. & STOKES J.K. (1964) The diagnosis of angina pectoris. *Am. Heart J.* **6,** 830.

G9 GEORGIEW H. & URBASZEK W. (1961) Modification of Wolff-Parkinson-White syndrome with ajmaline and possible resulting conclusion. *Z. Kresilaufforsch.* **50,** 19.

G10 GETTES L.S., SURAWICZ B. & SHIUE J.C. (1962) Effect of high K, low K, and quinidine on QRS duration and ventricular action potential. *Am. J. Physiol.* **203,** 1135.

G11 GIANELLY R., MAGLER F. & HARRISON D.C. (1968) Prinzmetal's variant angina with only slight coronary atherosclerosis. *Calif. Med.* **108,** 129.

G12 GILBERT J.L., LANGE G., POLEVOY J. & BROOKS C. McC. (1958) Effects of vasoconstrictor agents on cardiac irritability. *J. Pharm. Exp. Ther.* **123,** 9.

G13 GILLILAN R.E., HAWLEY R.R. & WARBASSE J.R. (1969) Second degree heart block occurring in a patient with Prinzmetal's variant angina. *Am. Heart J.* **77,** 380.

G14 GLOTZER S. & BARCHAN J. (1955) The effect of traction of the gallbladder on the electrocardiogram. *New York State J. Med.* **55,** 515.

G15 GODMAN M.J., LASSERS B.W. & JULIAN D.G. (1970) Complete bundle branch block complicating acute myocardial infarction. *N. Engl. J. Med.* **282,** 237.

G16 GOLDBERG H.H. & LEWIS S.M. (1950) Acute myocardial infarction and the Wolff-Parkinson-White syndrome. *Am. Heart J.* **40,** 614.

G17 GOLDBERGER E. (1947) Unipolar Lead Electrocardiography, p. 150. Philadelphia: Lea and Febiger.

G18 GOLDBERGER E. (1949) Unipolar Lead Electrocardiography, 2nd Edn. p. 246. Philadelphia: Lea and Febiger.

G19 GOLDBERGER E. & SCHWARTZ S.P. (1945) Electrocardiograms in which the main deflections are directed downward in the Standard leads. *Am. Heart J.* **29,** 62.

G20 GOLDBLOOM A.A. & DUMANIS A.A. (1946) Short P-R interval with prolongation of QRS complex and myocardial infarction. *Ann. Int. Med.* **25,** 362.

G21 GOLDHAMMER S. & SCHERF D. (1932) Elektrokardiographische untersuchungen bei kranken mit angina pectoris. *Z. Klin. Med.* **122,** 134.

G22 GOLDMAN M.J. (1953) RS-T segment elevation in mid and left precordial leads as a normal variant. *Am. Heart J.* **46,** 817.

G23 GOLDMAN M.J. (1960) Normal variants in the electrocardiogram leading to cardiac invalidism. *Am. Heart J.* **59,** 61.

G24 GONZALEZ VIDELA J. (1957) El sindrome de W.P.W. *Medicina Panamericana* **9,** 281. Cited by J. Laham, Ref. L1.

G25 GOODWIN J.F., HOLLMAN A., CLELAND W.P. & TEARE D. (1960) Obstructive cardiomyopathy simulating aortic stenosis. *Brit. Heart J.* **22,** 403.

G26 GORLIN R., KLEIN M.D. & SULLIVAN J. (1967) Prospective correlative study of ventricular aneurysm. *Am. J. Med.* **42,** 512.

G27 GOTTESMAN J., CASTEN D. & BELLER A.J. (1943) Changes in the electrocardiogram induced by acute pancreatitis. *JAMA* **123,** 892.

G28 GOTTSCHALK C.W. & CRAIGE E. (1956) A comparison of the precordial S-T and *T* wave in the electrocardiograms of 600 healthy young negro and white adults. *South med. J.* **49,** 453.

G29 GRANT R.P. (1950) Spatial vectorelectrocardiography. A method for calculating the spatial electrical vectors of the heart from conventional leads. *Circulation* **2,** 676.

G30 GRANT R.P. (1956) Left axis deviation. An electrocardiographic-pathological correlation study. *Circulation* **14,** 233.

G31 GRANT R.P. (1957) *Clinical Electrocardiography*, p. 116. New York: McGraw-Hill Book Co. Inc.

G32 GRANT R.P. (1957) *Clinical Electrocardiography*, p. 127. New York: McGraw-Hill Book Co. Inc.

G33 GRANT R.P. (1959) Peri-infarction block. *Prog. Cardiovasc. Dis.* **2,** 237.

G34 GRANT R.P. & DODGE H.I. (1956) Mechanisms of QRS complex prolongation in man. Left ventricular conduction disturbances. *Am. J. Med.* **20,** 834.

G35 GRANT R.P. & ESTES E.H. JR. (1952) *Spatial vector electrocardiography. Clinical electrocardiographic interpretation.* London: The Blakiston Div., McGraw-Hill Book Co. Ltd.

G36 GRANT R.P. & MURRAY R.H. (1954) QRS complex deformity of myocardial infarction in the human subject. *Am. J. Med.* **17,** 587.

G37 GRAYBIEL A. & ALLENBACH N.W. (1959) The work electrocardiogram. *Am. J. Cardiol.* **3,** 430.

G38 GRAYBIEL A., McFARLAND R.A., GATES D.C. & WEBSTER F.A. (1944) Analysis of the electrocardiograms obtained from 1000 young healthy aviators. *Am. Heart J.* **27,** 524.

G39 GRAYBIEL A. & WHITE P.D. (1935) Inversion of the T-wave in lead I or II in young individuals with neurocirculatory asthenia, with thyrotoxicosis in relation to certain infections and following paroxysmal ventricular tachycardia. *Am. Heart J.* **10**, 345.

G40 GRAYZEL J. (1958) Electrocardiographic criteria in the differential diagnosis of pre-excitation (W.P.W. syndrome) and arteriosclerotic heart disease. *N. Engl. J. Med.* **259**, 369.

G41 GRISHMAN A. & JAFFE H.L. (1951) Spatial vectorcardiography: wide QRS complexes with short P-R interval (W.P.W. syndrome). *J. Mt. Sinai. Hosp.* **18**, 208.

G42 GROEDEL F.M. & BORCHARDT P.R. (1948) *Direct Electrocardiography of the Human Heart.* New York: Brooklyn Medical Press Inc.

G43 GROSSMAN J.L. & DELMAN A.J. (1969) Serial P wave changes in acute myocardial infarction. *Am. Heart J.* **77**, 336.

G44 GROSSMAN M., WEINSTEIN W.W. & KATZ L.N. (1949) Use of exercise test in diagnosis of coronary insufficiency. *Ann. Int. Med.* **30**, 387.

G45 GRUSIN H. (1954) Peculiarities of the African's electrocardiogram and the changes observed in serial studies. *Circulation* **9**, 860.

G46 GUAZZI M., FIORENTINI C., POLESE A. & MAGRINI F. (1970) Continuous electrocardiographic recording in Prinzmetal's variant angina pectoris. *Brit. Heart J.* **32**, 611.

G47 GUBNER R. (1962) An appraisal of the exercise electrocardiogram test. *Ann. Life Insur. Med.* **1**, 111.

G48 GUERON M., STERN J. & COHEN W. (1967) Severe myocardial damage and heart failure in scorpion sting. *Am. J. Cardiol.* **19**, 719.

G49 GUTIERREZ M.R., CHANGFOOT G.H. & PERETZ D.I. (1968) Significance of T wave interruption by premature beats as a cause of sudden death. *Canad. Med. Ass. J.* **98**, 144.

H

H1 HAMPTON A.G., BECKWITH J.R. & WOOD J.E. (1959) The relationship between heart disease and gallbladder disease. *Ann. Intern. Med.* **50**, 1135.

H2 HAN J., DeFRAGLIA J., MILLET D. & MOE G.K. (1966) Incidence of ectopic beats as a function of basic rate in the ventricle. *Am. Heart J.* **72**, 632.

H3 HAN J., GARCIA DE JALON P. & MOE G.K. (1964) Adrenergic effects on ventricular vulnerability. *Circ. Res.* **14**, 516.

H4 HAN J. & MOE G.K. (1964) Non-uniform recovery of excitability in ventricular muscle. *Circ. Res.* **14**, 44.

H5 HANCOCK E.W. & COHN K. (1966) The syndrome associated with mid-systolic click and late-systolic murmur. *Am. J. Med.* **41**, 183.

H6 HARDEL M., BAJOLET A., GUERIN R., ELAERTS J. & GERARD J. (1969) Angor de Prinzmetal. A propos d'un cas complique d'infarctus du myocarde. *Arch. Mal Coeur* **62**, 1267.

H7 HARRIS A.S. (1950) Delayed development of ventricular ectopic rhythms following experimental coronary occlusion. *Circulation* **1**, 1318.

H8 HARRISON M.T. & GIBB B.II. (1964) Electrocardiographic changes associated with a cerebrovascular accident. *Lancet* **2**, 429.

H9 HARTOG M. & JOPLIN G.F. (1968) Effects of cortisol deficiency on the electrocardiogram. *Brit. Med. J.* **2**, 275.

H10 HARUMI K., BURGESS M.J. & ABILDSKOV J.A. (1966) Theoretic model of the T wave. *Circulation* **34**, 657.

H11 HAUSNER E. & SCHERF D. (1933) Ueber angina pectoris probleme. *Z. Klin. Med.* **126**, 166.

H12 HECHT H. (1946) Potential variations of the right auricular and ventricular cavities in man. *Am. Heart J.* **33**, 604.

H13 HECHT H.H. (1955) Research in electrocardiography. (Editorial). *Circulation Res.* **3**, 231.

H14 HEGGE F., TUNA N. & BURCHELL H. (1972): The correlation of S-T segment elevations and axis shifts in graded treadmill exercise tests with coronary arteriographic findings. *Am. J. Cardiol.* **29**, 269 (Abstr.).

H15 HEGGE F., TUNA N. & BURCHELL H. (1973) Coronary arteriographic findings in patients with axis shifts or S-T segment elevations on exercise-stress testing. *Am. Heart J.* **86**, 603.

H16 HEIM E. (1958) The electrocardiogram of long-distance runners (studied in 100 Olympic long-distance ski runners). *Schweij. Z. Sportmed.* **6**, 1.

H17 HEIMDAL A. & NORDENFELDT O. (1953) The effect of hydergine on the electrocardiogram. *Cardiologia* **23**, 359.

H18 HELLERSTEIN H.K. (1948) Atrial infarction with diagnostic electrocardiographic findings. *Am. Heart J.* **36**, 422.

H19 HELLERSTEIN H.K. & KATZ L.N. (1948) The electrical effects of injury at various myocardial locations. *Am. Heart J.* **36**, 184.

H20 HELLERSTEIN H.K. & MARTIN J.W. (1947) Incidence of thrombo-embolic lesions accompanying myocardial infarction. *Am. Heart J.* **33**, 443.

H21 HELLERSTEIN H.K., PROZAN G.B., LIBOW J.M., DOAN A.E. & HENDERSON J.A. (1961) Two-step exercise test as a test of cardiac function in chronic rheumatic heart disease and in arteriosclerotic heart disease with old myocardial infarction. *Am. J. Cardiol.* **7**, 234.

H22 HEYER H.E., WINANS H.M. & PLESSINGER V.J. (1947) Alterations in the form of the electrocardiogram in patients with mental disease. *Am. J. Med. Sci.* **214**, 23.

H23 HILAL H. & MASSUMI R. (1967) Variant angina pectoris. *Am. J. Cardiol.* **19**, 607.

H24 HINKLE L.E. JR., CARVER S.T. & STEVENS M. (1969) The frequency of asymptomatic disturbances of cardiac rhythm and conduction in middle-aged men. *Am. J. Cardiol.* **24**, 629.

H25 HISS R.G. & LAMB L.E. (1962) Electrocardiographic findings in 122,043 individuals. *Circulation* **25**, 947.

H26 HISS R.G., LAMB L.E. & ALLEN M.F. (1960) Electrocardiographic findings in 67,375 asymptomatic individuals. Part X. Normal values. *Am. J. Cardiol.* **6**, 200.

H27 HISS R.G., SMITH G.B., JR. & LAMB L.E. (1960) Pitfalls in interpreting electrocardiographic changes occurring while monitoring stress procedures. *Aerosp. Med.* **31**, 9.

H28 HODGE G.B. & MESSER A.L. (1948) The electrocardiogram in biliary tract disease and during experimental biliary distension. *Surg. Gynecol. Obstet.* **86**, 617.

H29 HOFFMAN B.F. (1961) Problems in cardiac electrophysiology. In *Biophysics of Physiological and Pharmacological Actions*, ed. Shanes A.M. Washington, D.C.: Am. A. Adv. Sc.,

H30 HOFFMAN B.F. & CRANEFIELD P.F. (1964) The physiologic basis of cardiac arrhythmias. *Am. J. Med.* **37**, 670.

H31 HOFFMAN I.R., TAYMOR C. & GOOTNICK A. (1964) Vectorcardiographic residua of inferior infarction. Seventy-eight cases studied with the Frank system. *Circulation* **29**, 562.

H32 HOLLMAN A., GOODWIN J.F., TEARE D. & RENWICK J.W. (1960) A family with obstructive cardiomyopathy (asymmetrical hypertrophy). *Brit. Heart J.* **22**, 449.

H33 HOLMGREN A. & MATTSSON K.H. (1954) A new ergometer with constant workload at varying pedalling rate. *Scand. J. Clin. Lab. Invest.* **6**, 137.

H34 HOLMGREN A. & STRANDELL T. (1961) On the use of chest-head leads for recording of electrocardiogram during exercise. *Acta Med. Scand.* **169**, 57.

H35 HOLTER N.J. (1957) Radioelectrocardiography: a new technique for cardiovascular studies. *Ann. N.Y. Acad. Sci.* **65**, 913.

H36 HOLTER N.J. & GENGERELLI J.A. (1949) Remote recording of physiological data by radio. *Rocky Mountain M.J.* **46**, 749.

H37 HOOGERWERF S. (1929–30) Elektrokardiographische untersuchungen der Amsterdamen Olympiakampfer. *Arbeits physiologie* **2**, 61.

H38 HORLICK L. (1959) A clinical re-evaluation of Master's two-step test. *Canad. M.A.J.* **80**, 9.

H39 HORWITZ O. & GRAYBIEL A. (1948) Prolongation of the Q-T interval in the electrocardiogram occurring as a temporary functional disturbance in healthy persons. *Am. Heart J.* **35**, 480.

H40 HUGENHOLTZ P.G., FORKNER C.E. & LEVINE H.D. (1961) A clinical appraisal of the vectorcardiogram in myocardial infarction. II Frank system. *Circulation* **24**, 825.

H41 HULBERT B. & MEYER H.M. (1949) Primary amyloidosis of the heart. *Am. Heart J.* **38**, 604.

H42 HUNT D. & SLOMAN G. (1969) Bundle branch block in acute myocardial infarction. *Brit. Med. J.* **1**, 85.

H43 HURWITZ M. & ELIOT R.S. (1964) Arrhythmias in acute myocardial infarction. *Dis. Chest* **45**, 616.

H44 HURWITZ M.M., LANGENDORF R. & KATZ L.N. (1943) The diagnostic QRS patterns in myocardial infarction. *Ann. Int. Med.* **19**, 924.

I

I1 IMAI S., RILEY A.L. & BERNE R.M. (1964) Effect of ischaemia on adenine nucleotides in cardiac and skeletal muscle. *Circulation Res.* **15**, 443.

I2 IMPERIAL E.S., CARBALLO R. & ZIMMERMAN H.A. (1960) Disturbances of rate, rhythm and conduction in acute myocardial infarction. *Am. J. Cardiol.* **5**, 24.

I3 IPPOLITO T.L., BLIER J.S. & FOX T.T. (1954) Massive T inversion. *Am. Heart J.* **48**, 88.

J

J1 JACKRELL J., MILLER J.A., SCHECHTER F.G., MINKOWITZ S. & STUCKEY J.H. (1967) A study of factors determining the development and persistence of A-V conduction defects following ligation of the anterior septal artery. *Bull. N.Y. Acad. Med.* **43**, 1214.

J2 JACOBSON D. & SCHRIRE V. (1966) Giant T-wave inversion. *Brit. Heart J.* **28**, 768.

J3 JAFFE H.L., CORDAY E. & MASTER A.M. (1948) Evaluation of the precordial leads of the electrocardiogram in obesity. *Am. Heart J.* **36**, 911.

J4 JAMES T.N. (1960) Coronary anatomy for the practising internist. *Minn. Med.* **43**, 847.

J5 JAMES T.N. (1961) Myocardial infarction and atrial arrhythmias. *Circulation* **24**, 761.

J6 JAMES T.N. (1961) Posterior myocardial infarction. *J. Mich. St. Med. Soc.* **60**, 1409.

J7 JAMES T.N. (1962) Arrhythmias and conduction disturbances in acute myocardial infarction. *Am. Heart J.* **64**, 416.

J8 JAMES T.N. (1968) The coronary circulation and conduction system in acute myocardial infarction. *Prog. Cardiovasc. Dis.* **10**, 410.

J9 JAMES T.N. & BURCH G.E. (1958) The blood supply of the human interventricular septum. *Circulation* **17**, 391.

J10 JAMES T.N. & GEOGHEGAN T. (1953) Sequential electrocardiographic changes following auricular injury. *Am. Heart J.* **46**, 830.

J11 JANSE M.J., VAN DER STEEN A.B.M., VAN DAM R.T. & DURRER D. (1969) Refractory period of the dog's ventricular myocardium following sudden changes in frequency. *Circ. Res.* **24**, 251.

J12 JEDLICKA J. & PANOS J. (1962) Die Rolle der negativen U-Wellen bei der entstehung der überdehnten T-negativitäten. *Cardiologia* **40**, 358.

J13 JENKINS J.S., BUCKELL M., CARTER A.B. & WESTLAKE S. (1969) Hypothalamic-pituitary-adrenal function after subarachnoid haemorrhage. *Brit. Med. J.* **4**, 707.

J14 JEWITT D.E., BALCON R., RAFTERY E.B. & ORAM S. (1967) Incidence and management of supraventricular arrhythmias after acute myocardial infarction. *Lancet* **2**, 734.

J15 JEZIERSKI W. (1936) Changes in the electrocardiogram after exercise in normals. *Polska Gazete Lekarska.* **15**, 677.

J16 JOHANSSON B. & VENDSALM A. (1957) The influence of adrenaline, nor-adrenaline, and acetylcholine on the electrocardiogram of the isolated perfused guinea-pig heart. *Acta Physiol. Scand.* **39**, 356.

J17 JOHNSON R.L., AVERILL K.H. & LAMB L.E. (1960) Electrocardiographic findings in 67,375 asymptomatic individuals. Part VI. Right bundle branch block. *Am. J. Cardiol.* **6**, 143.

J18 JOHNSTON F.D., WILSON F.N. & HECHT H.H. (1939): The precordial electrocardiogram in myocardial infarction complicated by bundle branch block. *J. Clin. Invest.* **18**, 476.

J19 LOUVE A., GUIRAN J.B., VIALLET H., GRAS A., BLANC M. ARNOUX M., ROUVIER M. & BRUNEL J.C. (1969) Les modifications electrocardiographiques au cours des crises d'angor spontane. A propos de la forme decrite par Prinzmetal. *Arch. Mal. Coeur* **62**, 331.

J20 JUHASZ-NAGY A. & SZENTIVANYI M. (1961) Localization of the receptors of the coronary chemo-reflex in the dog. *Arch. int. pharmacodyn.* **131**, 39.

J21 JULIAN D.G., VALENTINE P.A. & MILLER G.G. (1964) Disturbances of rate, rhythm and conduction in acute myocardial infarction. *Am. J. Med.* **37**, 915.

K

K1 KADISH A.H. (1953) Correlation of changes in body weight with electrocardiographic pattern. *Am. Practnr Dig. Treat.* **4**, 513.

K2 KAHN K.A. & SIMONSON E. (1957) Changes of mean spatial QRS and T vectors and of conventional electrocardiographic items in hard anaerobic work. *Circulation Res.* **5**, 629.

K3 KAIJSER L. (1966) EKG—förändringar vid koronarinsufficiens som funktion av arbetsintensitet och duration. *Läkartidningen* **63**, 3340.

K4 KALTER H.H. (1953) Reversal to normal of abnormal electrocardiograms following exercise tolerance tests in patients with coronary artery sclerosis and angina pectoris. *New York State J. Med.* **53**, 1548.

K5 KANNEL W.B., DAWBER T.R. & COHN M.E. (1958) The electrocardiogram in neurocirculatory asthenia (anxiety, neurosis or neurasthenia): a study of 203 neurocirculatory asthenia patients and 757 controls in the Framingham study. *Ann. Int. Med.* **49**, 1351.

K6 KARIV J. (1958) W.P.W. syndrome simulating myocardial infarction. *Am. Heart J.* **55**, 406.

K7 KARLEN W.S. & WOLFF L. (1956) The vectorcardiogram in pulmonary embolism. II. *Am. Heart J.* **51**, 839.

K8 KARPOVICH P. (1959) Physiology of Muscular Activity, 5th Edn. Philadelphia: W.B.Saunders.

K9 KATTUS A.A., JORGENSEN C.R., WORDEN R.E. & ALVARO A.B. (1971) S-T segment depression with near-maximal exercise in detection of preclinical coronary heart disease. *Circulation* **44**, 585.

K10 KATTUS A.A., MACALPIN R., LONGMIRE W.P., O'LOUGHLIN B.J. & BISHOP H. (1963) Coronary angiograms and the exercise electrocardiogram in the study of angina pectoris. *Am. J. Med.* **34**, 19.

K11 KATZ L.N. (1946) *Electrocardiography*. 2nd Edn. Philadelphia: Lea and Febiger.

K12 KATZ K.H., BERK M.S. & MAYMAN C.I. (1958) Acute myocardial infarction revealed in an isolated premature ventricular beat. *Circulation* **18**, 897.

K13 KATZ L.N. & LANDT H. (1935) The effect of standardized exercise on the four-lead electrocardiogram in the study of angina pectoris. *Am. J. Med. Sci.* **189**, 346.

K14 KAUFMAN J.M. & LUBERA R. (1967) Preoperative use of atropine and electrocardiographic changes. *JAMA* **200**, 197.

K15 KAYE H.B. (1948) Ventricular complexes in heart block. *Brit. Heart J.* **10**, 177.

K16 KEMP G.L. (1972) Value of treadmill stress testing in variant angina pectoris. *Am. J. Cardiol.* **30**, 781.

K17 KENNAMER R., BERNSTEIN J.L., MAXWELL M.H., PRINZMETAL M. & SHAW C.M. (1953) Studies on the mechanism of ventricular activity. V. Intramural depolarization potentials in the normal heart with a consideration of currents of injury in coronary artery disease. *Am. Heart J.* **46**, 379.

K18 KENNAMER R. & PRINZMETAL M. (1954) Depolarization of the ventricle with bundle branch block. Studies on the mechanism of ventricular activity. *Am. Heart J.* **47**, 769.

K19 KENNAMER R. & PRINZMETAL M. (1956) Myocardial infarction complicated by left bundle branch block. *Am. Heart J.* **51**, 78.

K20 KERNOHAN R.J. (1969) Post-paroxysmal tachycardia syndrome. *Brit. Heart J.* **31**, 803.

K21 KERT M.J. (1952) Electrocardiographic diagnosis of myocardial infarction in the presence of bundle branch block. *Ann. Western Med. & Surg.* **6**, 428.

K22 KERT M.J. & HOOBLER S.W. (1949) Observations on the potential variations of the cavities of the right side of the human heart. *Am. Heart J.* **38**, 97.

K23 KIESSLING C.E., SCHAAF R.S. & LYLE A.M. (1964) A study of T-wave changes in the electrocardiogram of normal individuals. *Am. J. Cardiol.* **13**, 598.

K24 KILLIP T. III (1967) In *Cardiac Pacing and Cardioversion*, ed.

Meltzer L.E. & Kitchell J.R. Philadelphia: The Charles Press Publishers Inc.

K25 KILLIP T. III & GAULT H.J. (1965) Mode of onset of atrial fibrillation in man. *Am. Heart J.* **70**, 172.

K26 KILLIP T. III & KIMBALL J.T. (1967) Treatment of myocardial infarction in a coronary care unit. A two-year experience with 250 patients. *Am. J. Cardiol.* **29**, 457.

K27 KINCAID D.T. & BOTTI R.E. (1972) Significance of isolated left anterior hemiblock and left axis deviation during acute myocardial infarction. *Am. J. Cardiol.* **30**, 797.

K28 KISTIN A.D. & ROBB G.C. (1949) Modification of the electrocardiogram of myocardial infarction by anomalous atrioventricular excitation (Wolff-Parkinson-White syndrome). Report of a case. *Am. Heart J.* **37**, 249.

K29 KITCHELL J.R. (1966) In *The Current Status of Intensive Coronary Care*. New York: The Charles Press.

K30 KITCHIN A.H. & NEILSON J.M. (1972) The *T* wave of the electrocardiogram during and after exercise in normal subjects. *Cardiovasc. Res.* **6**, 143.

K31 KLAKEG C.H., PRUITT R.D. & BURCHELL H.B. (1955) Study of electrocardiograms recorded during exercise tests on subjects in fasting state and after ingestion of heavy meal. *Am. Heart J.* **49**, 614.

K32 KLASS M. & HAYWOOD L.J. (1970) Atrial fibrillation associated with acute myocardial infarction. A study of 34 cases. *Am. Heart J.* **79**, 752.

K33 KLEMOLA E. (1942) Untersuchungen über das belastungselektrokardiogramm bei myokardschädigungen nach akuten infektionskrankheiten. *Acta Societatis Medicorum Fennicae 'Duodecim'* **32**, 59.

K34 KONECKE L.L. & KNOEBEL S.B. (1972) Nonparoxysmal junctional tachycardia complicating acute myocardial infarction. *Circulation* **45**, 367.

K35 KOSKELO P., PUNSAR S. & SIPILA W. (1964) Subendocardial haemorrhage and ECG changes in intracranial bleeding. *Brit. Med. J.* **1**, 1479.

K36 KOSOVICZ J. & ROGUSKA J. (1963) Electrocardiogram in hypopituitarism: reversibility of changes during treatment. *Am. Heart J.* **65**, 17.

K37 KOSSMANN C.E. (1956) The electrocardiogram and vectorcardiogram in coronary heart disease. *J. Chron. Dis.* **4**, 434.

K38 KOSSMANN C.E. (1958) Endocardial, myocardial and epicardial leads in man: current concepts of the spread of excitation and recovery in the ventricular wall. In *Advances in Electrocardiography*, ed. Kossmann C.E. p. 103. New York: Grune and Stratton.

K39 KOSSMANN C.E. (1958) Electrocardiographic effects of myocardial injury: electrical images. In *Advances in Electrocardiography*, ed. Kossmann C.E. p. 189. New York: Grune and Stratton.

K40 KOSSMANN C.E., BERGER A.R., RADER B., BRUMLIK J., BRILLER S.A. & DONNELLY J.H. (1950) Intracardiac and intravascular potentials resulting from electrical activity of the normal human heart. *Circulation* **2**, 10.

K41 KOSSMANN C.E., BURCHELL H.B., PRUITT R.D. & SCOTT R.C. (1962) The electrocardiogram in ventricular hypertrophy and bundle branch block. A panel discussion. *Circulation* **26**, 1337.

K42 KOSSMANN C.E. & DE LA CHAPELLE C.E. (1938) The precordial electrocardiogram in myocardial infarction I. Observations on cases with infarction principally of the anterior wall of the left ventricle and adjacent septum. *Am. Heart J.* **15,** 700.

K43 KOSTUK W.J. & BEANLANDS D.S. (1970) Complete heart block associated with acute myocardial infarction. *Am. J. Cardiol.* **26,** 380.

K44 KRIKLER D.M. & LEFEVRE D. (1970) Intermittent left bundle branch block without obvious heart disease. *Lancet* **1,** 498.

K45 KROOP I.G., JAFFE H.L. & MASTER A.M. (1949) The significance of RS-T elevation in acute coronary insufficiency. *Bull. NY Acad. Med.* **25,** 465.

K46 KRUMBHAAR E.B. & CROWELL C. (1925) Spontaneous rupture of the heart: clinicopathologic study based on 22 unpublished cases and 632 from the literature. *Am. J. Med. Sci.* **170,** 828.

K47 KULBERTUS H.E. & COLLIGNON P.G. (1969) Ventricular pre-excitation simulating anteroseptal infarction. *Dis. Chest* **56,** 461.

K48 KULBERTUS H.E., COLLIGNON P.G. & HUMBERT L. (1969) Vectorcardiographic study of QRS loop in patients with superior axis deviation and right bundle branch block. *Brit. Heart J.* **32,** 386.

K49 KULBERTUS H.E., COYNE J.J. & HALLIDIE-SMITH K.A. (1969) Conduction disturbances before and after surgical closure of ventricular septal defect. *Am. Heart J.* **77,** 123.

K50 KULBERTUS H.E. & HUMBERT L. (1972) Transient hemiblock: an abnormal type of response to the Master two-step exercise test. *Am. Heart J.* **83,** 574.

L

L1 LAHAM J. (1953) Infarctus du myocarde compliques de W.P.W. In *Etudes Electrocardiographiques.* Paris: Librairie Maloine.

L2 LAHAM J. (1969) In *Actualites Electrocardiographiques Le Syndrome de Wolff-Parkinson-White.* Paris: Librairie Malione.

L3 LAMB L.E. (1959) Multiple variations of W.P.W. conduction in one subject. Intermittent normal conduction and a false positive exercise tolerance test. *Am. J. Cardiol.* **4,** 346.

L4 LANGENDORF R. (1939) Elektrokardiogramm bei Vorhof-Infarkt. *Acta Med. Scand.* **100,** 136.

L5 LANGENDORF R. & PICK A. (1938) Zur diagnose des myokardinfarktes mit hilfe von brustwandableitungen. *Acta Med. Scand.* **96,** 80.

L6 LANGENDORF R. & PICK A. (1968) Atrioventricular block, Type II (Mobitz)—its nature and clinical significance. *Circulation* **38,** 819.

L7 LANGENDORF R., PICK A. & WINTERNITZ M. (1955) Mechanisms of intermittent ventricular bigeminy. I. Appearance of ectopic beats dependent upon the length of the ventricular cycle, the 'rule of bigeminy'. *Circulation* **11,** 422.

L8 LAPIN A.W. & SPRAGUE H.B. (1948) Respiratory movement as a factor in the production of Q waves in lead I and in unipolar leads from the left of the precordium in human left bundle branch block. *Am. Heart J.* **35,** 962.

L9 LASCANO E.F. (1943) Irrigacion normal del nodulo de Tawara, haz de His y sus ramas. *Rev. Arg. Cardiol.* **10,** 23.

L10 LASSERS B.W. & JULIAN D.G. (1968) Artificial pacing in management of complete heart block complicating myocardial infarction. *Brit. Med J.* **2,** 142.

L11 LAWRIE D.M. (1968) Ventricular fibrillation. In *Acute Myocardial Infarction,* ed. Julian D.G. & Oliver M.F., p. 99. Edinburgh: E. & S. Livingstone.

L12 LAWRIE D.M., GREENWOOD T.W., GODDARD M., HARVEY A.C., DONALD K.W., JULIAN D.G. & OLIVER M.F. (1967) A coronary-care unit in the routine management of acute myocardial infarction. *Lancet* **2,** 109.

L13 LAWRIE D.M., HIGGINS M.R., GODMAN M.J., OLIVER M.F., JULIAN D.G. & DONALD K.W. (1968) Ventricular fibrillation complicating acute myocardial infarction. *Lancet* **2,** 523.

L14 LEEDS M.F. & KROOPF S.S. (1953) Exercise test in electrocardiography: detection of coronary artery disease. *Calif. Med.* **79,** 36.

L15 LEGNANI L., NASI C. & RIMONDINI R. (1970) La sindrome post-tachicardica. *Minerva Cardioangiologica.* **18,** 487.

L16 LEITNER ST. J. & STEINLIN H. (1943) Untersuchungen über den einfluss des vegetativen nervensystems auf das elektrokardiogramm. *Arch. Kresilauflorsch.* **13,** 62.

L17 LEMBERG L., CASTELLANOS A. JR. & ARCEBAL A.G. (1971) The vectorcardiogram in acute left anterior hemiblock. *Am. J. Cardiol.* **28,** 483.

L18 LENEGRE J. (1958) *Contribution à l'étude des Blocs de Branche.* Paris: J.B.Balliere et fils.

L19 LENEGRE J. (1964) Etiology and pathology of bilateral bundle branch block in relation to complete heart block. *Prog. Cardiovasc. Dis.* **6,** 409.

L20 LENGYEL L., CARAMELL Z., MONFORT J. & GUERRA J.C. (1957) Initial electrocardiographic changes in experimental occlusion of the coronary artery in non-anaesthetized dogs with closed thorax. *Am. Heart J.* **53,** 334.

L21 LEPESCHKIN E. (1940) Der monophasische aktionsstrom des herzens und das elektrokardiogram bei erstilkung. *Ztschr. f.d. ges. exper. Med.* **107,** 478.

L22 LEPESCHKIN E. (1950) Slide for direct determination of corrected relative Q-T duration, heart rate, and percentamplitudes of electrocardiographic deflection. *Exper. Med. & Surg.* **8,** 240.

L23 LEPESCHKIN E. (1960) Exercise tests in the diagnosis of coronary artery disease. *Circulation* **22,** 986.

L24 LEPESCHKIN E. (1964) The electrocardiographic diagnosis of bilateral bundle branch block in relation to heart block. *Prog. Cardiovasc. Dis.* **6,** 445.

L25 LEPESCHKIN E. (1969) *Modern Electrocardiography,* 2nd printing. Ann Arbor, Michigan: Edward Bros.

L26 LEPESCHKIN E. Unpublished observations. Cited by E. Lepeschkin (1960).

L27 LEPESCHKIN E. & SURAWICZ B. (1952) Measurement of duration of QRS interval. *Am. Heart J.* **44,** 80.

L28 LEPESCHKIN E. & SURAWICZ B. (1953) New criteria for recognition 'false-positive' electrocardiographic exercise test. Presented at the 26th Scientific Session of the American Heart Association.

L29 LEPESCHKIN E. & SURAWICZ B. (1953) Duration of Q-U interval and its components in electrocardiograms of normal persons. *Am. Heart J.* **46,** 9.

L30 LEPESCHKIN E. & SURAWICZ B. (1958) Characteristics of true-positive and false-positive results of electrocardiographic Master two-step exercise tests. *New Engl. J. Med.* **258,** 511.

L31 LEPESCHKIN E., SURAWICZ B. & TERRIEN C.M. (1959) incidence provoked by electrocardiographic exercise tests. Presented at the Symposium on Electrocardiographic Exercise Tests. Burlington, Vermont.

L32 LESBRE J.P., ANE M. & SALVADOR M. (1968) L'angor de Prinzmetal. *Ann. Cardiol. Angeiol.* **17,** 215.

L33 LEV M. (1964) Anatomic basis for atrioventricular block. *Am. J. Med.* **37,** 742.

L34 LEV M., KINARE S.G. & PICK A. (1970) The pathogenesis of atrioventricular block in coronary disease. *Circulation* **42,** 409.

L35 LEV M., SODI-PALLARES D. & FRIEDLAND CH. (1962) Estudio histopatologico de comunicaciones auriculoventriculares en nu caso de sindrome de W.P.W. con bloqueo completo de la rama izquierda del fasciculo de His. *Proceedings of the IVth World Congress of Cardiology, Mexico,* p. 228.

L36 LEVANDER-LIUDGREN M. (1962) Studies in neurocirculatory asthenia (Da Costa's syndrome). *Acta Med. Scand.* **172,** 665.

L37 LEVENSTEIN J. & SCHAMROTH L. (1974) Myocardial infarction diagnosed from the ectopic beats of idioventricular tachycardia. *Heart and Lung* **3,** 129.

L38 LEVINE H.D. (1953) Non-specificity of the electrocardiogram associated with coronary artery disease. *Am. J. Med.* **15,** 344.

L39 LEVINE H.D. (1958) Static and dynamic electrocardiographic phenomena in coronary artery disease. *JAMA* **167,** 964.

L40 LEVINE H.D. & BURGE J.C. JR. (1948) Septal infarction with complete heart block and intermittent anomalous atrioventricular excitation (W.P.W. syndrome): Histologic demonstration of a right lateral bundle. *Am. Heart J.* **36,** 431.

L41 LEVINE H.D. & FORD R.V. (1950) Subendocardial infarction: Report of six cases and critical survey of the literature. *Circulation* **1,** 246.

L42 LEVINE H.D., LOWN B. & STREEPER R.B. (1952) The clinical significance of post-extrasystolic *T* wave changes. *Circulation* **6,** 538.

L43 LEVINE H.D., YOUNG E. & WILLIAMS R.A. (1972) Electrocardiogram and vectorcardiogram in myocardial infarction. *Circulation* **45,** 457.

L44 LEVINE H.J. & WHITE N.W. (1962) Unusual ECG patterns in rupture of vertebral artery aneurysm. *Arch. Int. Med.* **110,** 523.

L45 LEVINE S.A. (1945) *Clinical Heart Disease.* 3rd Edn. p. 398. Philadelphia: W.B.Saunders.

L46 LEVINTHAL J. & PURDY A. (1951) Electrocardiogram with deep *S* waves in all three Standard leads. Report of ten cases. *Am. J. Dis. Child.* **81,** 59.

L47 LEVY L. II, JACOBS H.J., CHASTAUT H.P. & STRAUSS H.B. (1950) Prominent *R* wave and shallow *S* wave in lead V1 as a result of lateral myocardial infarction. *Am. Heart J.* **40,** 447.

L48 LEWIS B.I. (1964) Mechanism and management of hyperventilation syndrome. *Biochem. Clin.* **4,** 89.

L49 LEWIS T. & ROTHSCHILD M.A. (1915) The excitatory process in the dog's heart. II. The ventricles. *Phil. Trans. R. Soc., B (Lond.)* **206,** 181.

L50 LIEBERMAN J.S., TAYLOR A. & WRIGHT J.S. (1954) The effect of intravenous trypsin administration on the electrocardiogram of the rabbit. *Circulation* **10,** 338.

L51 LIEBOW I.M. & FEIL H. (1941) Digitalis and normal work electrocardiogram. *Am. Heart J.* **22,** 683.

L52 LINDSAY S. (1946) The heart in primary systemic amyloidosis. *Am. Heart J.* **32,** 419.

L53 LINN H. & PICK A. (1963) Antero-septal myocardial infarction developing in stages. *Dis. Chest.* **43,** 644.

L54 LIPPESTAD C.T. & MARTON P.F. (1967) Sinus arrest in proximal right coronary artery occlusion. *Am. Heart J.* **74,** 551.

L55 LITTMAN D. (1946) Persistence of the juvenile pattern in precordial leads of healthy adult negroes, with report of electrocardiographic survey on three hundred negro and two hundred white subjects. *Am. Heart J.* **32,** 370.

L56 LITTMAN D. (1948) Abnormal electrocardiograms in the absence of demonstrable heart disease. *Am. J. Med.* **5,** 337.

L57 LITTMAN D. & BLAND E.F. (1953) Some pitfalls in electrocardiography. *M. Clin. North America.* **37,** 1341.

L58 LITTMAN D. & RODMAN M.H. (1951) An exercise test for coronary insufficiency. *Circulation* **3,** 875.

L59 LIU C.K., GREENSPAN G. & PICCIRILLO R.T. (1961) Atrial infarction of the heart. *Circulation* **23,** 331.

L60 LJUNG O. (1951) Alterations in the electrocardiogram as a result of emotionally stimulated respiratory movement especially with reference to the so-called 'fright electrocardiogram'. *Acta Med. Scand.* **141,** 221.

L61 LOGIC J.R., MORROW D.H. & GATZ R.N. (1969) Idioventricular tachycardia complicating experimental myocardial infarction. *Dis. Chest.* **56,** 477.

L62 LOGUE R.B., HANSON J.F. & KNIGHT W.A. (1944) Electrocardiographic studies in neurocirculatory asthenia. *Am. Heart J.* **28,** 574.

L63 LOMBARDI M. & MASINI G. (1966) *La pre-eccitazione ventricolare. Contributo clinico-sperimentale.* Milan: Recordati.

L64 LOOP F.D. (1971) Ventricular aneurysmectomy. *Surg. Clin. North America* **51,** 1071.

L65 LOVE W.S. JR. & BRUGLER G.W. (1937) Electrocardiograms similar to those of coronary thrombosis with especial reference to those obtained in pulmonary infarction. *South Med. J.* **30,** 371.

L66 LOWN B. (1966) In *The Current Status of Intensive Coronary Care.* ed. Meltzer L.E. & Kitchell J.R. p. 44. Philadelphia: The Charles Press Publishers Inc.

L67 LOWN B. (1967) Electrical reversion of cardiac arrhythmias. *Brit. Heart J.* **29,** 469.

L68 LOWN B. (1967) In *Cardiac Pacing and Cardioversion.* ed. Meltzer L.E. & Kitchell J.R. p. 77. Philadelphia: The Charles Press Publishers Inc.

L69 LOWN B., FAKHRO A.M. & HOOD W.B. JR. (1967) The coronary care unit. *J. Am. Med. Ass.* **199,** 188.

L70 LOWN B., KLEIN M.D. & HERSHBERG P. (1969) Coronary and precoronary care. *Am. J. Med.* **46,** 705.

L71 LOWN B., VASSAUX C., HOOD W.J. JR., FAKHRO A.M., KAPLINSKY E. & ROBERGE G. (1967) Unresolved problems in coronary care. *Am. J. Cardiol.* **20,** 494.

M

M1 MACALPIN R. (1970) Variant angina pectoris (letter). *N. Engl. J. Med.* **282,** 1491.

M2 MACALPIN R.N. & KATTUS A.A. (1967) Angina pectoris at rest with preservation of exercise capacity—angina inversa. *Circulation* **35–36** (*Supp. II*), 176 (Abstr.).

M3 MACALPIN R.N., WEIDNER W.A., KATTUS A.A. & HANAFEE W.N. (1966) Electrocardiographic changes during selective coronary cineangiography. *Circulation* **34,** 627.

M4 MACMILLAN R.L., BROWN K.W.G., PECKHAM G.B., KAHN O., HUTCHISON D.B. & PATON M. (1967) Changing perspectives in coronary care. A five-year study. *Am. J. Cardiol.* **20,** 451.

M5   MAGENDAIITZ H. & SHORTSLEEVE J. (1951) Electrocardiographic abnormalities in patients exhibiting anxiety. *Am. Heart J.* **42**, 849.

M6   MAHEIM I. (1931) *Les maladies organiques du faisceau de His-Tawara.* Paris: Nasson et Cie.

M7   MAHEIM I., HATT P.Y. & RIVIER J.L. (1954) L'infarctus septal et les lesions du tissu specifique ventriculaire. *Arch. Mal. Coeur* **47**, 465.

M8   MAINZER F. (1958) L'influence de l'anxiete sur l'electrocardiogramme: son importance dans l'electrocardiographie pratique. *Cardiologia.* **32**, 362.

M9   MALLACH J.F., FINKELMAN I., ARIEFF A.J. & ROBERTS R.C. (1943) Electrocardiographic changes resulting from dilantin medication. *Quart. Bull. Northwestern Univ. Med. School* **17**, 97.

M10   MALLORY G.K., WHITE P.D. & SALCEDO-SALGAR J. (1939) The speed of healing of myocardial infarction. A study of the pathologic anatomy in 72 cases. *Am. Heart J.* **18**, 647.

M11   MANDEL W.J., BURGESS M.J., NEVILLE J. JR. & ABILDSKOV J.A. (1968) Analysis of *T* wave abnormalities associated with myocardial infarction using a theoretic model. *Circulation* **38**, 178.

M12   MANN R.H. & BURCHELL H.B. (1954) The significance of *T* wave inversion in sinus beats following ventricular extrasystoles. *Am. Heart J.* **47**, 504.

M13   MANNING G.W. (1957) The electrocardiogram of the two-step exercise stress test. *Am. Heart J.* **54**, 823.

M14   MARRIOTT H.J.L. (1960) Coronary mimicry: normal variants, and physiologic, pharmacologic and pathologic influences that simulate coronary patterns in the electrocardiogram. *Ann. Int. Med.* **52**, 411.

M15   MARRIOTT H.J.L. (1969) Arrhythmias in acute myocardial infarction. In *Coronary Heart Disease.* ed. Brest A.N. Philadelphia: F.A.Davis Co.

M16   MARRIOTT H.J.L. (1972) *Practical Electrocardiography*, 4th Edn. Baltimore: Williams and Wilkens Co.

M17   MARRIOTT H.J.L. (1972) *Workshop in electrocardiography.* Oldmar, Florida: Tampa Tracings.

M18   MARRIOTT H.J.L. & FOGG E. (1970) Constant monitoring for cardiac dysrrhythmias and blocks. *Mod. Conc. Cardiovasc. Dis.* **39**, 103.

M19   MARRIOTT H.J.L. & FOGG E. (1970) Unpublished observations. Cited by H.J.L.Marriott & E.Fogg.

M20   MARRIOTT H.J.L. & HOGAN P. (1970) Hemiblock in acute myocardial infarction. *Chest* **58**, 342.

M21   MARRIOTT H.J.L. & MENDENEZ M.M. (1969) AV dissociation revisited. *Progr. Cardiovasc. Dis.* **8**, 522.

M22   MARSHALL R.M., BLOUNT S.G. & GENTON E. (1968) Acute myocardial infarction: influence of a coronary care unit. *Arch. intern. Med.* **122**, 472.

M23   MARUFFO C.A. (1967) Fine structural study of myocardial changes induced by isoproterenol in rhesus monkey (macaca mulatta). *Am. J. Pathol.* **50**, 27.

M24   MASON R.E. (1959) The Master test in patients with coronary heart disease and in normal subjects. *Heart Bull.* **8**, 67.

M25   MASON R.E. & LIKAR I. (1966) A new system of multiple-lead exercise electrocardiography. *Am. Heart J.* **71**, 196.

M26   MASON R.E., LIKAR I., BIERN R.O. & ROSS R.S. (1967) Multiple lead exercise electrocardiography. *Circulation* **36**, 517.

M27   MASON R.E., LIKAR I.N. & ROSS R.S. (1964) New system of multiple leads in exercise electrocardiography. Comparison with coronary arteriography. *Circulation* **30** (Suppl. **3**), 123 (Abstr.).

M28   MASSUMI R.A., GOLDMAN A., RAKITA L., KURAMOTO K. & PRINZMETAL M. (1955) Studies on the mechanism of ventricular activity. XVI. Activation of the human ventricle. *Am. J. Med.* **19**, 832.

M29   MASTER A.M. (1933) *P* wave changes in acute coronary occlusion. *Am. Heart J.* **8**, 462.

M30   MASTER A.M. (1935) The two-step test of myocardial function. *Am. Heart J.* **10**, 495.

M31   MASTER A.M. (1944) Electrocardiogram and 'two-step' exercise: test of cardiac function and coronary insufficiency. *Am. J. Med. Sci.* **207**, 435.

M32   MASTER A.M. (1953) 'Two-step' exercise electrocardiogram: its use in heart diseases, including valvular heart disease of adults. *Bull. St. Francis Sanat. Cardiol. Child.* **18**, 1.

M33   MASTER A.M. (1958) Iproniazid (Marsilid) in angina pectoris. *Am. Heart J.* **56**, 570.

M34   MASTER A.M. (1964) 'Silent' coronary artery disease. *Med. Tribune* **5**, 15 (Abstr.).

M35   MASTER A.M. (1968) The Master two-step test. *Am. Heart J.* **75**, 837.

M36   MASTER A.M. (1970) Is the highest rate attained in the Master 'two-step' test sufficient? *Circulation* **41**, (Suppl. **3**) (Abstr.).

M37   MASTER A.M. (1970): 'Augmented' two-step test. *Trans. Ass. Life Ins. Med. Dir. Amer.* **54**, 52.

M38   MASTER A.M. (1972) Exercise testing for evaluation of cardiac performance. *Am. J. Cardiol.* **30**, 718.

M39   MASTER A.M., DACK S. & JAFFE H.L. (1938) Bundle branch block and intraventricular block in acute coronary artery occlusion. *Am. Heart J.* **16**, 283.

M40   MASTER A.M., DACK S. & JAFFE H.L. (1941) Premonitory symptoms of acute coronary occlusion. A study of 260 cases. *Ann. Intern. Med.* **14**, 1155.

M41   MASTER A.M. & DONOSO E. (1959) A symposium: The two-step exercise test. *Heart Bull.* **8**, 63.

M42   MASTER A.M., FIELD L.E. & DONOSO E. (1957) Coronary artery disease and the 'two-step exercise test'. *New York J. Med.* **57**, 1051.

M43   MASTER A.M., FRIEDMAN R. & DACK S. (1942) The electrocardiogram after standard exercise as a functional test of the heart. *Am. Heart J.* **24**, 777.

M44   MASTER A.M. & GELLER A.J. (1964) Magnitude of silent coronary disease. *New York J. Med.* **64**, 2865.

M45   MASTER A.M. & GELLER A.J. (1969) The extent of complete asymptomatic coronary artery disease. *Am. J. Cardiol.* **23**, 173.

M46   MASTER A.M. & JAFFE H.L. (1941) The electrocardiographic changes after exercise in angina pectoris. *J. Mt. Sinai Hosp.* **7**, 629.

M47   MASTER A.M. & OPPENHEIMER E.T. (1929) A simple tolerance test for circulatory efficiency with standard tables for normal individuals. *Am. J. Med. Sci.* **177**, 223.

M48   MASTER A.M., PORDY L. & CHESKY K. (1953) Two-step exercise electrocardiogram: follow-up investigation in patients with chest pain and normal resting electrocardiogram. *JAMA* **151**, 458.

M49   MASTER A.M. & ROSENFELD I. (1959) The Master two-step electrocardiographic test brought up to date. *Tr. A Life Insur. M. Dir. America* **43**, 70.

M50   MASTER A.M. & ROSENFELD I. (1961) The 'two-step' exercise test brought up to date. *New York State J. Med.* **61**, 1850.

M51   MASTER A.M. & ROSENFELD I. (1962) The Master two-step test. Use in diagnosis of 'incipient' coronary artery disease. *Ohio State Med. J.* **58**, 1011.

M52 MASTER A.M. & ROSENFELD L. (1965) Silent coronary heart disease. *Mod. Med.* **33,** 78.

M53 MASTER A.M. & ROSENFELD I. (1967) Exercise electrocardiography as an estimation of cardiac function *Chest* **51,** 347.

M54 MASTER A.M. & ROSENFELD I. (1967) Two-step exercise test: current status after 25 years. *Mod. Conc. Cardiovasc. Dis.* **36,** 19.

M55 MASTER A.M. & ROSENFELD I. (1968) Current status of the two-step exercise test. *J. Electrocardiol.* **1,** 5.

M56 MATHISON A.K. & PALMER J.D. (1947) Diffuse scleroderma with involvement of the heart. *Am. Heart J.* **33,** 366.

M57 MATTINGLY T.W. (1962) The postexercise electrocardiogram. Its value in the diagnosis and prognosis of coronary arterial disease. *Am. J. Cardiol.* **9,** 395.

M58 MATTINGLY T.W., FANCHER P.S., BAUER F.L. & ROBB G.P. (1954): The value of the double standard two-step tolerance test in detecting coronary disease in a follow-up study of 1000 military personnel. Research report. Army Medical Service Graduate School, Walter Reed Army Medical Center, Washington, D.C.

M59 MATTINGLY T.W., ROBB G.P. & MARKS H.H. (1957) The electrocardiographic stress tests in suspected coronary disease: a long-term statistical evaluation of the types of responses to the double standard two-step exercise test and the anoxemia test. Walter Reed Army Institute Research, No. **75,** 1.

M60 MAYER J.W., CASTELLANOS A. JR. & LEMBERG L. (1963) The spatial vectorcardiography in peri-infarction block. *Am. J. Cardiol.* **11,** 613.

M61 MAYERSON H.S. & DAVIS W.D. (1942) The influence of posture on the electrocardiogram. *Am. Heart J.* **24,** 593.

M62 MAYTIN O., CASTILLO C. & CASTELLANOS A. JR. (1970) The genesis of QRS changes produced by selective coronary arteriography. *Circulation* **41,** 247.

M63 MAZER M. & REISINGER J.A. (1944) Electrocardiographic study of cardiac aging based on records at rest and after exercise. *Ann. Int. Med.* **21,** 645.

M64 McARTHUR S.W. & WAKEFIELD H. (1945) Observations on the human electrocardiogram during experimental distension of the gallbladder. *J. Lab. Clin. Med.* **30,** 349.

M65 McCONAHAY D.R., McCALLISTER B.D. & SMITH R.E. (1971) Postexercise electrocardiography: correlations with coronary arteriography and left ventricular hemodynamics. *Am. J. Cardiol.* **28,** 1.

M66 McGINN S. & WHITE P.D. (1935) Acute cor pulmonale resulting from pulmonary embolism: its clinical recognition. *JAMA* **114,** 1473.

M67 McGURL F.J. & ROSS R.L. (1957) The double Master test; a study of 247 normal men. *Tr. A. Life Insur.* **40,** 40.

M68 MEDRANO G.A., BISTENI A., BRANCATO R.W., PILEGGI F., and Sodi-Pallares D. (1957) The activation of the interventricular septum in the dog's heart under normal conditions and in bundle branch block. *Bull. N.Y. Acad. Sci.* **65,** 804.

M69 MEDRANO G.A., BRENES P.C., DE MICHELI A. & SODI-PALLARES D. (1969) El bloqueo de la subdivision anterior de la rama izquierda solo o asociado al bloqueo de la rama derecha. *Arch. Inst. Cardiol. Mexico* **39,** 672.

M70 MEDRANO G.A., BRENES C. & SODI-PALLARES, D. (1970) Necrosis posteroinferior del ventriculo izquierdo aislada y asociada a bloqueo de la subdivision posterior de la rama izquierda del haz de His. *Arch. Inst. Cardiol. Mexico* **40,** 645.

M71 MEDRANO G.A., DE MICHELI A., BISTENI A. & SODI-PAL-LARES, D. (1962) Infartos septales anteriores complicados con bloqueo de rama (estudio experimental electro-vectocardiografico). *IVth World Congress of Cardiology, Mexico* p. 250.

M72 MEDRANO G.A., DE MICHELI A., CISNEROS F. & SODI-PALLARES D. (1970) The anterior subdivision block of the left bundle branch of His. I. The ventricular activation process. *J. Electrocardiol.* **3,** 7.

M73 MEDRANO G.A., PILEGGI F., BISTENI A. & SODI-PALLARES, D. (1958) Nuevas investigaciones sobre la activacion del tabique interventricular en condiciones normales y con bloqueo de rama. IV. Estudio de la porcion posterior del tercio medio. *Arch. Inst. Cardiol. Mexico* **28,** 812.

M74 MEDRANO G.A., PILEGGI F., SOTOMAYOR A., BISTENI A. & SODI-PALLARES D. (1956) Nuevas investigaciones sobre la activacion del tabique interventricular en condiciones normales y con bloqueo de rama. I. Estudio de la porcion postero-basal. *Arch. Inst. Cardiol. Mexico* **26,** 616.

M75 MEDRANO G.A., PILEGGI F., SOTOMAYOR A., BISTENI A. & SODI-PALLARES D. (1957) Nuevas investigaciones sobre la activacion del tabique interventricular en condiciones normales y con bloqueo de rama. II. Estudio de la porcion antero-basal. *Arch. Inst. Cardiol. Mexico* **27,** 299.

M76 MEDRANO G.A., PILEGGI F., SOTOMAYER A., BISTENI A. & SODI-PALLARES D. (1957) Nuevas investigaciones sobre la activacion del tabique interventricular en condiciones normales y con bloqueo de rama. III. Estudio del tercio medio del tabique. Prociones anterior y media. *Arch. Inst. Cardiol. Mexico* **27,** 609.

M77 MELLVILLE K.I., BLUM B., SHISTER H. & SILVER M.D. (1963) Cardiac ischemic changes and arrhythmias induced by hypothalamic stimulation. *Am. J. Cardiol.* **12,** 781.

M78 MELTZER L.E. & COHEN H.E. (1972) The incidence of arrhythmias associated with acute myocardial infarction. In *Textbook of Coronary Care*, ed. Meltzer L.E. & Dunning A.J., Amsterdam: Excerpta Medica.

M79 MELTZER L.E. & KITCHELL J.R. (1966) The incidence of arrhythmias associated with acute myocardial infarction. *Prog. Cardiovasc. Dis.* **9,** 50.

M80 MELTZER L.E., PINNEO R. & KITCHELL J.R. (1965) *Intensive Coronary Care—A Manual for Nurses*, p. 180. Philadelphia: The Charles Press Publishers Inc.

M81 MEYER P. & SCHMIDT C. (1949) Troubles post-extrasystoliques de la repolarisation. *Arch. Mal Coeur* **42,** 1175.

M82 MILLAR K. & ABILDSKOV J.A. (1968) Notched *T* waves in young persons with central nervous system lesions. *Circulation* **37,** 597.

M83 MIROWSKI M., NEILL C.A. & TAUSSIG H.B. (1963) Left atrial ectopic rhythm in mirror-image dextrocardia and in normally placed malformed hearts. Report of 12 cases with 'dome and dart' *P* waves. *Circulation* **27,** 864.

M84 MISSAL M.E. (1938) Exercise tests and the electrocardiograph in the study of angina pectoris. *Ann. Int. Med.* **11,** 2018.

M85 MITCHELL J.H. & SHAPIRO A.P. (1954) The relationship of adrenalin and *T*-wave changes in the anxiety state. *Am. Heart J.* **48,** 323.

M86 MOGENSON L. (1970) Ventricular tachyarrhythmias and lignocaine prophylaxis in acute myocardial infarction (a clinical and therapeutic study). *Acta Med. Scand.* Suppl. **188,** 513.

M87 MOIA B. & ACEVEDO H.T. (1945) El diagnostico Electrocardiographico del infarto de miocardio complicado por bloqueo de rama. *Rev. Argent. de Cardiol.* **11,** 341.

M88 MOLL A. & LUTTEROTTI M. (1951) Die Beursteilung des 'Diskrepantztypus der R-Zacke' (rI, SII, SIII—Bild des EKG). *Z. fur Kreislaufforsch.* **40,** 737.

M89 MOSS A.J., SCHNITZLER R., GREEN R. & DeCAMILLA, J. (1971) Ventricular arrhythmias 3 weeks after acute myocardial infarction. *Ann. Intern. Med.* **75,** 837.

M90 MURAYAMA M., HARUMI K., CHEN C. & MURAO S. (1971) Post-extrasystolic ST, T changes in the exercise vectorcardiogram with Frank's lead. *Japanese Heart J.* **12,** 185.

M91 MURNAGHAN D., McGINN S. & WHITE P.D. (1943) Pulmonary embolism with and without acute cor pulmonale, with especial reference to the electrocardiogram. *Am. Heart J.* **25,** 573.

M92 MYERS G.B., KLEIN H.A. & STOFER B.E. (1948) Correlation of electrocardiographic and pathologic findings in anteroseptal infarction. *Am. Heart J.* **36,** 535.

M93 MYERS G.B., KLEIN H.A., STOFER B.E. & HIRATZKA T. (1957) Normal variations in multiple precordial leads. *Am. Heart J.* **34,** 785.

M94 MYERS G.B., SEARS C.H. & HIRATZKA T. (1951) Correlation of electrocardiographic and pathologic findings in ring-like subendocardial infarction of the left ventricle. *Am. J. Med. Sci.* **222,** 417.

M95 MYERS G.B. & TALMERS F.N. (1955) The electrocardiographic diagnosis of acute myocardial ischemia. *Ann. Int. Med.* **43,** 361.

N

N1 NADAS A., ALIMURUNG M. & SIERACKI L.A. (1951) Cardiac manifestations of Friedreich's ataxia. *N. Engl. J. Med.* **244,** 239.

N2 NAHUM L.H., HAMILTON W.F. & HOFF H.E. (1943) The injury current in the electrocardiogram. *Am. J. Physiol.* **139,** 202.

N3 NARULA O.S. & SAMET P. (1970) Wenkebach and Mobitz type II A-V block due to block within the His bundle and bundle branches. *Circulation* **41,** 947.

N4 NATHAN D. & BEELER G.W. JR. (1970) The effect of isoproterenol on ventricular action potentials and contraction. *Physiologist* **13,** 269.

N5 NELSON C.V. (1955) Effect of the finite boundary on potential distributions in volume conductors. *Circulation Res.* **3,** 236.

N6 NELSON C.V. (1965) Determination of the resultant dipole moment of the heart in the human and the animal. In *Electrophysiology of the Heart*, ed. Taccardi B. & Marchetti G., p. 281. Oxford: Pergamon Press.

N7 NELSON C.V., LANGE R.L., HECHT H.H., CARLISLE R.P. & RUBY A.S. (1956) Effect of intracardiac blood, and of fluids of different conductivities on the magnitude of surface vectors. *Circulation* **14,** 977.

N8 NEUFELD H.N., ONGLEY P.A. & EDWARDS J.E. (1960) Combined congenital subaortic stenosis and infundibular pulmonary stenosis. *Brit. Heart J.* **22,** 403.

N9 NEUMAN A. (1972) Intermittent regional delay of left ventricular activation. The influence of such a delay on the standard electrocardiogram; report of 33 cases. *Chest* **61,** 633.

N10 NICOLAI G.F. & SIMONS A. (1909) Zur klinik des elektrokardiogramms. *Med. Klin.* **5,** 160.

N11 NIELSEN B.L. (1973) S-T segment elevation in acute myocardial infarction. Prognostic importance. *Circulation* **48,** 338.

N12 NIEMI T. (1955) Master's two-step tolerance test: application to series of 104 normal old people. *Ann. med. int. Fenniae* **44,** 99.

N12 NORDENFELDT O. (1965) Orthostatic ECG changes and the andrenergic beta receptor blocking agent propranolol (Inderal). *Acta Med. Scand.* **178,** 393.

N14 NORRIS R.M. (1969) Heart block in posterior and anterior myocardial infarction. *Brit. Heart J.* **31,** 352.

N15 NORRIS R.M. (1970) Arrhythmias in acute myocardial infarction. In *Symposium on Cardiac Arrhythmias*, ed. Sandøe E., Flensted-Jensen E. & Olesen K.H., p. 734. Södertälje, Sweden: A.B.Astra.

N16 NORRIS R.M. & CROXON M.S. (1970) Bundle branch block in acute myocardial infarction. *Am. Heart J.* **79,** 728.

N17 NORRIS R.M., MERCER C.J. & YEATES S.E. (1970) Idioventricular rhythm complicating acute myocardial infarction. *Brit. Heart J.*, **32,** 617.

O

O1 OAKLEY C.M. (1970) Diagnosis of pulmonary embolism. *Brit. Med. J.* **2,** 773.

O2 OLIVER M.F. (1968) In *Acute Myocardial Infarction*, ed. Julian D.G. & Oliver M.F. Edinburgh: E. & S. Livingstone.

O3 ONGLEY P.A. & duSHANE J.W. (1966) Counterclockwise superiorly displaced frontal plane loops of the vectorcardiogram in children. In *Vectorcardiography—1965*, ed. Hoffman L. & Taymor R.C., p. 329. Amsterdam: North Holland Publishing Co.

O4 OPDYKE D.F. & SELKURT E.E. (1948) A study of alleged reflexes following coronary occlusion. *Am. Heart J.* **36,** 73.

O5 OSHER H.L. & WOLFF L. (1953) Electrocardiographic pattern simulating myocardial injury. *Am. J. Med. Sci.* **226,** 541.

O6 OSTRANDER L.D. JR. (1971) Left axis deviation: prevalence, associated conditions, and prognosis. An epidemiologic study. *Ann. Int. Med.* **75,** 23.

P

P1 PALAGI L., SONNINO S., PULETTI M., JACOBELLIS G.F. & BISCHIERI L. (1966) Indagini su l'importanza del ritardo di attivanzione del miocardio 'ischemico' nella genesi della corrente di lesione. *Cuore Circ.* **50,** 248.

P2 PALMER D.G. (1962) Interruption of *T* waves by premature QRS complexes and the relationship of this phenomenon to ventricular fibrillation. *Am. Heart J.* **63,** 367.

P3 PANTRIDGE J.F. (1951) Observations on the electrocardiogram and ventricular gradient in complete left bundle branch block. *Circulation* **3,** 589.

P4 PANTRIDGE J.F. & GEDDES J.S. (1967) A mobile intensive-care unit in the management of myocardial infarction. *Lancet* **2,** 271.

P5 PAPP C. & SMITH K.S. (1951) Electrocardiographic patterns in slight coronary attacks. *Brit. Heart. J.* **13,** 17.

P6 PARE J.A.P., FRASER R.G., PIROZYNSKI W.J., SHANK J.A. & STUBBINGTON D. (1961) Hereditary cardiovascular dysplasia. *Am. J. Med.* **31,** 37.

P7   PARISI A.F., BECKMANN C.H. & LANCASTER M.C. (1971) The spectrum of S-T segment elevation in the electrocardiograms of healthy adult men. *J. Electrocardiol.* **4,** 137.

P8   PARKER C.S., BREAKELL C.G. & CHRISTOPHERSON F. (1953) The radioelectrocardiogram. Radiotransmission of electrophysiological data from the ambulant and active patient. *Lancet* **1,** 1285.

P9   PARKER R.L., ODEL H.M., LOGAN A.H., KELSEY J.R. & EDWARDS J.E. (1950) Primary systemic amyloidosis. *M. Clin. North America.* **34,** 1119.

P10 PAYNE C.A. & GRENNFIELD J.C. (1963) Electrocardiographic abnormalities associated with myotonic dystrophy. *Am. Heart J.* **65,** 436.

P11 PENTECOST B.L. & MAYNE N.M.C. (1968) Results of a general hospital coronary care service. *Brit. Med. J.* **1,** 830.

P12 PENTIMONE F., PESOLA A., L'ABBATE A., SMORFA A. & GIUSTI C. (1967) Effetto del propranololo sulle modifica elettocardiografiche secondarie alla prova de iperventilarione volontaria ed alla prova ortostatica. *Cuore Circ.* **51,** 79.

P13 PERELMAN J.S. & MILLER R. (1947) Atrio-nodal rhythm with ventricular bigeminy. Report of a case with unusual mechanism. *Am. Heart J.* **33,** 34.

P14 PERLMAN M.M. (1972) Electrocardiographic changes in acute pulmonary embolism. *Heart and Lung* **1,** 831.

P15 PERLOFF J.K. (1964) The recognition of strictly posterior myocardial infarction by conventional scalar electrocardiography. *Circulation* **30,** 706.

P16 PERLOFF J.K., ROBERTS W.C. & DE LEON A.C. JR. (1967) The distinctive electrocardiogram of Duchenne's progressive muscular dystrophy. An electrocardiographic-pathologic correlative study. *Am. J. Med.* **42,** 179.

P17 PICCOLO E., DE MICHELI A., COCCO F. & SODI-PALLARES, D. (1960) Etude electrocardiographique de l'infarctus du myocarde sur les bases d'une nouvelle classification. *Mal. Cardiovasc.* **1,** 365.

P18 PICCOLO E., MIORI R. & FURLANELLO F. (1965) Diagnostic aspects of peri-infarction block. *Cardiovasc. Comp.* **1,** 23.

P19 PICK A. & DOMINGUEZ P. (1957) Nonparoxysmal A-V nodal tachycardia. *Circulation* **16,** 1022.

P20 PICK A., LANGENDORF R. & KATZ L.N. (1961) A-V nodal tachycardia with block. *Circulation* **24,** 12.

P21 PIPBERGER H.V., STALLMAN F.W. & BERSON A.S. (1962) Automatic analysis of the P-QRS-T complex of the electrocardiogram by digital computer. *Ann. Int. Med.* **57,** 776.

P22 PLAVSIC C., MARIC D. & ZIMOLO A. (1956) Infarctus du myocarde et syndrome de Wolff-Parkinson-White. *Acta Cardiol.* **11,** 190.

P23 POGGI, L., BORY M., PINAS E., D'JOUNO J., DJIANE P., FRANCOIS G., SERRADIMIGNI A. & AUDIER M. (1969) L'enregistrement electrographique continu dans l'angor de Prinzmetal. *Arch. Mal. Coeur* **62,** 1241.

P24 POLLOCK A.V. & BERTRANS C.A. (1956) Electrocardiographic changes in acute pancreatitis. *Surgery* **40,** 951.

P25 PORTER R.W., KAMIKAWA K. & GREENHOOT J.H. (1962) Persistent electrocardiographic abnormalities experimentally induced by stimulation of the brain. *Am. Heart J.* **64,** 815.

P26 POZZI L.L. & FANTINI F. (1961) Difficolta diagnostiche nella sindrome di W.P.W. *Cardiologia Practica* **12,** 43. Quoted in Reference L1.

P27 PRESCOTT R., QUINN J.S. & LITTMAN D. (1963) Electrocardiographic changes in hypertrophic subaortic stenosis which simulate myocardial infarction. *Am. Heart J.* **66,** 43.

P28 PRINZMETAL M., EKMEKCI A., KENNAMER R., KWOCZYNSKI J.K., SHUBIN H. & TOYOSHIMA H. (1960) Variant form of angina pectoris; previously undelineated syndrome. *JAMA* **1,** 794.

P29 PRINZMETAL M., EKMEKCI A., TOYOSHIMA H. & KWOCZYNSKI J.K. (1959) Angina pectoris. III. Demonstration of a chemical origin of S-T deviation in classic angina pectoris, its variant form, early myocardial infarction, and some non-cardiac conditions. *Am. J. Cardiol.* **3,** 276.

P30 PRINZMETAL M., KENNAMER R., MERLISSS R., WADA T. & BOR N. (1959) Angina pectoris. I. A variant form of angina pectoris. *Am. J. Med.* **27,** 374.

P31 PRINZMETAL, M., SHAW C., MAXWELL M., FLAMM E., GOLDMAN A., KIMURA N., RAKITA L., BORDUAS J., ROTHMAN S. & KENNAMER R. (1954) Studies on mechanism of ventricular activity; depolarisation complex in pure subendocardial infarction; role of subendocardial region in normal electrocardiogram. *Am. J. Med.* **16,** 469.

P32 PRUITT R.D., BARNES A.R. & ESSEX H.E. (1945) Electrocardiographic changes associated with lesions in the deeper layers of the myocardium. An experimental study. *Am. J. Med. Sci.* **210,** 100.

P33 PRUITT R.D., DENNIS E.W. & KINARD S.A. (1963) The difficult electrocardiographic diagnosis of myocardial infarction. *Prog. Cardiovasc. Dis.* **6,** 85.

P34 PRUITT R.D., KLALEG C.H. & CHAPIN L.E. (1955) Certain clinical states and pathologic changes associated with deeply inverted *T* waves in the precordial electrocardiogram. *Circulation* **11,** 517.

P35 PRUITT R.D. & VALENCIA F. (1948) The immediate electrocardiographic effects of circumscribed myocardial injuries; an experimental study. *Am. Heart J.* **35,** 161.

P36 PRYOR R. & BLOUNT S.G. (1966) The clinical significance of true left axis deviation. *Am. Heart J.* **72,** 391.

P37 PUDDU V. & SIBILIA D. (1960) Contributo clinico alla conoscenza dell'angina di tipo Prinzmetal. *Proceedings of the 3rd European Congress of Cardiology.*

P38 PUECH P., LATOUR H., HERTAULT J. & GROLLEAU R. (1964) L'ajmaline injectable dans les tachycardies paroxystiques et le syndrome W.P.W. Comparaison avec la procainamide. *Arch. Mal. Coeur* **57,** 867.

Q

Q1   QUERIDO A., VAN DER WERFFTEN BOSCH J.J., BLOM P.S. & GILSE H.A. (1954) Post-partum hypopituitarism. *Acta Med. Scand.* **149,** 291.

R

R1   RAKITA L., BORDUAS J.L., ROTHMAN S. & PRINZMETAL M. (1954) Studies on the mechanism of ventricular activity. XII. Early changes in the RS-T segment and QRS complex following acute coronary artery occlusion. Experimental study and clinical applications. *Am. Heart J.* **48,** 351.

R2   RANDLES F.S. & FRADKIN N.F. (1948) Electrocardiographic alterations resembling those produced by myocardial infarction observed during a spontaneous attack of angina pectoris. *Ann. Int. Med.* **28,** 671.

R3 RAYNAUD R., BROCHIER M., MORAND P., FAUCHIER J.P., RAYNAUD P. & CHATELAIN B. (1969) Une forme clinique de L'angine de poitrine: l'angor de Prinzmetal. *Sem. Hôp. Paris* **45**, 2662.

R4 REINDELL H. (1938) Kymographische und elektrokardiographische befunde am sportherzen. *Deutsch. Arch. Klin. Med.* **181**, 485.

R5 REINDELL H. (1939) Die herzbeurteilung beim sportsmann und die differentialdiagnostische bewertung der befunde im de EKG und kymogramm. *Deutsch. med. Wchnschr.* **65**, 1369.

R6 REMINGTON J.W. & AHLQUIST R.P. (1953) Effect of sympathomimetic drugs on the Q–T interval and on the duration of ejection. *Am. J. Physiol.* **174**, 165.

R7 REYNOLDS E.W., JR., VAN DER ARK R. & JOHNSTON F.D. (1960) Effect of acute myocardial infarction on electrical recovery and transmural temperature gradient in the left ventricular wall of dogs. *Circ. Res.* **8**, 730.

R8 RHOADS D.V., EDWARDS J.E. & PRUITT R.D. (1961) The electrocardiogram in the presence of myocardial infarction and intraventricular block of the left bundle branch block type. *Am. Heart J.* **62**, 735.

R9 RICHARDSON J.A., WOODS E.F. & BAGWELL E.E. (1960) Circulating epinephrine and norepinephrine in coronary occlusion. *Am. J. Cardiol.* **5**, 613.

R10 RICHMAN J.L. & WOLFF L. (1954) Left bundle branch block masquerading as right bundle branch block. *Am. Heart J.* **47**, 383.

R11 RIHL J., HUTTMANN A. & SPIEGL E. (1935) Uber das arbeitselektrokardiogramm. *Ztschr. Kreislaufforsch.* **27**, 659.

R12 RINZLER S.H. & TRAVELL J. (1947) The electrocardiographic diagnosis of acute myocardial infarction in the presence of the Wolff-Parkinson-White syndrome. *Am. J. Med.* **3**, 106.

R13 RISEMAN, J.E.F. & STERN B. (1934) A standardized exercise tolerance test for patients with angina pectoris on exertion. *Am. J. Med. Sci.* **188**, 646.

R14 RISEMAN J.E.F., WALLER J.V. & BROWN M.G. (1940) The electrocardiogram during attacks of angina pectoris: Its characteristics and diagnostic significance. *Am. Heart J.* **19**, 683.

R15 RIVERA-DIAZ R.S., RAMOS-MORALES F. & GARCIA-PARLMIERI E.A. (1961) The electrocardiographic changes in acute phosphorus poisoning in man. *Am. J. Med. Sci.* **241**, 758.

R16 ROBB G.P. (1951) Coronary artery disease, stress tests. *Med. Ann. District of Columbia* **20**, 313.

R17 ROBB G.P. (1959) Value of the electrocardiographic Master exercise test as determined from a follow-up of one thousand consecutive tests in military personnel and in life insurance applicants. *Seminar on the Electrocardiographic Exercise Test.* Burlington, Vermont: Vermont Heart Association.

R18 ROBB G.P. & MARKS H.H. (1960) Evaluation of type and degree of change in post-exercise electrocardiogram in detecting coronary artery disease. *Proc. Soc. Exper. Biol. and Med.* **103**, 450.

R19 ROBB G.P. & MARKS H.H. (1962) The post-exercise electrocardiogram in the detection of coronary disease: a long-term evaluation. *Tr. A. Life Insur. M. Dir. America* **45**, 81.

R20 ROBB G.P. & MARKS H.H. (1964) Latent coronary artery disease. Determination of its presence and severity by the exercise electrocardiogram. *Am. J. Cardiol.* **13**, 603.

R21 ROBB G.P. & MARKS H.H. (1967) Post-exercise ECG in arteriosclerotic heart disease. *JAMA* **200**, 918.

R22 ROBB G.P., MARKS H.H. & MATTINGLY T.W. (1957) The value of the double standard two-step exercise test in the detection of coronary disease. *Tr. A. Life Insur. M. Dir. America* **40**, 52.

R23 ROBB G.P., MARKS H.H. & MATTINGLY T.W. (1958) Stress tests in the detection of coronary disease. *Postgrad. Med.* **24**, 419. (Suppl. to p. 7). N.Y.C., New York: Metropolitan Life Insurance Co.

R24 ROBIN C., MENUET J.C., BABIN-CHEVAYE L. & HOREAU J. (1968) L'angor de Prinzmetal. *Coeur Med. Int.* **7**, 221.

R25 ROBINSON J.S. (1965) Prinzmetal's variant of angina pectoris. *Am. Heart J.* **70**, 797.

R26 ROBINSON J.S., SLOMAN G. & MCRAE C. (1964) Continuous electrocardiographic monitoring in the early stages after acute myocardial infarction. *Med. J. Aust.* **1**, 427.

R27 ROBINSON S. (1938) Experimental studies of physical fitness in relation to age. *Arb. Physiol.* **10**, 251.

R28 ROCHLIN I. & EDWARDS W.L.J. (1954) The misinterpretation of electrocardiograms with post-prandial T-wave inversion. *Circulation* **10**, 843.

R29 RODRIGUEZ M.I., ANSELMI A. & SODI-PALLARES D. (1953) The electrocardiographic diagnosis of septal infarctions. *Am. Heart J.* **45**, 525.

R30 RODRIGUEZ M.I. & SODI-PALLARES D. (1952) The mechanism of complete and incomplete bundle branch block. *Am. Heart J.* **44**, 715.

R31 ROESLER H. (1960) An electrocardiographic study of high take-off of the R (R′)–T segment in right precordial leads. *Am. J. Cardiol.* **6**, 920.

R32 ROKSETH R. & HATLE L. (1971) Sinus arrest in acute myocardial infarction. *Brit. Heart J.* **33**, 639.

R33 ROKSETH R., HATLE L., GEDDE-DAHL D. & FOSS P.O. (1970) Pacemaker therapy in sino-atrial block complicated by paroxysmal tachycardia. *Brit. Heart J.* **32**, 93.

R34 ROOS J.C. & DUNNING A.J. (1970) Right bundle-branch block and left axis deviation in acute myocardial infarction. *Brit. Heart J.* **32**, 847.

R35 ROSEN I.L. & GARDBERG M. (1957) Effects of non-pathologic factors on electrocardiogram. I. Results of observations under controlled conditions. *Am. Heart J.* **53**, 494.

R36 ROSEN K.M., LOEB H.S., CHUQUIMA R., ZIAD S.M., RAHIMTOOLA S.H. & GUNNAR R.M. (1970) Site of heart block in acute myocardial infarction. *Circulation* **42**, 925.

R37 ROSENBAUM F.F. (1957) Anomalous atrioventricular excitation. Panel discussion. *Ann. New York Acad. Sci.* **65**, 832.

R38 ROSENBAUM F.F., ERLANGER H., COTRIM N., JOHNSTON F.D. & WILSON F.N. (1944) The effects of anterior infarction complicated by bundle branch block upon the form of the QRS complex of the canine electrocardiogram. *Am. Heart J.* **27**, 783.

R39 ROSENBAUM F.F., HECHT H.H., WILSON F.N. & JOHNSTON F.D. (1945) The potential variations of the thorax and the oesophagus in anomalous atrioventricular excitation (Wolff-Parkinson-White syndrome). *Am. Heart J.* **29**, 281.

R40 ROSENBAUM F.F. & LEVINE S.A. (1941) Acute myocardial infarction. *Arch. Intern. Med.* **68**, 913.

R41 ROSENBAUM F.F., JOHNSTON F.D. & ALZAMORA V.V. (1944) Persistent displacement of the RS-T segment in a case of metastatic tumour of the heart. *Am. Heart J.* **27**, 667.

R42 ROSENBAUM M.B. (1964) Chagasic myocardiopathy. *Prog. Cardiol. Dis.* **7**, 199.

R43 ROSENBAUM M.B. (1968) Types of right bundle branch block and their clinical significance. *J. Electrocardiol.* **1**, 221.

R44 ROSENBAUM M.B. (1969) Types of left bundle branch block and their clinical significance. *J. Electrocardiol.* **2**, 197.

R45 ROSENBAUM M.B. (1970) In *Symposium on Cardiac Arrhythmias*, ed. Sandøe E., Flensted-Jensen E. & Olesen K.H. Södertalje, Sweden: A.B.Astra.

R46 ROSENBAUM M.B. & ALVAREZ A.J. (1955) The electrocardiogram in chronic chagasic myocarditis. *Am. Heart J.* **50**, 492.

R47 ROSENBAUM M.B., CORRADO G. & OLIVERA R. (1970) Right bundle branch block with left anterior hemiblock surgically induced in tetralogy of Fallot. *Am. J. Cardiol.* **26**, 12.

R48 ROSENBAUM M.B., ELIZARI M.V. & LAZZARI J.O. (1970) *The Hemiblocks.* Oldsmar, Florida: Tampa Tracings.

R49 ROSENBAUM M.B., ELIZARI M.V. & LAZZARI J.O. (1968) *Los Hemibloqueos.* Beunos Aires, Argentina: Paidos.

R50 ROSENBAUM M.B., ELIZARI M.V. & LAZZARI J.O. (1969) The mechanism of bidirectional tachycardia. *Am. Heart J.* **78**, 4.

R51 ROSENBAUM M.B., ELIZARI M.V., LAZZARI J.O., NAU G.J., LEVI R.J. & HALPERN M.S. (1969) Intraventricular trifascicular blocks. The syndrome of right bundle branch block with intermittent left anterior and posterior hemiblock. *Am. Heart J.* **78**, 306.

R52 ROSENBAUM M.B., ELIZARI M.V., LAZZARI J.O., NAU G.J., LEVI R.J. & HALPERN M.S. (1969) Intraventricular trifascicular blocks. Review of the literature and classification. *Am. Heart J.* **78**, 450.

R53 ROSENBAUM M.B., ELIZARI M.V. & LEVI R.J. (1969) Five cases of intermittent left anterior hemiblock. *Am. J. Cardiol.* **24**, 1.

R54 ROSS R.S. & FRIESINGER G.C. (1968) *Coronary arteriography. Symposium on coronary heart disease.* 2nd Edn. Monograph No. 2, p. 59. American Heart Association.

R55 ROTHBERGER C.J. & WINTERBERG H. (1917) Experimentelle beitrage zur kenntnis der reizleitungstorungen in den kammern des saugetiorherzens. *Ges. Exp. Med.* **5**, 264.

R56 ROTHFELD E.L., BERNSTEIN A., CREWS A.H., PARSONNET V. & ZUCKER I.R. (1965) Telemetric monitoring of arrhythmias in acute myocardial infarction. *Am. J. Cardiol.* **15**, 38.

R57 ROTHFELD E.L., BERNSTEIN A., PARSONNET V., ZUCKER I.R. & ALINSONORIN C.A. (1967) Telemetric monitoring of the electrocardiogram in acute myocardial infarction. *Dis. Chest.* **51**, 193.

R58 ROTHFELD E.L. & ZUCKER I.R. (1967) Non-paroxysmal ventricular tachycardia. *Clin. Res.* **15**, 220.

R59 ROTHFELD R.L., ZUCKER I.R. & ALINSONORIN C. (1967) Non-paroxysmal ventricular tachycardia. *Circulation* **35**, 227.

R60 ROTHFELD E.L., ZUCKER I.R., PARSONNET V. & ALINSONORIN C.A. (1968) Idioventricular rhythm in acute myocardial infarction. *Circulation* **37**, 203.

R61 ROTHFELD E.L., ZUCKER I.R. & TIU R. (1969) The electrocardiographic syndrome of superior axis and right bundle branch block. *Dis. Chest* **55**, 306.

R62 ROTMAN M., WAGNER G.S. & WALLACE A.G. (1972) Bradyarrhythmias in acute myocardial infarction. *Circulation* **45**, 703.

R63 ROVETTO M.J. & LEFER A.M. (1970) Electrophysiologic properties of cardiac muscle in adrenal insufficiency. *Am. J. Physiol.* **218**, 1015.

R64 RUMBALL A. & ACHESON E.D. (1963) Latent coronary heart disease detected by electrocardiogram before and after exercise. *Brit. Med. J.* **1**, 423.

R65 RUSER H.R. (1970) Prinzmetalische angina pectoris. *Ztschr. Kreislaufforsch.* **9**, 849.

R66 RUSSEK H.I. (1957) Master two-step test in coronary artery disease. *JAMA* **165**, 1772.

R67 RUSSEK H.I. (1960) Evaluation of nitrites in the treatment of angina pectoris. *Am. J. Med. Sci.* **239**, 478.

R68 RUSSEK H.I., ZOHMAN B.L. & DORSET V.F. (1955) Objective evaluation of coronary vasodilator drugs. *Am. J. Med. Sci.* **229**, 46.

S

S1 SAID S.I. & BRYANT J.M. (1955) Right intraventricular block in normal subjects. *Clin. Res. Proc.* **3**, 197.

S2 SAID S.I. & BRYANT J.M. (1956) Right and left bundle branch block in young healthy subjects. *Circulation* **14**, 993.

S3 SAID S.I., McLAUGHLIN H.M. & BRYANT J.M. (1956) Prominent Q waves in electrocardiograms simulating posterolateral myocardial infarction. *Clin. Res. Proc.* **4**, 10.

S4 SALAZAR J. & McKENDRICK C.S. (1970) Ventricular parasystole in acute myocardial infarction. *Brit. Heart J.* **32**, 377.

S5 SALTZMAN P., LINN H. & PICK A. (1966) Right bundle branch block with left axis deviation. *Brit. Heart J.* **28**, 703.

S6 SALVETTI A., CELLA P.L., ARRIGONI P. & BIANCALANA D. (1964) Comportamento della fase di ripolarizzazione ventricolare dopo sforzo e dopo iperventilazine volontaria in giovani sani. *Cuore Circ.* **48**, 192.

S7 SAMSON W.E. & SCHER A.M. (1960) Mechanism of S-T segment alteration during myocardial injury. *Circ. Res.* **8**, 780.

S8 SANDBERG L. (1957) EKG undersokning under och after graderad arbetsbleastning. *Nord. Med.* **58**, 1719.

S9 SANDBERG L. (1961) Studies on electrocardiographic changes during exercise tests. *Acta Med. Scand. Suppl.* **169**, 365.

S10 SANDERS A. (1939) Experimental localized auricular necrosis: Electrocardiographic study. *Am. J. Med. Sci.* **198**, 690.

S11 SANDLER I.A. & MARRIOTT H.J.L. (1965) Differential morphology of anomalous ventricular complexes of right bundle branch block type in lead. VI. Ventricular ectopy versus aberration. *Circulation* **31**, 551.

S12 SAPHIR O. (1942) Isolated myocarditis. *Am. Heart J.* **24**, 167.

S13 SATAKE K. & KIMURA E. (1962) On the electrocardiographic findings in the gastrointestinal diseases, especially on the changes in the RS-T segment and the T wave. *Jap. Heart J.* **3**, 167.

S14 SAYER W.J., MOSER M. & MATTINGLY T.W. (1954) Pheochromocytoma and the abnormal electrocardiogram. *Am. Heart J.* **48**, 42.

S15 SCANDINAVIAN COMMITTEE ON ECG CLASSIFICATION (1967) The 'minnesota Code' for ECG classification. Adaptation to CR leads and modification of the code for ECGs recorded during and after exercise. *Acta Med. Scand. Suppl.* **481**.

S16 SCHAEFER H. (1951) *Das Elektrokardiogramm, Theorie und Klinik.* Berlin: Springer Verlag.

S17 SCHAMROTH L. The QRS:S-T ratio in lead V2 in left bundle branch block. Unpublished observations.

S18 SCHAMROTH L. The non-delta QRS axes in the W.P.W. syndrome. Unpublished observations.

S19 SCHAMROTH L. (1961) An appraisal of the electrocardiographic exercise test. *S.A. Med. J.* **35**, 865.

S20   SCHAMROTH L. (1965) Concealed extrasystoles and the 'Rule of Bigeminy'. *Cardiologia* **46,** 51.

S21   SCHAMROTH L. (1965) The genesis and evolution of ectopic ventricular rhythm. M.D. Thesis, University of the Witwatersrand, Johannesburg.

S22   SCHAMROTH L. (1966) The genesis and evolution of ectopic ventricular rhythm. *Brit. Heart J.* **28,** 244.

S23   SCHAMROTH L. (1967) The electrocardiographic manifestations of right ventricular dominance. *S.A. Med. J.* **41,** 119.

S24   SCHAMROTH L. (1968) Idioventricular tachycardia. *J. Electrocardiol.* **1,** 205.

S25   SCHAMROTH L. (1969) Idioventricular tachycardia. *Dis. Chest* (Editorial) **56,** 466.

S26   SCHAMROTH L. (1969) Fundamental mechanisms in the genesis and evolution of myocardial fibrillation. *S.A. Med. J.* **43,** 631.

S27   SCHAMROTH L. (1971) *The Disorders of Cardiac Rhythm.* Oxford: Blackwell Scientific Publications Ltd.

S28   SCHAMROTH L. (1971) The physiological basis of ectopic ventricular rhythm: a unifying concept. *S.A. Med. J. Suppl.* (December).

S29   SCHAMROTH L. (1971) *An Introduction to Electrocardiography.* 4th Edn. Oxford: Blackwell Scientific Publications Ltd.

S30   SCHAMROTH L. (1972) The electrocardiographic diagnosis of acute myocardial infarction. In *Textbook of Coronary Care,* ed. Meltzer L.E. & Dunning A.J. Amsterdam: Excerpta Medica.

S31   SCHAMROTH L. (1974) The pathogenesis and mechanism of ventricular arrhythmias. In *Progress in Cardiology,* ed. Goodwin J.F. & Yu P. Philadelphia: Lea & Febiger.

S32   SCHAMROTH L. & BRADLOW B.A. (1964) Incomplete left bundle branch block. *Brit. Heart J.* **26,** 285.

S33   SCHAMROTH L. & CHESLER E. (1963) Phasic aberrant ventricular conduction. *Brit. Heart J.* **2,** 219.

S34   SCHAMROTH L. & JASPAN J.B. (1973) Variant angina pectoris: atypical—Prinzmetal's—angina pectoris. *Heart and Lung* **2,** 431.

S35   SCHAMROTH L. & KRIKLER D.M. (1967) Location of the pre-excitation areas in the Wolff-Parkinson-White syndrome *Am. J. Cardiol.* **19,** 892.

S36   SCHAMROTH L. & LAPINSKY G.B. (1972) The Wolff-Parkinson-White syndrome associated with myocardial infarction and right bundle branch block. *J. Electrocardiol.* **5,** 299.

S37   SCHAMROTH L. & LEVENSTEIN J. (1974) The electrocardiographic characteristics of the variant—Prinzmetal's—atypical form of angina pectoris manifesting in complicating ventricular extrasystoles. *S.A. Med. J.* **48,** 1146.

S38   SCHAMROTH L. & PERLMAN M.M. (1972) The electrocardiographic manifestations of acute true posterior myocardial infarction. *Heart and Lung* **1,** 658.

S39   SCHER A.M. (1965) Newer data on myocardial infarction. In *Electrophysiology of the Heart,* ed. Taccardi B. & Marchetti G. p. 217. London: Pergamon Press.

S40   SCHER A.M. & YOUNG A.C. (1955) Spread of excitation during premature ventricular systoles. *Circulation Res.* **3,** 535.

S41   SCHER A.M. & YOUNG A.C. (1956) The pathway of ventricular depolarization in the dog. *Circulation Res.* **4,** 461.

S42   SCHER A.M. & YOUNG A.C. (1957) Ventricular depolarization and the genesis of QRS. *Ann. N.Y. Acad. Sci.* **65,** 768.

S43   SCHER A.M., YOUNG A.C., MALMGREN A.L. & ERICKSON R.V. (1955) Activation of the interventricular septum. *Circulation Res.* **3,** 56.

S44   SCHER A.M., YOUNG A.C., MALMGREM A.L. & PATON R.R. (1953) Spread of electrical activity through the wall of the ventricle. *Circulation Res.* **1,** 539.

S45   SCHERF D. (1935) Koronarerkrankungen. *Erg. Ges. Med.* **20,** 237.

S46   SCHERF D. (1944) Alterations in the form of the *T* waves with changes in heart rate. *Am. Heart J.* **28,** 332.

S47   SCHERF D. (1947) Fifteen years of electrocardiographic exercise test in coronary disease. *New York State J. Med.* **47,** 2420.

S48   SCHERF D. (1960) Development of the electrocardiographic exercise test. Standardized versus non-standardized tests. *Am. J. Cardiol.* **5,** 433.

S49   SCHERF D. (1968) The electrocardiographic exercise test. *J. Electrocardiol.* **1,** 141.

S50   SCHERF D. & GOLDHAMMER S. (1933) Zur Frühdiagnose der angina pectoris mit hilfe des elektrokardiogramms. *Ztschr. Klin. Med.* **124,** 111.

S51   SCHERF D. & SCHAFFER A.I. (1952) Electrocardiographic exercise test. *Am. Heart J.* **43,** 927.

S52   SCHERF D. & SCHLACHMAN M. (1948) Electrocardiographic and clinical studies on the action of ergotamine tartrate and dihydro-ergotamine 45. *Am. J. Med. Sci.* **216,** 673.

S53   SCHERF D. & SCHOTT A. (1953) *Extrasystoles and Allied Arrhythmias.* London: William Heinemann.

S54   SCHERF D. & WEISSBERG J. (1941) The alterations of the *T*-waves caused by a change of posture. *Am. J. Med. Sci.* **210,** 693.

S55   SCHERF D., YILDIZ M. & JODY A. (1958) Electrocardiographic changes during hyperventilation tetany. *Am. J. Med. Sci.* **236,** 369.

S56   SCHERLIS L., SANDBERG A.A., WENER J., DVORKIN Y. & MASTER A.M. (1950) Effects of single and double '2-step' exercise tests upon electrocardiograms of 200 normal persons. *J. Mt. Sinai Hosp.* **17,** 242.

S57   SCHINDLER S.C. & SURAWICZ B. (1967) Clinical significance of the ECG pattern with prolonged Q-Tc interval, and increased T or U amplitude, CVA pattern. *Am. J. Cardiol.* **19,** 148. (Abstr.)

S58   SCHNEIDER R.G. & LYON A.F. (1969) Use of oral potassium salts in the assessment of *T*-wave abnormalities in the electrocardiogram: a clinical test. *Am. Heart J.* **77,** 721.

S59   SCHWANN H.P. & KAY C.F. (1956) Specific resistances of body tissues. *Circulation Res.* **4,** 664.

S60   SCHWEITZER P., HILDEBRAND T., KLVANOVA H., SIMKO S., GALAJDOVA E. & GREGOROVA J. (1967) De einfluss der adrenergen blockade auf die orthostatischen veraenderungen der inted lalvektoren von QRS, T so ie des ventrikelgradienten bei patienten mit neurozirkulatorischer asthenie und thyreotoxikose. *Z. Kreislaufforsch.* **56,** 316.

S61   SCOTT R.C. (1965) Left bundle branch block—a clinical assessment. *Am. Heart J.* **70,** 535.

S62   SCOTT R.C., MANITSAS G.T., KIM O.J. & SPITZ H.B. (1971) Left posterior hemiblock: a new diagnostic sign in dissecting aneurysm? *J. Electrocardiol.* **4,** 261.

S63   SEARS G.A. & MANNING G.W. (1956) Routine electrocardiography: postprandial *T*-wave changes. *Am. Heart J.* **56,** 591.

S64   SHABETAI R., SURAWICZ B. & HAMMILL W. (1968) Monophasic action potentials in man. *Circulation* **38,** 341.

S65   SHADAKSHARAPPA K.S., KLABFLEISCH J.M., CONRADD L.L. & SARKAR N.K. (1968) Recognition and significance of intraventricular block due to myocardial infarction (peri-infarction block). *Circulation* **37**, 20.

S66 SHAFFER C.F. & CHAPMAN D.W. (1951) Exercise electrocardiogram: aid in diagnosis of arteriosclerotic heart disease in persons exhibiting abnormally large Q3 waves. *Am. J. Med.* **11**, 26.

S67 SHAPIRO H.S., RIBEILIMA J. & WENDT V.E. (1964) Myocardial infarction in progressive muscular dystrophy. *Am. J. Cardiol.* **14**, 232.

S68 SHARPEY-SCHAFER E.P. (1943) Potassium effects on the electrocardiogram of thyroid deficiency. *Brit. Heart J.* **5**, 85.

S69 SHEEHAN H.L. & SUMMERS V.K. (1949) The syndrome of hypopituitarism. *Q. J. Med.* **18**, 319.

S70 SHEFFIELD L.T. & REEVES T.J. (1965) Graded exercise in the diagnosis of angina pectoris. *Mod. Conc. Cardiovasc. Dis.* **34**, 1.

S71 SHERLAG B.J., LAU S.H., HELFANT R.H., BERKOWITZ W.D., STEIN E. & DAMATO A.N. (1969) Catheter technique for recording His bundle activity in man. *Circulation* **39**, 13.

S72 SHIELDS P.L. (1957) Auricular infarction. *J. Indiana State M.A.* **50**, 177.

S73 SHIPLEY R.A. & HALLARAN W.R. (1936) The four-lead electrocardiogram in two hundred normal men and women. *Am. Heart J.* **11**, 325.

S74 SHUSTER S. (1960) The electrocardiogram in subarachnoid haemorrhage. *Br. Heart J.* **22**, 316.

S75 SILVER H.M. & LANDOWNE M. (1953) Relation of age to certain electrocardiographic responses of normal adults to standardized exercise. *Circulation* **8**, 510.

S76 SILVERMAN J.J. & SALOMON S. (1959) Myocardial infarction pattern discovered by ventricular extrasystoles. *Am. J. Cardiol.* **4**, 695.

S77 SILVERMAN M.E. & FLAMM M.D. (1971) Variant angina pectoris. Anatomic findings and prognostic implications. *Ann. Intern. Med.* **75**, 339.

S78 SILVERTSSEN E., HOEL B., BAY G. & JÖRGENSEN L. (1973) Electrocardiographic atrial complex and acute atrial myocardial infarction. *Am. J. Cardiol.* **31**, 450.

S79 SIMONSON E. (1953) Effect of moderate exercise on electrocardiogram in healthy young and middle-aged men. *J. Appl. Physiol.* **5**, 584.

S80 SIMONSON E. (1963) Use of the electrocardiogram in exercise tests. *Am. Heart J.* **66**, 552.

S81 SIMONSON E., BAKER C., BURNS N., KEIPER C., SCHMITT O.H. & STACKHOUSE S. (1968) Cardiovascular stress electrocardiographic changes produced by driving an automobile. *Am. Heart J.* **75**, 125.

S82 SIMONSON E., ENZER N. & GOODMAN J.S. (1945) Coronary insufficiency, revealed by ectopic nodal and ventricular beats in the presence of left bundle branch block. *Am. J. M. Sci.* **209**, 349.

S83 SIMONSON E. & KEYS A. (1950) The effect of an ordinary meal on the electrocardiogram. Normal standards in middle-aged men and women. *Circulation* **1**, 1000.

S84 SIMONSON E. & KEYS A. (1956) Electrocardiographic exercise test: changes in scalar ECG and in mean spatial QRS and T vectors in two types of exercise: effect of absolute and relative body weight and comment on normal standards. *Am. Heart J.* **52**, 83.

S85 SIMONSON E. & McKINLAY C.A. (1950) The meal test in clinical electrocardiography. *Circulation* **1**, 1000.

S86 SITZ-HUGH T. & WOLFERTH C.C. (1935) Cardiac improvement following gall-bladder surgery. *Ann. Surg.* **101**, 478.

S87 SJÖSTRAND T. (1947) Changes in the respiratory organs of workmen at an ore smelting works. *Acta Med. Scand. Suppl.* **196**, 687.

S88 SJÖSTRAND T. (1950) The relationship between the heart frequency and the S-T level of the electrocardiogram. *Acta Med. Scand.* **138**, 201.

S89 SJÖSTRAND T. (1951) The electrocardiographic work and hypoxemia tests. *Scand. J. Clin. Lab. Invest.* **3**, 1.

S90 SLEEPER J.C. & ORGAIN E.S. (1963) Differentiation of benign from pathologic T waves in the electrocardiogram. *Am. J. Cardiol.* **11**, 338.

S91 SLOMAN G., DOWLING J. & VOHRA J. (1971) Prevention and treatment of ventricular dysrhythmias. *Brit. Heart J.* **33**, Suppl., 165.

S92 SMIRK F.H., NOLLA-PANADES J. & WALLIS T. (1964) Experimental ventricular flutter and ventricular paroxysmal tachycardia. *Am. J. Cardiol.* **14**, 79.

S93 SMIRK F.H. & PALMER D.G. (1960) A myocardial syndrome with particular reference to the occurrence of sudden death and of premature systoles interrupting antecedent T waves. *Am. J. Cardiol.* **6**, 620.

S94 SMITH J.E. (1950) Electrocardiographic response in exercise tolerance tests. *J. Aviation Med.* **21**, 470.

S95 SMITH L.A., KENNAMER R. & PRINZMETAL M. (1954) Ventricular excitation in segmental and diffuse types of experimental bundle-branch block. *Circulation Res.* **2**, 221.

S96 SMITH M. & RAY C.T. (1970) Electrocardiographic signs of early right ventricular enlargement in acute pulmonary embolism. *Chest* **58**, 205.

S97 SMITH R.F., HARTHORNE J.W. & SANDERS C.A. (1967) Vectorcardiographic changes during intracoronary injections. *Circulation* **36**, 63.

S98 SODEMAN W.A. (1940) A study of the T wave of the electrocardiogram in left bundle branch block. *J. Clin. Invest.* **19**, 784.

S99 SODEMAN W.A., JOHNSTON F.D. & WILSON F.N. (1944) The QI deflection of the electrocardiogram in bundle branch block and axis deviation. *Am. Heart J.* **28**, 271.

S100 SÖDERHOLM B., THULESIUS O., HEYMAN F., MALMCRONA R. & BJÖRNTORP P. (1962) Myocardial infarction in the younger age groups. III. Follow-up observations with special reference to exercise tolerance tests. *Acta Med. Scand.* **172**, 585.

S101 SODERSTROM N. (1948) Myocardial infarction and mural thrombosis in the atria of the heart. *Acta Med. Scand. Suppl.* **217**, 1.

S102 SODI-PALLARES D. (1957) Fusion beats and anomalous atrioventricular excitation. *Ann. New York Acad. Sci.* **65**, 845.

S103 SODI-PALLARES D. (1962) Electrografia deductiva. *Arch. Inst. Cardiol Mexico* **32**, 679.

S104 SODI-PALLARES D., ANSELMI G., CONTRERAS R. & MEDRANO G.A. (1959) Proceso de activacion y correlacion anatomica en cortes seriados, como base de una nueva classificacion de los infartos. *Primer Symposium Internacional Sobre Arteroesclerosis y Enfermedad Coronaria.* Mexico: Ed. Interamericana S.A.

S105 SODI-PALLARES D., BARBATO E., ESTANDIA A. & ESPINO-VELA J. (1949) La activacion ventricular en el corazon del perro. *Arch. Inst. Cardiol. Mexico* **19**, 688.

S106 SODI-PALLARES D., BISTENI A. & HERMANN G.R. (1952) Some views on the significance of qR and QR type complexes in right precordial leads in the absence of myocardial infarction. *Am. Heart J.* **43**, 716.

S107 SODI-PALLARES D., BISTENI A., MEDRANO G.A. & AYALA C. (1960) Electrocardiography and vectorcardiography. In *Clinical Cardiopulmonary Physiology*. New York: Grune and Stratton.

S108 SODI-PALLARES D., BISTENI A., MEDRANO G.A. & CISNEROS F. (1955) The activation of the free left ventricular wall in the dog's heart in normal conditions and in left bundle branch block. *Am. Heart J.* **49**, 587.

S109 SODI-PALLARES D., BISTENI A., MEDRANO G.A., GINEFRA P., PORTILLO B. & DEL RIO R. (1958) La 'barrera fisiologica' del tabique interventricular. Volume des Communications. III, p. 32. Bruxelles: Congres Mondial de Cardiologie.

S110 SODI-PALLARES D., BISTENI A., PILEGGI F. & MEDRANO G.A. (1957) Acerca del tejido electricamente muerto. *Principia Cardiologica.* **4**, 163.

S111 SODI-PALLARES D., BRANCATO R.S., PILEGGI F., BISTENI A., MEDRANO G.A. & BARBATO E. (1957) The ventricular activation and the vectorcardiographic curve. *Am. Heart J.* **54**, 498.

S112 SODI-PALLARES D. & CALDER R.M. (1956) *New Bases of Electrocardiography*. St. Louis: C.V.Mosby and Co.

S113 SODI-PALLARES D., CISNEROS F., MEDRANO G.A., BISTENI A., TESTELLIE M.R. & MICHELI A.D. (1963) Electrocardiographic diagnosis of myocardial infarction in the presence of bundle branch block (right and left), ventricular premature beats, and Wolff-Parkinson-White syndrome. *Prog. Cardiovasc. Dis.* **6**, 107.

S114 SODI-PALLARES D., MEDRANO G.A., BISTENI A. & PONCE DE LEON G.G. (1970) *Deductive and Polyparametric Electrocardiography*. The Instituto Nacional de Cardiologia de Mexico.

S115 SODI-PALLARES D., MEDRANO G.A. & CISNEROS A.F. (1955) The activation of the free left ventricular wall in the dog's heart in normal conditions and in left bundle branch block. *Am. Heart J.* **49**, 587.

S116 SODI-PALLARES D. & RODRIGUEZ M.I. (1952) Morphology of the unipolar leads recorded at the septal surfaces. Its application to the diagnosis of left bundle branch block complicated by myocardial infarction. *Am. Heart J.* **43**, 27.

S117 SODI-PALLARES D., RODRIGUEZ M.I. & BISTENI A. (1952) Diagnostico electrocardiografico de bloqueo de rama izquierda complicado con infarto del miocardio. *Arch. Inst. Cardiol. Mexico* **22**, 1.

S118 SODI-PALLARES D., RODRIGUEZ M.I., CHAIT L.O. & ZUCKER-MAN R. (1951) The activation of the ventricular septum. *Am. Heart J.* **41**, 569.

S119 SOMMERVILLE W., LEVINE H.D. & THORN G.W. (1951) The electrocardiogram in Addison's disease. *Medicine* **30**, 43.

S120 SOMMERVILLE W. & WOOD P. (1949) Cardiac infarction with bundle branch block. *Brit. Heart J.* **11**, 305.

S121 SONES F.M. JR & SHIREY E.K. (1962) Cine coronary arteriography. *Mod. Conc. Cardiovasc. Dis.* **31**, 735.

S122 SPANG K. (1957) *Rhythmusstörungen des Herzens*. Stuttgart: Georg Thieme Verlag.

S123 SPANN J.F., MOELLERING R.C., HABER E. & WHEELER E.O. (1964) Arrhythmias in acute myocardial infarction. *New Engl. J. Med.* **271**, 427.

S124 SPARKS H.V., HOLLENBERG M., CARRIERE S., FUNKENSTEIN D., ZAKHEIM R.M. & BARGER A.C. (1970) Sympathomimetic drugs and repolarization of ventricular myocardium of the dog. *Cardiovasc. Res.* **4**, 363.

S125 SPODICK D.H. (1972) Electrocardiographic responses to pulmonary embolism. Mechanisms and source of variability. *Am. J. Cardiol.* **30**, 695.

S126 SPRAGUE H.B. & ORGAIN E.S. (1935) Electrocardiographic study of cases of coronary occlusion proved at autopsy at the Massachussetts General Hospital, 1914–1934. *New Engl. J. Med.* **212**, 903.

S127 SPRITZ N., COHEN B.D., FRIMPTER G.W. & RUBIN A.L. (1958) Electrographic interrelationship of the pre-excitation (W.P.W.) syndrome and myocardial infarction. *Am. Heart J.* **56**, 715.

S128 SPRITZER H.W., PETERSON C.R., JONES R.C. & OVERHOLT E.L. (1969) Electrocardiographic abnormalities in acute pancreatitis: two patients studied by selective coronary arteriography. *Milit. Med.* **134**, 687.

S129 STANEREN D.C. & TECULESCU D.B. (1967) Isolated atrial infarction. *Dis. Chest* **51**, 643.

S130 STANNARD M., SLOMAN J.G., HARE W.S.C. & GOBLE A.J. (1967) Prolapse of the posterior leaflet of the mitral valve: a clinical, familial and cine-angiographic study. *Brit. Med. J.* **3**, 71.

S131 STAPLETON J.F., SEGAL J.P. & HARVEY W.F. (1970) The electrocardiogram of myocardopathy. *Prog. Cardiovasc. Dis.* **13**, 217.

S132 STEIN I. & WROBLEWSKI F. (1951) Myocardial infarction in Wolff-Parkinson-White syndrome. *Am. Heart J.* **42**, 624.

S133 STEPHAN E., LAHAM E., PANIER M. & SALEH J. (1965) Coeur et hypopituitarisme. *Arch. Mal Coeur* **58**, 1493.

S134 STEWART C.B. & MANNING G.W. (1944) A detailed analysis of the electrocardiograms of five hundred R.C.A.F. aircrew. *Am. Heart J.* **27**, 502.

S135 STOCK E., GOBLE A. & SLOMAN G. (1967) Assessment of arrhythmias in myocardial infarction. *Brit. Med. J.* **2**, 719.

S136 STOCK R.J. & MACKEN D.L. (1968) Observations on heart block during continuous electrocardiographic monitoring in myocardial infarction. *Circulation* **38**, 993.

S137 STOKES W. (1946) The effect of nitrite and exercise on the inverted *T* wave. *Brit. Heart J.* **8**, 62.

S138 STORCH S. & MASTER A.M. (1951) RS-T segment, *T* wave and heart rate after two-step and 10 per cent anoxemia tests. *JAMA* **146**, 1011.

S139 STRIVASTAVA S.C. & ROBSON A.D. (1964) Electrocardiographic abnormalities associated with subarachnoid haemorrhage. *Lancet* **2**, 431.

S140 STUCKEY J.H. & HOFFMANN B.F. (1961) Direct studies of the *in situ* specialised conducting system. In *The Specialised Tissues of the Heart*. Amsterdam: Elsevier.

S141 SURAWICZ B. (1966) Electrocardiographic pattern of cerebrovascular accident. *JAMA* **197**, 913.

S142 SURAWICZ B. (1972) The pathogenesis and clinical significance of primary *T*-wave abnormalities. In *Advances in Electrocardiography*, ed. Schlant R.C. & Hurst J.W. New York: Grune and Stratton.

S143 SURAWICZ B., DAOUD F.S. & GETTES L.S. (1970) Effect of isoproterenol on primary and secondary *T*-wave abnormalities. *Circulation* **12**, Suppl. III, 46.

S144 SURAWICZ B. & LASSETER K.C. (1970) Effect of drugs on the electrocardiogram. *Prog. Cardiovasc. Dis.* **13**, 26.

S145 SURAWICZ B. & LASSETER K.C. (1970) Electrocardiogram in pericarditis. *Am. J. Cardiol.* **26**, 471.

S146 SUTTON R. & DAVIES M. (1968) The conduction system in acute myocardial infarction complicated by heart block. *Circulation* **38**, 987.

S147 SZILAGYI N. & GINSBURG M. (1962) Acute myocardial infarction revealed in the presence of right bundle branch block and ventricular extrasystoles. *Am. J. Cardiol.* **9,** 232.

S148 SZILAGYI N. & SOLOMAN S.L. (1959) Variations in the form of the *T* wave in a case of partial heart block. *Am. Heart J.* **58,** 637.

T

T1 TAGGART P. & GIBBONS D. (1967) Motor-car driving and the heart rate. *Brit. Med. J.* **1,** 411.

T2 TALBOT F.J. & LEONARD J.J. (1958) Severe left axis deviation in the presence of pulmonary emphysema. *Circulation* **18,** 787.

T3 TALBOT S.A., LIKAR I. & HARRISON W.K. JR. (1966) Exercise escalator for electrocardiographic studies in patients with coronary heart disease. *Am. Heart J.* **72,** 35.

T4 TAMAGNA I.G., BUTTERWORTH J.S. & POINDEXTER C.A. (1948) Wolff-Parkinson-White syndrome with myocardial infarction. An experimental study. *Am. Heart J.* **35,** 948.

T5 TEARE R.D. (1958) Asymmetrical hypertrophy of the heart in young adults. *Brit. Heart J.* **20,** 1.

T6 TESTONI F., NARBONE N.B. & TOMMASELLI A. (1968) Aspetti vettocardiographici nei blocki focali sinistri con electro-cardiogramma di tipo R1-S2-S3. *Mal. Cardiovasc.* **9,** 379.

T7 THOMAS C.B. (1951) Cardiovascular response of normal young adults to exercise as determined by double Master two-step test. *Bull. Johns Hopkins Hosp.* **89,** 181.

T8 THOMPSON W.P. (1943) The electrocardiogram in the hyperventilation syndrome. *Am. Heart J.* **25,** 372.

T9 THOMPSON S.P. (1910) *The life of William Thomson, Baron Kelvin of Largs.* London: MacMillan Co.

T10 THOMSON W. (LORD KELVIN) (1884) *Reprints of papers on electrostatics and magnetism.* 2nd Edn. London: MacMillan.

T11 THOREN C. (1964) Cardiomyopathy in Friedreich's ataxia. With studies of cardiovascular and respiratory function. *Acta Paediatrics. Suppl.* **53,** 153.

T12 THORN G.W., DORRANCE S.S. & DAY E. (1942) Addison's disease: evaluation of synthetic desoxycorticosterone acetate therapy in 158 patients. *Ann. Intern. Med.* **16,** 1054.

T13 TREVINO A., RAZI B. & BELLER B.M. (1971) The characteristic electrocardiogram of accidental hypothermia. *Arch. Intern. Med.* **127,** 470.

T14 TUCKER H.S.G., MOSS L.F. & WILLIAMS J.P. (1948) Hemochromatosis with death from heart failure. *Am. Heart J.* **35,** 993.

T15 TULLOCH J.A. (1952) The electrocardiographic features of high posterolateral myocardial infarction. *Brit. Heart J.* **14,** 379.

T16 TWISS A. & SOKOLOW, M. (1942) Angina pectoris: significant electrocardiographic changes following exercise. *Am. Heart J.* **23,** 498.

U

U1 UHLEY H.N. & RIVKIN L.M. (1964) Electrocardiographic patterns following interruption of the main and peripheral branches of the canine left bundle of His. *Am. J. Cardiol.* **13,** 41.

U2 UNGER P.N., LESSER M.E., KUGEL V.H. & LEV M. (1958) The concept of 'masquerading' bundle branch block. An electrocardiographic-pathologic correlation. *Circulation* **17,** 397.

U3 UNTERMAN D. & DEGRAFF A.C. (1948) Effect of exercise on electrocardiogram (Master '2-step' test) in diagnosis of coronary insufficiency. *Am. J. Med. Sci.* **215,** 671.

U4 URSCHEL D. & GATES G.E. (1953) The T-vector changes in hypothyroidism. *Am. Heart J.* **45,** 611.

U5 USHIYAMA K., KIMURA E., KIKUCHI H. & MABUCHI G. (1969) Effects of nitroglycerin and propranolol on angina pectoris induced by intravenous infusion of isoproterenol. *Isr. J. Med. Sci.* **5,** 736.

V

V1 VAN BOGAERT A., VAN CENEBEEK A., VANDEL J., ARNOLDI M. & VAN DER HENST H. (1958) Dextrodeviation de QRS dans les deviation cliniques par lesion ventriculaire gauche (etude esperimentale). *Arch. Mal. Coeur* **51,** 513.

V2 VAN DAM R.T. & DURRER D. (1961) Experimental study on the intramural distribution of the excitability cycle and on the form of the epicardial *T* wave in the dog heart *in situ*. *Am. Heart J.* **61,** 537.

V3 VAN MUIJDEN N.H. (1934) Das Kammerelectrokardiogramm nach arbeit, bei herzgesunden mit dem spannungs—electrokardiographen registriert. *Ztschr. Klin. Med.* **127,** 192.

V4 VARRIALE P. & KENNEDY R.J. (1972) Right bundle branch block and left posterior fascicular block. Vectorcardiographic and clinical features. *Am. J. Cardiol.* **29,** 459.

V5 VAZIFDAR J.P. & LEVINE S.A. (1966) Rarity of atrial tachycardia in acute myocardial infarction and thyrotoxicosis. *Arch. Intern. Med.* **118,** 41.

V6 VEDIN J.A., WILHELMSSON C.E., WILHELMSEN L., BJURE J. & EKSTRÖM-JODAL B. (1972) Relation of resting and exercise-induced ectopic beats to other ischaemic manifestations and to coronary risk factors. *Am. J. Cardiol.* **30,** 25.

V7 VEDOYA R., NESSI C.T. & COPELLO C.E. (1950) Duracion del intervalo QT despues de la prueba de esfuerzo en la angina de pecho. *Rev. Argent. Cardiol.* **17,** 325 & 340.

V8 VIDELA J.G. (1957) El diagnostico del infarcto de miocardio en presencia del sindrome de Wolff-Parkinson-White. *Rev. Argent. Cardiol.* **24,** 18.

V9 VILLAMIL A., BUZZI R., FRANCO R. & MARTINEZ, ZUVIRIA E. (1954) Modificaciones de la sistole electrica y del grandiente ventriculaire producidas por la prueba de esfuerzo (Master) en sujetos normales y con cardiopatia coronaria. *Rev. Argent. Cardiol.* **21,** 258.

V10 VISCIDI P.C. & GEIGER A.J. (1943) Electrocardiographic observations on 500 unselected young adults at work. *Am. Heart J.* **26,** 763.

W

W1 WAGNER R. & ROSENBAUM M.B. (1972) Transient left posterior hemiblock. Association with acute lateral myocardial infarction. *Am. J. Cardiol.* **29,** 558.

W2 WAHLUND H. (1948) Determination of the physical working

capacity. A physiological and clinical study with special reference to standardization of cardiopulmonary functional tests. *Acta Med. Scand. Suppl.* **215.**

W3 WALSTON II A., BOINEAU J.P., SPACH M.S., AYERS C.P. & ESTES E.H. (1968) Relationship between ventricular depolarisation and QRS in right and left bundle branch block. *J. Electrocardiol.* **1,** 155.

W4 WANKA J. & LAJOS T.Z. (1969) Prognosis of right bundle-branch block with left axis deviation. *Circulation* 40, *Suppl.* **3,** 212.

W5 WARTMAN W.B. & HELLERSTEIN H.K. (1948) Heart disease in 2,000 consecutive autopsies. *Ann. Int. Med.* **28,** 41.

W6 WASSERBURGER R.H. (1955) Observations on the 'juvenile pattern' in adult Negro males. *Am. J. Med.* **18,** 428.

W7 WASSERBURGER R.H. (1958) The riddle of the labile *T* wave. *Am. J. Cardiol.* **2,** 179.

W8 WASSERBURGER R.H., ALT W.J. & LLOYD C.J. (1961) The normal RS-T segment elevation variant. *Am. J. Cardiol.* **8,** 184.

W9 WASSERBURGER R.H. & CORLISS R.J. (1962) Value of oral potassium salts in differentiation of functional and organic *T*-wave changes. *Am. J. Cardiol.* **10,** 673.

W10 WASSERBURGER R.H. & CORLISS R.J. (1965) Prominent precordial *T* waves as an expression of coronary insufficiency. *Am. J. Cardiol.* **16,** 195.

W11 WASSERBURGER R.H. & LORENZ T.H. (1956) The effect of hyperventilation and pro-banthine on isolate RS-T segment and *T* wave abnormalities. *Am. Heart J.* **51,** 666.

W12 WASSERBURGER R.H., SIEBECKER K.L. & LEWIS W. (1956) The effect of hyperventilation on the normal adult electrocardiogram. *Circulation* **13,** 850.

W13 WASSERBURGER R.H., WHITE D.H. & LINDSAY E.R. (1962) Non-infarctional QS in II, III and AVF complexes. *Am. Heart J.* **46,** 617.

W14 WATT J.B., FREUD G.D. & DURRER D. (1958) Left anterior arborization block combined with right bundle branch block in canine and primate hearts. An electrocardiographic study. *Circulation Res.* **22,** 57.

W15 WATT T.B., MURAO S. & PRUITT R.D. (1965) Left axis deviation induced experimentally in a primate heart. *Am. Heart J.* **70,** 381.

W16 WATT T.B. & PRUITT R.D. (1965) Electrocardiographic findings associated with experimental arborization block in dogs. *Am. Heart J.* **69,** 642.

W17 WEBER D.M. & PHILLIPS J.H. JR. (1966) A re-evaluation of electrocardiographic changes accompanying acute pulmonary embolism. *Am. J. Med. Sci.* **251,** 381.

W18 WECHSLER R.L., BELLET S., KAPLAN A.K. & NEMIR P. JR. (1954) Electrocardiographic changes following biliary and gastric distention in freshly infarcted unanesthetized dogs. *Surg. Forum* **5,** 131.

W19 WEGRIA R., SEGERS M., KEATING R.P. & WARD H.P. (1949) Relationship between the reduction in coronary flow and the appearance of electrocardiographic changes. *Am. Heart J.* **38,** 90.

W20 WEINBERG S.L., GROVE G.R., ZIPF R.E., DANIELS D.C. & MURPHY J.P. (1959) Normal response curve to exercise of relative cardiac output measured with radio-iodinated serum albumin. *Circulation* **19,** 590.

W21 WEINBERG S.L., REYNOLDS R.W., ROSENMAN R.H. & KATZ L.N. (1950) Electrocardiographic changes associated with patchy myocardial fibrosis in the absence of confluent myocardial infarction. *Am. Heart J.* **40,** 745.

W22 WEISENFELD S. & MESSINGER W.J. (1952) Cardiac involvement in progressive muscular dystrophy. *Am. Heart J.* **43,** 170.

W23 WEISS M.M. & HAMILTON J.E. (1939) The effect of gallbladder disease on the electrocardiogram. *Surgery* 6, 893.

W24 WEISS S., STEAD E.A., WARREN J.V. & BAILEY O.T. (1943) Scleroderma heart disease. *Arch. Int. Med.* **71,** 749.

W25 WENDKOS M.H. (1944) The influence of autonomic imbalance on the human electrocardiogram. *Am. Heart J.* **28,** 549.

W26 WENDKOS M.H. (1963) The Pharmacodynamics of Organic Nitrates in Relation to Cardiac Diagnosis and Treatment in Man. A.M.A. Exhibit, June.

W27 WENDKOS M.H. (1965) The effects of a potassium mixture on abnormal cardiac repolarization in hospitalized psychiatric patients. *Am. J. Med. Sci.* **249,** 76.

W28 WENDKOS M.H. & LOGUE R.B. (1946) Unstable *T* waves in leads II and III in persons with neurocirculatory asthenia. *Am. Heart J.* **31,** 711.

W29 WENER J., SANDBERG A.A., SCHERLIS L., DVORKIN J. & MASTER A.M. (1953) The electrocardiographic response to the standard two-step exercise test. *Canad. med. Ass. J.* **68,** 368.

W30 WESSLER S. & FREEDBERG A.S. (1948) Cardiac amyloidosis. *Arch. Int. Med.* **82,** 63.

W31 WEYN A.S. & MARRIOTT H.J.L. (1962) The T-V1 taller than T-V6 pattern. Its potential value in early recognition of myocardial disease. *Am. J. Cardiol.* **10,** 764.

W32 WHEELER E.O. (1970) Emotional stress: Cardiovascular disease and cardiovascular symptoms. In *The Heart*, ed. Hurst J.W. & Logue R.B. p. 1414. New York: McGraw-Hill.

W33 WHITE P.D. (1934) Electrocardiographic evidence of recent coronary thrombosis superimposed on bundle branch block resulting from previous coronary disease. *Am. Heart J.* **10,** 260.

W34 WHITE N.K., EDWARDS J.E. & DRY T.J. (1950) The relationship of the degree of coronary sclerosis with age in men. *Circulation* **1,** 645.

W35 WHITE P.D., CHAMBERLAIN F.L. & GRAYBIEL A. (1941) Inversion of the *T* waves in lead II caused by a variation in position of the heart. *Brit. Heart J.* **3,** 233.

W36 WHITE P., COHEN M.E. & CHAPMAN W.P. (1947) The electrocardiogram in neurocirculatory asthenia anxiety neurosis and effort syndrome. *Am. Heart J.* **34,** 390.

W37 WHITING R.B., KLEIN M.D. & VAN DER VEER, J. (1970) Variant angina pectoris. *N. Engl. J. Med.* **282,** 709.

W38 WIGGERS C.J. & WEGRIA R. (1940) Ventricular fibrillation due to single localised induction and condensor shocks applied during the vulnerable phase of ventricular systole. *Am. J. Physiol.* **128,** 500.

W39 WIGGERS H.C. & WIGGERS C.J. (1935) The interpretation of monophasic action potentials from the mammalian ventricle indicated by changes following coronary occlusion. *Am. J. Physiol.* **113,** 683.

W40 WIGLE E.D., HEIMBECKER R.O. & GUNTON R.W. (1962) Idiopathic ventricular septal hypertrophy causing muscular subaortic stenosis. *Circulation* **26,** 325.

W41 WILLARD J.H. (1950) Cardiac symptoms secondary to gastrointestinal tract disturbances. *Am. Practnr. Dig. Treat.* **1,** 376.

W42 WILSON F.N. (1936) *Diseases of the Coronary Arteries and Cardiac Pain*, p. 316. New York: MacMillan Co.

W43 WILSON F.N. (1936) The electrocardiogram in diseases of the coronary arteries. In *Diseases of the Coronary Arteries and Cardiac Pain*, p. 281. New York: MacMillan Co.

W44 WILSON F.N. (1936) The electrocardiogram in diseases of the coronary arteries. In *Diseases of the Coronary Arteries and Cardiac Pain*, p. 320. New York: MacMillan Co.

W45 WILSON F.N. (1938) Recent progress in electrocardiography and the interpretation of borderline electrocardiograms. *Proc. Am. Life Insur. Dir.* **24**, 96.

W46 WILSON F.N. (1941–42) Concerning the form of the QRS deflection of the electrocardiogram in bundle branch block. *J. Mt. Sinai Hosp.* **8**, 1110.

W47 WILSON F.N. & HERRMANN G.R. (1920) Bundle branch block and arborization block. *Arch. Intern. Med.* **26**, 153.

W48 WILSON F.N., HILL I.G.W. & JOHNSTON F.D. (1934) The interpretation of the galvanometric curves obtained when one electrode is distinct from the heart and the other near or in contact with its surface. II. Observations on the mammalian heart. *Am. Heart J.* **10**, 176.

W49 WILSON F.N., HILL I.G.W. & JOHNSTON F.D. (1934) The form of the electrocardiogram in experimental myocardial infarction. *Am. Heart J.* **9**, 596.

W50 WILSON F.N., HILL I.G.W. & JOHNSTON F.D. (1935) The form of the electrocardiogram in experimental myocardial infarction. III. The later effects produced by legation of the anterior descending branch of the left coronary artery. *Am. Heart J.* **10**, 1025.

W51 WILSON F.N., JOHNSTON F.D. & HILL I.G.W. (1935) The form of the electrocardiogram in experimental myocardial infarction. IV. Additional observations on the later effects produced by ligation of the anterior descending branch of the left coronary artery. *Am. Heart J.* **10**, 1025.

W52 WILSON F.N. & JOHNSTON F.D. (1941) The occurrence in angina pectoris of electrocardiographic changes similar in magnitude and in kind to those produced by myocardial infarction. *Am. Heart J.* **22**, 64.

W53 WILSON F.N., JOHNSTON F.D., ROSENBAUM F.F., ERLANGER H., KOSSMANN C.E., HECHT H., COTRIM N., DE OLIVEIRA R.M., SCARSI R. & BARKER P.S. (1944) The precordial electrocardiogram. *Am. Heart J.* **27**, 19.

W54 WILSON F.N., ROSENBAUM F.F. & JOHNSTON F.D. (1947) Interpretation of the ventricular complex of the electrocardiogram. In *Advances in Internal Medicine*, **2**, 1. New York: Interscience Publishers Inc.

W55 WILSON F.N., ROSENBAUM F.F., JOHNSTON F.D. & BARKER P.S. (1945) The electrocardiographic diagnosis of myocardial infarction complicated by bundle branch block. *Arch. Inst. Cardiol. Mexico* **14**, 201.

W56 WILSON G.M. & MILLER H. (1953) Exchangeable sodium in Addison's disease in relation to the electrocardiogram and the action of cortisone. *Clin. Sci.* **12**, 113.

W57 WILSON J.L. & KNUDSON K.P. (1957) Infarction of the cardiac atria. *N. Engl. J. Med.* **251**, 559.

W58 WINDESHEIM J.H. & PARKIN T.W. (1958) Electrocardiograms of ninety patients with acrosclerosis and progressive diffuse sclerosis. *Circulation* **17**, 874.

W59 WINTON S.S. & WALLACE L. (1946) An electrocardiographic study of psychoneurotic patients. *Psychosom. Med.* **8**, 332.

W60 WOLFF L. (1959) Anomalous atrioventricular excitation (W.P.W. syndrome). *Circulation* **19**, 14.

W61 WOLFF L. & RICHMAN J.L. (1953) The diagnosis of myo-

cardial infarction in patients with anomalous atrioventricular excitation (Wolff-Parkinson-White Syndrome). *Am. Heart J.* **45**, 545.

W62 WOOD F.C. & WOLFERTH C.C. (1931) Angina pectoris. The clinical and electrocardiographic phenomena of the attack, and their comparison with the effects of experimental temporary coronary occlusion. *Arch. Intern. Med.* **47**, 33.

W63 WOOD F.C., WOLFERTH C.C. & LIVEZEY M.M. (1931) Angina pectoris. *Arch. Intern. Med.* **47**, 339.

W64 WOOD P. (1941) Pulmonary embolism: diagnosis by chest lead electrocardiography. *Brit. Heart J.* **3**, 21.

W65 WOOD P. (1948) Electrocardiographic appearances in acute and chronic pulmonary heart disease. *Brit. Heart J.* **10**, 87.

W66 WOOD P. (1956) *Diseases of the Heart and Circulation*. 2nd Edn, p. 813. London: Eyre and Spottiswoode.

W67 WOOD P., McGREGOR M., MAGIDSON O. & WHITTAKER W. (1950) The effort test in angina pectoris. *Brit. Heart J.* **12**, 363.

W68 WOOD R.S., TAYLOR W.J., WHEAT M.W. JR. & SCHIEBLER, G.L. (1962) Muscular subaortic stenosis in childhood. *Pediatrics* **30**, 749.

Y

Y1 YANOWITZ F., PRESTON J.B. & ABILDSKOV J.A. (1966) Functional distribution of right and left stellate innervation to the ventricles: Production of neurogenic electrocardiographic changes by unilateral alteration of sympathetic tone. *Circ. Res.* **18**, 416.

Y2 YATER W.M., WALSH P.P., STAPLETON J.F. & CLARK M.L. (1951) Comparison of clinical and pathologic aspects of coronary artery disease in men of various age groups: a study of 950 autopsied cases from the Armed Forces Institute of Pathology. *Ann. Intern. Med.* **34**, 352.

Y3 YOUNG E.W. & KOENIG B.S. (1944) Auricular infarction. *Am. Heart J.* **28**, 287.

Y4 YOUNG E. & WILLIAM C. (1968) The frontal plane vectorcardiogram in old inferior myocardial infarction. *Circulation* **37**, 604.

Y5 YU P.N.G., BRUCE R.A., LOVEJOY F.W. JR. & McDOWELL M.E. (1951) Variations in electrocardiographic responses during exercise. Studies of normal subjects under unusual stresses and of patients with cardiopulmonary diseases. *Circulation* **3**, 368.

Y6 YU P.N.G., BRUCE R.A., LOVEJOY F.W. JR. & PEARSON R. (1950) Observations on the changes of the ventricular systole (QR interval) during exercise. *J. Clin. Invest.* **29**, 279.

Y7 YU P.N.G. & SOFFER A. (1952) Studies of electrocardiographic changes during exercise (modified double two-step test). *Circulation* **6**, 183.

Y8 YU P.N.G. & STEWART J.M. (1950) Subendocardial myocardial infarction with special reference to the electrocardiographic changes. *Am. Heart J.* **39**, 862.

Y9 YU P.N.G., YIM B.J.B. & STANDFIELD A. (1959) Hyperventilation syndrome. *Arch. Intern. Med.* **103**, 902.

Z

Z1 ZAO Z.Z., HERMANN G.R. & HEJTMANCIK M.R. (1958) A

vector study of the delta wave in 'non-delayed' conduction. *Am. Heart J.* **56,** 920.

Z2   ZATUCHNI J., AEGENTER E.E., MOLTHAN L. & SHUMAN C.R. (1951) The heart in progressive muscular dystrophy. *Circulation* **3,** 846.

Z3   ZEH E. (1950) Vergleichende Untersuchungen über den einfluss von Gynergen und Hydergin auf das elektrokardiogramm. *Z. Kreislaufforsch.* **39,** 675.

Z4   ZOLL P.M. & SACKS D.R. (1945) Myocardial infarction superimposed on short P-R, prolonged QRS complex; case report. *Am. Heart J.* **30,** 527.

Z5   ZONDEK H. (1964) The electrocardiogram in myxoedema. *Brit. Heart J.* **26,** 227.

Z6   ZUCKERMAN R., RODRIQUEZ M.I. & SODI-PALLARES D. (1950) Electropathology of acute cor pulmonale. *Am. Heart J.* **40,** 805.

Z7   ZWILLINGER L. (1935) Die digitaliseinwirkung auf das arbeits-elektrokardiogramm. *Med. Klin.* **30,** 977.

General Index

341